'Over the last decade the scope of the h̶ significantly, with a growing amount of m understand the contested politics, treatments, anu ᴜ̶ᴠ̶ᴜ̶ illness. In this volume, Chris Millard and Jennifer Wallis bring together an outstanding collection of researchers to map out these new territories. Together they have created an indispensable guide for practitioners, students, historians, policy makers, and family researchers exploring the complex and often obscure roots of our current understandings of mental health.'

Rhodri Hayward, *Queen Mary University of London, UK*

'This book is an indispensable resource for anyone writing on the history of mental health, from students and academics to those writing local, family, and survivor histories. Chris Millard and Jennifer Wallis have assembled a Who's Who of current experts in the field to guide us through institutional and medical sources for the history of psychiatry. But this collection goes beyond the clinical territory, to include activist and radical histories, literary sources, and the sensitivities and ethics of oral histories. By incorporating the voice of lived experience and marginalised individuals, this handbook will help us move towards a more democratic and representative history of mental health.'

Sarah Marks, *Birkbeck, University of London, UK*

'Chris Millard and Jennifer Wallis have created the first port of call for any historian interested in doing original research in the history of psychiatry. Featuring contributions from historians doing innovative, cutting-edge research, *Sources in the History of Psychiatry* will help historians from all career stages navigate the many fascinating primary sources that can reveal how mental health has been experienced and understood since 1800.'

Matthew Smith, *University of Strathclyde, UK*

'Given the growing interest in the history of mental illness and the institutions dedicated to looking after mental patients in the past, this is a timely and incredibly useful book. With their overviews and illustrative examples, the chapters in this collection show readers where sources can be found and demonstrate how these can be turned into engaging histories. Whether you are an academic teaching "Madness and Society", a student studying the history of mental health, or an amateur historian interested in the history of your local mental hospital, this book is for you.'

Carsten Timmerman, *University of Manchester, UK*

SOURCES IN THE HISTORY OF PSYCHIATRY, FROM 1800 TO THE PRESENT

This book offers a general introduction to historical sources in the history of psychiatry, delving into the range of sources that can be used to investigate this dynamic and exciting field.

The chapters in this volume deal with physical sources that might be encountered in the archive, such as asylum casebooks, artwork, material artefacts, post-mortem records, more general types of source including medical journals, literature, public enquiries, and key themes within the field such as feminist sources, activist and survivor sources. Offering practical advice and examples for the novice, as well as insightful suggestions for the experienced scholar, the authors provide worked-through examples of how various source types can be used and exploited and reflect productively on the limits and constraints of different kinds of source material. In so doing it presents readers with a comprehensive guide on how to 'read' such sources to research and write the history of psychiatry.

Methodically rigorous, clear and accessible, this is a vital reference for students just starting out within the field through to more experienced scholars experimenting with new and unfamiliar sources in the history of medicine and history of psychiatry more specifically.

Chris Millard is Senior Lecturer in the History of Medicine and Medical Humanities at the University of Sheffield, UK. He is interested in the history of self-harm, illness deception, child abuse, and the uses of 'personal experience' in scholarly writing.

Jennifer Wallis is Lecturer in the History of Science and Medicine, and Medical Humanities Teaching Fellow, at Imperial College London, UK. Her publications include *Investigating the Body in the Victorian Asylum* (2017) and the co-authored volume *Anxious Times: Medicine & Modernity in Nineteenth-Century Britain* (2019).

The Routledge Guides to Using Historical Sources

How does the historian approach primary sources? How do interpretations differ? How can such sources be used to write history?

The *Routledge Guides to Using Historical Sources* series introduces students to different sources and illustrates how historians use them. Titles in the series offer a broad spectrum of primary sources and, using specific examples, examine the historical context of these sources and the different approaches that can be used to interpret them.

Reading Primary Sources
The Interpretation of Texts from Nineteenth and Twentieth Century History, 2nd edition
Edited by Miriam Dobson and Benjamin Ziemann

Sources for the History of Emotions
A Guide
Edited by Katie Barclay, Sharon Crozier-De Rosa and Peter N. Stearns

Games of History
Games and Gaming as Historical Sources
Apostolos Spanos

Doing Spatial History
Edited by Riccardo Bavaj, Konrad Lawson and Bernhard Struck

Sources in the History of Psychiatry, from 1800 to the Present
Edited by Chris Millard and Jennifer Wallis

For more information about this series, please visit: https://www.routledge.com/Routledge-Guides-to-Using-Historical-Sources/book-series/RGHS

SOURCES IN THE HISTORY OF PSYCHIATRY, FROM 1800 TO THE PRESENT

Edited by Chris Millard and Jennifer Wallis

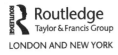

Routledge
Taylor & Francis Group

LONDON AND NEW YORK

First published 2022
by Routledge
4 Park Square, Milton Park, Abingdon, Oxon OX14 4RN

and by Routledge
605 Third Avenue, New York, NY 10158

Routledge is an imprint of the Taylor & Francis Group, an informa business

British Library Cataloguing-in-Publication Data
A catalogue record for this book is available from the British Library

Library of Congress Cataloging-in-Publication Data
Names: Millard, Chris, 1983- editor. | Wallis, Jennifer, 1983- editor.
Title: Sources in the history of psychiatry, from 1800 to the present / edited by Chris Millard and Jennifer Wallis.
Description: Milton Park, Abingdon, Oxon ; New York, NY : Routledge Taylor & Francis Group, 2022. |
Series: Routledge guides to using historical sources | Includes bibliographical references and index.
Identifiers: LCCN 2021049135 (print) | LCCN 2021049136 (ebook) | ISBN 9780367541231 (hardback) | ISBN 9780367541217 (paperback) | ISBN 9781003087694 (ebook) | ISBN 9781000557169 (adobe pdf) | ISBN 9781000557176 (epub)
Subjects: LCSH: Psychiatry--History.
Classification: LCC RC438 .S54 2022 (print) | LCC RC438 (ebook) | DDC 616.89/14--dc23/eng/20211103
LC record available at https://lccn.loc.gov/2021049135
LC ebook record available at https://lccn.loc.gov/2021049136

ISBN: 978-0-367-54123-1 (hbk)
ISBN: 978-0-367-54121-7 (pbk)
ISBN: 978-1-003-08769-4 (ebk)

DOI: 10.4324/9781003087694

Typeset in Bembo
by MPS Limited, Dehradun

CONTENTS

FIGURES

TABLES

CONTRIBUTORS

Steffan Blayney is a historian at the University of Sheffield and a co-organiser of History Acts, which connects activists and historians. He is currently working on a history of mental health activism and radical left politics in Britain.

Sarah Chaney is a historian of medicine, with a background in curating medical museums and research interests in the history of psychiatry and nursing. She is a Research Fellow at Queen Mary University of London Centre for the History of the Emotions and Events and Exhibitions Manager at the Royal College of Nursing. Her monograph, *Psyche on the Skin: A History of Self-Harm* (Reaktion Books, 2017) explores the history of self-injury as a psychiatric category.

Sarah Crook is a History lecturer at Swansea University. She researches the history of feminism, medical histories, and the history of universities. Her work has been published in a range of academic journals, including *Women's History Review*, *Contemporary British History*, *Medical Humanities*, and the *Journal of the History of Medicine and Allied Sciences*. Prior to joining Swansea she held the Sir Christopher Cox Junior Fellowship at New College, Oxford, and completed her PhD at Queen Mary University of London.

Melissa Dickson is Lecturer in Victorian Literature at the University of Birmingham. She has published on the interactions between literature, science, and medicine in Victorian literature and culture, and on nineteenth-century constructions of the Orient and industrial modernity. She is the author of *Cultural Encounters with the Arabian Nights in Nineteenth-Century Britain* (Edinburgh University Press, 2019), a co-author of *Anxious Times: Medicine & Modernity in Nineteenth-Century Britain* (University of Pittsburgh Press, 2019), and a co-editor of *Progress and Pathology: Medicine and Culture in the Nineteenth Century* (Manchester University Press, 2020).

Louise Hide is a social historian of psychiatry and its institutions. She is a Wellcome Trust Fellow in Medical Humanities (grant reference: 205417/Z/16/ Z) based in the Department of History, Classics and Archaeology at Birkbeck, University of London. Her research project is titled 'Cultures of Harm in Residential Institutions for Long-term Adult Care, Britain 1945–1980s'. She has co-edited a special issue of *Social History of Medicine* ('Cultures of Harm in Institutions of Care', 2018) and has published on the histories of pain, delusions, and institutional cultures. Her first monograph, *Gender and Class in English Asylums, 1890–1914*, was published in 2014 by Palgrave Macmillan.

Victoria Hoyle is Lecturer in Public History at the University of York. Her research engages with twentieth- and twenty-first-century histories of health and social care using participatory and co-productive action methodologies. Her recent work on the memory and identity needs of care-experienced adults has been published in the *British Journal of Social Work*, *Child and Family Social Work*, and *Archival Science*. Her current research explores the ways in which histories of child sexual abuse have been constructed and presented in the context of transitional justice processes in Britain and Ireland.

Katie Joice is a doctoral student at Birkbeck, University of London and a member of the Wellcome-funded Hidden Persuaders project. She is currently researching the relationship between the post-war psychological sciences and visual culture, the anti-psychiatry movement, and the history of death in the twentieth century.

Sloan Mahone is Associate Professor of the History of Medicine at the University of Oxford. She specialises in the history of psychiatry and neurology in East Africa. Her recent work has focused on psychiatry and photography in Kenya and Zanzibar, modern day trepanation surgery, and material and visual culture. Her new research engages with neurologists in Africa, India, and Brazil in developing embedded oral history projects within clinical and public health research on epilepsy and stigma in resource-poor settings in Africa and globally.

Cheryl McGeachan is Lecturer in Human Geography at the University of Glasgow. Her research explores the lived experiences of mental ill-health in historical and contemporary contexts. Grounded in uncovering worldly encounters with people, place, and objects, she has worked with numerous archives, collections, and community partners to develop stories of mental ill-health that are often overlooked and ignored. She has written extensively about asylum and post-asylum spaces, Scottish psychiatrist R.D. Laing, and the Art Extraordinary collection.

Chris Millard is Senior Lecturer in the History of Medicine and Medical Humanities at the University of Sheffield. He has published on the history of 'self-harm' in Britain (Palgrave, 2015), and on the relationship between anthropology, experience, history, medicine, and selfhood. He remains committed to a book on the history of Munchausen Syndrome and Munchausen by Proxy, which during the near-decade of research and writing, has become fused with a project on the politics of using personal experience in academic work.

Chris Philo is Professor of Geography at the University of Glasgow. He has long researched what he calls the historical geography of, to paraphrase Foucault, 'the space reserved for insanity', reconstructing the spaces, places, environments, locations, and landscapes integral to the where of 'madness'. His book, *A Geographical History of Institutional Provision for the Insane* (Edward Mellen Press, 2004), brought together his primary research on the English and Welsh experience in this respect from the medieval period to the 1860s. He has also researched the historical and contemporary geographies of learning disability. Additionally, he has worked extensively on the history and theory of geography (as both academic discipline and more diffuse form of knowledge), as well as in the interdisciplinary subfields of rural geography, animal geography, children's geography, and urban studies.

Beatriz Pichel is Senior Lecturer in Photographic History (VC2020) at the Photographic History Research Centre, De Montfort University, Leicester. Her work across photographic history, medical history, the history of emotions, and cultural history seeks to understand how photographic practices shape experiences and inform knowledge. Her current project, 'Photography and the Making of Modern Medicine in France, 1840–1914', examines how photography became a tool in the making and dissemination of medical knowledge at a time when medical specialisms were emerging. This project is funded by a British Academy/ Leverhulme Small Research Grant and will be published as a monograph by Palgrave Macmillan. Beatriz is the co-editor of *Emotional Bodies: The Historical Performativity of Emotions* (University of Illinois Press, 2019). Her first monograph, *Picturing the Western Front: Photography, Practices and Experiences in First World War*, was published in 2021 with Manchester University Press.

Cris Sarg is an early career researcher. Her overall research interests focus on medical ethics and medical history in a transnational context. To date she has focused on psychiatric patient experiences, the migration/immigration of patients, gender (its expression, ideals, and stereotypes), medical ideas, and medical personnel in the Scottish context in the late nineteenth and early twentieth centuries. Her future research will build upon this foundation, comparing and contrasting the Scottish context with the wider British Empire, especially the Australian, Canadian, and South African contexts.

Nicholas Tromans is an independent historian based in London. He has taught at Kingston University, was Curator of the Watts Gallery in Surrey 2013–2018, and has worked at both Sotheby's and Christie's auction houses. A specialist in nineteenth-century British painting, Tromans is the author or editor of books on David Wilkie, G.F. Watts, Orientalist painting, Richard Dadd, and (with Susan Owens) Christina Rossetti. He has contributed chapters and articles to a wide range of books, catalogues, and journals. His latest publications include an essay on the alienist Daniel Hack Tuke and his artist son, Henry Scott Tuke, 'Pruning a Genius: Marginalia by Richard Dadd' in *History of Psychiatry*, and a book, *The Private Lives of Pictures: Art at Home in Britain 1800–1940* (all 2021).

Jennifer Wallis is Lecturer in the History of Science and Medicine, and Medical Humanities Teaching Fellow, at Imperial College London. Her publications include *Investigating the Body in the Victorian Asylum: Doctors, Patients, and Practices* (Palgrave Macmillan, 2017) and the co-authored volume *Anxious Times: Medicine & Modernity in Nineteenth-Century Britain* (University of Pittsburgh Press, 2019).

Janet Weston is a historian of health and law, currently based at the Centre for History in Public Health at the London School of Hygiene and Tropical Medicine. Her first book, *Medicine, the Penal System and Sexual Crime in England, 1919–1960s*, was published by Bloomsbury in 2018. She is currently working on a second book which will explore the history of mental incapacity and the Court of Protection.

ACKNOWLEDGEMENTS

Chris Millard gratefully acknowledges the insight of Sarah Marks' comments on his chapter, and the love and support of his family.

Jennifer Wallis would like to thank Nicol Ferrier and Rebecca Wynter for their generous and helpful comments.

Both Chris and Jennifer would like to thank all the contributors to this book for their patience and dedication as the volume has come together. It has been a pleasure to work with such an insightful group of people, each of whom has encouraged us to think about the history of psychiatry in new ways.

INTRODUCTION

Chris Millard and Jennifer Wallis

Psychiatry is perhaps the branch of medicine most self-consciously concerned with its own history. Psychiatrists are often explicitly aware of, and active participants in, making the history of their discipline.[1] In *Our Necessary Shadow* (2013), Consultant Psychiatrist Tom Burns asks: 'Does this history matter? I think it does… [C]urrent controversies, and especially the vehemence with which they are argued, are hopelessly baffling without some grasp of this history and how it has shaped attitudes and thinking.'[2] But psychiatry's history is not simply the preserve of interested practitioners (current or retired). Since the 1960s serious and sustained academic interest in psychiatry has been pursued by historians (Kathleen Jones), philosophers (Michel Foucault), sociologists (Andrew Scull), anthropologists (Erving Goffman), as well as disaffected psychiatric practitioners (the most famous of whom are Ronald D. Laing and David Cooper in Britain).

The history of psychiatry, like any other history, resembles its sources; in the case of psychiatry, the available sources have undergone transformations in both institutional and conceptual ways. A recognisably modern kind of psychiatry begins in the courtroom, at the trial of James Hadfield in 1800, and legal frameworks have been central to psychiatric practice ever since. Mental health law, criminal law, compulsory treatment, patients' rights, and ideas of competence and responsibility all straddle this medico-legal divide. However, court documents have been underused in histories of psychiatry (as Janet Weston's chapter in this volume discusses). The history of psychiatry instead becomes inseparable from a colossal building project that begins in the early nineteenth century, and accelerates after the 1840s. Lunatic asylums are built to house and treat increasing numbers of patients. The asylums grow in size until the middle of the twentieth century when there are approximately 150,000 psychiatric inpatients in 1955.[3] By this point, asylums have been renamed 'psychiatric hospitals', but they remain hulking Victorian structures, usually built outside large population centres.

DOI: 10.4324/9781003087694-1

Asylums have been explored in histories of psychiatry for decades.[4] They contain a huge amount of documentation and bureaucratic traces of psychiatric practice. These documents – casebooks, reception orders, patient notes, institutional reports, inspection records, and more – remain central to histories of psychiatry in the nineteenth, and early twentieth, centuries (see Cris Sarg, Cheryl McGeachan and Chris Philo's chapter in this volume, for example). Roy Porter's call for a 'medical history from below', attempting to recapture 'The Patient's View' (1985),[5] has been influential, and more recent works have gone beyond these institutional histories to consider the multi-faceted nature of psychiatric practice both inside and outside the asylum's walls. During the early twentieth century, psychiatry came to prominence in multiple fields, including education, industry, criminal justice, social work, and child guidance. Thus, the potential for a history of psychiatry beyond asylum records (and practitioner biographies) has increased exponentially in recent years.[6]

From the 1950s onwards the picture shifts as asylum provision itself begins to be scaled back. New psychiatric medication (such as chlorpromazine) enables the management of some of the more florid psychiatric symptoms in outpatient facilities and clinics. Work by psychiatrists such as Russell Barton, John Wing, and George Carstairs focuses on the negative psychological effects of large institutions compared to domestic or other community environments, often in close collaboration with anthropologists such as Elizabeth Monck and George Brown (Carstairs was trained in both disciplines).[7] The Conservative governments of the 1950s and early 1960s are able to fold this anti-institutionalism into a fiscal strategy that reduces expenditure on the vast asylums. Most famously, Enoch Powell's 1961 'Water Tower' speech heralds the active role the government seeks to play in the closure of these institutions:

> nothing less than the elimination of by far the greater part of this country's mental hospitals as they exist today... it is our duty to err on the side of ruthlessness. For the great majority of these establishments there is no appropriate future use.[8]

This double movement – with psychiatric thinking and practice emerging across more diverse fields, and the closure of the asylums – transforms the number and location of available sources for historians of psychiatry. The asylums prove quite recalcitrant, but begin to close from the 1980s onwards, vividly described from the inside by Barbara Taylor, among others.[9] These closures thus bring many challenges, including the dispersal and destruction of many institutional records as asylums are converted into luxury accommodation (Friern in North London, for example, or Middlewood just outside of Sheffield) or demolished. But the other side of the historiographical coin is an opportunity to diversify the sources that underpin histories of psychiatry – including sources that have existed for many years prior to asylum closure.[10] Today, any historian of psychiatry must be adept at excavating psychiatric influence and practice from a vast range of disparate sources that no longer necessarily have a strong institutional unity. Greg Eghigian notes in 2011 that 'recent psychiatric knowledge is not being made or housed simply in the hospital or the clinic. It has become a technoscience that operates in numerous settings' including offices, courtrooms, prisons, schools, and professional sports.[11] This volume is an attempt to guide those who want to exploit this chaotic, rich, and often confusing jumble of sources in order to construct reflective, robust, and responsible histories. The examples in this volume focus primarily on the British context because that is the expertise of the editors and contributors, but many of the issues raised, and questions to be asked, will be pertinent in different national contexts.

Historians of psychiatry can now draw upon a wide range of primary and archival sources, from post-mortem records, to probation reports, to films, artworks, and anti-capitalist pamphlets. This is in addition to the photographs, hospital casebooks, professional journals, and legal proceedings that have long buttressed the history of psychiatry. The range of sources widens as more public records come into use following the closure period (for clinical records in the UK this is normally after 100 years). The advent of digitisation has also significantly expanded the range of sources that the historian has at their fingertips. The Wellcome Library's digitised mental healthcare archives are freely available online to anyone wanting to browse nineteenth-century casebooks and admission registers (see Sarg et al.'s chapter in this volume);[12] professional journals have been digitised for decades, and PubMed Central and Europe PubMed Central are dedicated online repositories for many kinds of documents in the history of medicine, including psychiatry (on journals, see Chris Millard's chapter in this volume).[13]

This transformation in psychiatric source bases, whether the historian is working with primary material in an archive search room, or perusing digitised documents from the comfort of their living room, has been a growing focus of discussion in recent years. A special issue of *Rethinking History* journal in 2018, for example, examined 'Bureaucracy, archive files and knowledge production', with many contributing authors emphasising the 'curated' nature of the archive. Some authors, such as Sally Swartz, have addressed these difficulties with specific reference to the history of psychiatry. Swartz calls for historians to 'try to find multiple perspectives on patients' experience' by using a variety of source types that will allow them to explore multiple contemporary 'representations' of madness.[14] Catharine Coleborne notes that '[i]nstitutional closures ... created other ways to represent and access these worlds and experiences for the former inmates of institutions' and takes David Wright's observation about the 'primacy of the mental hospital' in order to foreground 'the overwhelming amount of institutional source material for the institutions of the nineteenth century, these sites for confinement have loomed large in both public imaginations, and in the scholarship of the history of mental health'.[15]

Each of Swartz's 'multiple perspectives' is based upon varied documentary foundations in this effort to get out from underneath the potentially suffocating weight of the asylum and its documentary footprint. Each source type comes with its own set of opportunities and constraints, exclusions and emphases. It has become more common in recent years to stress the geographical connections that influence psychiatric practice. In the case of Britain, the use of psychiatry (and particularly psychiatric taxonomies) within the British Empire is an important field of study.[16] Imperial records have their own set of ethical and practical problems, as is shown in Sloan Mahone's chapter in this volume.

A burgeoning interest in the practice of photography within institutional settings also presents the researcher with myriad ethical considerations (such as how best, and indeed whether, to reproduce such images), alongside practical questions about authorship, production technologies, and contemporary aesthetic conventions.[17] As Beatriz Pichel's chapter in this volume demonstrates, such questions are vital when dealing with the 'inherently unstable' medium of the photograph, the meanings of which change over time in a continuous dialogue with viewers. The history of art, too, has long been established as a valuable sub-discipline in history, and paintings have much to contribute to discussions in the history of psychiatry (on which, see Nicholas Tromans' chapter in this volume). Students and academics need to know how to 'read' such sources if we are to produce such histories accurately and responsibly.

The discipline of history, no less than the discipline of psychiatry, has undergone substantial change over the twentieth century. Most prominent have been the moves into social and cultural history (often buttressed by anthropological and ethnographic techniques and insights), and the advent of what used to be called the 'linguistic turn' and is now more commonly bunched under the imprecise (and often derogatory) term 'postmodernism'. The move towards social history can be traced back to a group of French scholars of the *Annales* school, named after the journal they founded for their scholarship in 1929. These scholars, including Marc Bloch, Emmanuel Le Roy Ladurie, and Fernand Braudel, sought to broaden history's focus on the elites of monarchs and battles and diplomacy, to the history of ways of thinking, and social life – the history of *mentalities*. In Britain, this social history was influentially fused with Marxism by E.P. Thompson, in his toweringly influential *The Making of the English Working Class* (1963). This was further developed by scholars from departments of literature – most notably Hayden White – who focused upon the literary nature of historical work, and how various narrative conventions structured historical accounts.[18]

Cultural history – which includes material culture and popular culture – has been influential in stressing the way that communities of people are held together by certain assumptions and conventions that mesh to form a worldview. Any object, any conversation, any practice, can form evidence for this worldview; this means that the number of available sources balloons from the traditional official documents of state to include almost anything. Concerns with objects can inform myriad discussions (including those in and around psychiatry as Sarah Chaney shows in this volume), and this conversation around objects has been going on for many years in history and across the human sciences – from the history of consumerism to the sociologists involved in Actor Network Theory.[19]

History and historians have also been caught up in social movements and influenced by activist communities. Feminist historians in the 1970s first began to return women to the historical record, before broadening out and analysing gender relations – the various social and political aspects of *masculinity* and *femininity* – in history. Key among these scholars was Joan W. Scott, who began her career as a historian of factory workers and published the influential *Gender and the Politics of History* in 1988.[20] Scholars of sexuality have also for the past 30 or 40 years been uncovering different ideas of selfhood and different conceptions of sexuality and attraction throughout history.[21] Indeed one of the more influential early historians of madness, Michel Foucault, was also a scholar of sexuality later in his career.[22] It is clear that sexuality has been managed, interpreted, and pathologised by psychiatry more than any other medical speciality in the last two centuries. Finally, historians of science and sociologists of scientific knowledge have produced an influential body of scholarship on medicine. Psychiatry's troubled status as a branch of medicine (and indeed as a scientific pursuit *at all*), means that there is yet another angle from which it can be investigated.[23] Historians of psychiatry must not only pick their way through the metaphorical (and literal) rubble of the asylum system, the dispersed chaos of various psychologically-inflected disciplines and practices, but also the changing landscape of history itself. It is not just the 'psychiatry' in 'the history of psychiatry' that has been transformed, but the 'history' too.

It is good to end on a couple of reflective notes, thinking about the borders of psychiatry and the limitations of this volume. As the asylums were run down and sold off, and many patients unceremoniously dumped on an underfunded patchwork of community and outpatient services, the porous boundaries and multifaceted nature of 'psychiatry' became more obvious – but this issue has a much longer history. Nikolas Rose popularised the use of the term 'psy disciplines' to throw a blanket over the ragged disciplinary contests and cooperations between psychiatry, psychology, psychoanalysis, psychometrics, and various kinds of counselling.[24] But even outside of these disciplines, there are pertinent questions about what makes a particular practice or institution 'psychiatric'. This comes to the fore in Louise Hide's chapter in this volume, which deals with various kinds of institutions, including care homes and institutions for those with 'mental handicap', where the presence of doctors, let alone those with any psychiatric training, was scarce. Histories seem to latch first onto the more prestigious and established disciplines; we must be careful that historians do not unthinkingly reproduce their boundaries and exacerbate their exclusions.

In the past few decades historians have become increasingly self-conscious about their work, reflecting upon its limitations and exclusions in print. The work of constructing this volume has been an active project since 2018, and from our present vantage point in Spring 2021 the world looks rather different, specifically regarding the salience and prominence of racial inequality. This is a guide to historical sources, and is written by and for historians. History-writing cannot exist outside of the contexts and networks within which it is embedded; it reflects (and reproduces) the partiality and inequality of its networks and its present. Whilst there is significant commentary on issues of race and racism in this volume (especially in Mahone's chapter on imperial sources, but also in Sarah Crook's on feminist sources), the changes of the past few years have thrown the limitations of the discussions around sources and racism into much sharper relief for us as editors. It is indicative of the privilege that underpins this project – and the homogeneity of our contributors – that race did not appear to us a fundamental omission when planning and executing the early stages of this project. It is much more obvious now. History in general is always indelibly marked by the conditions of its present production, and all the inequalities that structure the present. The present, of course, shifts and transforms – sometimes slowly and imperceptibly, at other times with sudden ruptures. We think such a rupture has happened with regard to race and racism, at least to us, in our small corner of psychiatric history, but also more broadly across academic disciplines more generally. Indeed, it is to be hoped that the growing field of Black British history will come to bear more explicitly on the history of psychiatry, and its sources, as well as vice versa. Racism and psychiatry have a long and intertwined history, and those in Britain who see racism in the Anglophone world as an essentially North American problem are seriously misguided. There is a much more established historical field dealing with race and psychiatry in the United States, and this should be taking root in British history departments too.

Layout of the book

In the first chapter, Cris Sarg, Cheryl McGeachan, and Chris Philo explore three principal kinds of records found in asylums: case files (admission/reception papers), case notes (casebooks), and patient registers. These materials formed the backbone of nineteenth-century institutional psychiatry. This chapter gives an example of how these records can shine a careful light on the practices of scientific racism, with the association of 'Jewishness' and various mental pathologies, for example 'persecution complex'. They emphasise that the records contain ample material for both quantitative study as well as qualitative material, and, if used carefully, can be the basis for robust accounts of patient experiences inside the asylum's walls, but also offer plenty of evidence about the families of those committed to, and treated within, the asylum.

Beatriz Pichel discusses the importance of photographs within the history of psychiatry in the second chapter, but also considers how photographs can be ethically charged sources. Pichel sketches the possibilities for using photographs in the history of psychiatry, for both works that have them as their principal focus, and for those that use photographs in a more peripheral manner. There is also a discussion of photographs' historiographies, mapping changes in how these images have been utilised by historians of psychiatry. Finally, there is a practical and ethical guide to using photographs in history – which not only touches upon how to navigate institutional ethics clearance, but also opens up broader ethical questions around the uses of photographs and the possibilities for responsible consent and acknowledgement.

In the third chapter, Jennifer Wallis explores the post-mortem records that documented an important aspect of psychiatric practice in the nineteenth century: the search for the physiological causes and effects of mental illnesses. As well as documents that attest to the scientific aspirations and activities of psychiatry in this period, Wallis shows how post-mortem records can also shed light on relationships between institutions, doctors, and families, and the everyday lives and bodily experiences of patients within the asylum. Her chapter offers practical advice for dealing with these complex and sometimes confusing records, including how to use them in conjunction with other source types such as contemporary textbooks. Post-mortem records are noted to be unusually 'resonant' sources, containing photographs, diagrams, and sometimes even physical traces of pathological work. Thus, the researcher is encouraged to carefully consider their engagement with such records, which can constitute a particularly emotionally charged encounter with the dead.

In a chapter that exemplifies the longstanding concern that history has with material objects, Sarah Chaney's exploration of the material culture of psychiatry centres around a number of particularly iconic objects. The status of objects (as opposed to written texts) has rapidly changed in history over the last 30 years, and these sources need careful attention and contextualisation, as much as the provenance of any document. Chaney shows, through the example of the straitjacket, how objects might productively play a full part in the history of psychiatry. Teasing out the symbolism of the straitjacket across a number of registers shows the complexity of objects, alongside a practical guide for finding objects, and how to appraise what is found. Crucially, Chaney shows how psychiatry's material culture can enrich and enter into dialogue with the various other source materials available to historians.

In Chapter 5, Chris Millard returns us to texts, and extremely conventional ones at that, in an assessment of medical journals. Millard shows that despite these sources being extremely official and readily accessible (being mostly online and keyword searchable), there are still enormous hidden complexities within them. They contain many different kinds of source – from peer-reviewed science to snark-filled correspondence – and are often excellent for initial orientation in a topic. 'Official' attitudes can be gauged from editorials, and different kinds of report across different kinds of journal, can contribute huge amounts of information whether looking at changing treatments, technical innovations, or new diagnostic labels.

Melissa Dickson shows in Chapter 6 how fictional accounts can be used as sources in the history of psychiatry. Dickson shows how works of fiction that involve descriptions of mental life were influenced by the psychiatric thought of their day, but also how these imaginative works had an impact upon the work of psychiatrists and alienists. Using fictional works in history requires a significant amount of caution and contextualisation, but as Dickson shows, these texts can be invaluable sources for historians of psychiatry and the mind sciences more generally. The interconnections between literary and scientific worlds have been studied for many decades, and fiction is a crucial source to draw upon.

In Chapter 7, Sloan Mahone shows how important imperial and colonial records can be in the history of psychiatry. Issues of power, abuse, marginalisation, and often frank violence are a significant part of psychiatry's history. In imperial and colonial contexts, the researcher must deal with multiple, simultaneous kinds of marginalisation, silencing and oppression, with records produced by an administrative system that is essentially exploitative. The practical constraints of access to archives combine with the need to read sources extremely carefully, and often 'against the grain', in order to gain valuable insight. For historians, the issue of contextual sensitivity is crucial, and Mahone shows how debates over historical and cross-cultural diagnosis must be reckoned with if the historian is to use these records responsibly. Especially if doing 'fieldwork' *from* a former colonial power in a former colonial territory, there are legacies of inequality that must be considered with sensitivity, caution, and respect in the present at least as much as in the past. This is of course in addition to the power imbalances that structure psychiatric institutions and their patients more generally. Within these complicated, crisscrossing networks of power relations and subjugations, between a traumatic past and an uncertain present, is a key part of psychiatry's history, just as relevant to the metropole as it is to the colony.

Given the inextricable nature of psychiatry from legal matters such as mental capacity, criminal responsibility, and consent to treatment, legal sources have been relatively neglected within the history of psychiatry. In Chapter 8, Janet Weston shows how legal documents can be used to illuminate important issues in this field. These sources are described by Weston, who also takes us through some specific readings of case law – detailed legal judgements – to show how important issues in the history of psychiatry can be illuminated. The history of Victorian psychiatry's relationship with the legal profession is a relatively well-tilled field, but as we move into the twentieth century, Weston shows how ideas of responsibility and capability circulated in courtrooms and legal proceedings, and how legal, psychiatric, and lay understandings confirmed or conflicted with one another in productive and vital ways.

Louise Hide's chapter on public inquiries shows how scandal, abuse, and mistreatment have impacted the history of psychiatry. The chapter also demonstrates how these sources can challenge ideas of what the history of psychiatry can encompass. Hide shows how these public legal forums open up questions of professional advancement, responsibility, and welfare, as they relate to notions of care and institutional provision, not just for those designated 'mentally ill' but also those considered to have 'mental handicap' or 'learning difficulties'. Hide draws a detailed history of the emergence of scandals in the twentieth century in Britain, and how inquiries into instances of alleged mistreatment produced complicated and rich documents. These documents contain individual testimony, but also a focus on institutional culture that is extremely difficult to get at from other sources. Various local conventions, or the neglect of certain rules or safeguards, usually only emerge in the historical record in investigations like these, and Hide shows how they can be exploited.

In Chapter 10, Steffan Blayney opens up the field of survivor and activist sources, a place where the boundaries of the archive are far from set. Ephemera, pamphlets, posters, and leaflets all feature here, and are difficult to find. One of the most important stories in the history of psychiatry is how people who are subject to psychiatry have carved out a place and a platform from which to speak. Once considered 'patients', many now self-define as 'service users' or 'survivors' of psychiatry, and their history is one that needs much ethical caution and practical effort to tell in a robust and responsible manner. The variety of sources that survive needs careful contextualisation, and much attention to what might have been lost, rather than simply what has been haphazardly preserved. Blayney highlights the crucial role of individual collectors in this preservation, also offering hints on how the development of service user or survivor movements might be traced through contemporary radical publications and audiovisual materials. In writing the history of the survivor movement, Blayney asks us to consider our own position as historians in the research process. Engaging in participatory research and co-production with survivors, for example, can be a means of enriching our historical understanding, at the same time seeking to avoid the replication of the unequal power structures that have long characterised psychiatry.

In Chapter 11, Sarah Crook brings a variety of sources into focus that can elucidate the relationship between feminism and psychiatric practice. In doing so, Crook charts the feminist historiography of psychiatry, and shows how psychiatry in the twentieth century has been inextricably bound up with the maintenance of gendered, patriarchal norms, and also subject to various strategies of feminist resistance against those norms. Taking in magazines such as *Spare Rib* and *Shrew*, alongside efforts to record and preserve oral histories of participants and activists in the Women's Liberation Movement, there is a huge number of archival sources that can be utilised in feminist histories. Crook develops this account of the sources with several examples of feminist critiques that centre around psychiatric practices and diagnostics.

Nicholas Tromans brings the possibilities of works of art into the history of psychiatry in Chapter 12. Famous works, including Charles-Louis Müller's painting of Philippe Pinel striking the chains from the mad, and Jean-Martin Charcot demonstrating hysteria at the Salpêtrière Hospital in Paris, are considered for what they might tell us about the professional identity of those who ministered to and treated the mad. The influence of paintings is also charted in various textbooks, and the way that paintings and images affected diagnostic practice is considered. Tromans also shows how the art produced by psychiatric patients (whether produced for therapeutic reasons or not) might usefully be brought into the analysis of the history of psychiatry.

In Chapter 13, Katie Joice explores the potential of audiovisual sources in the history of psychiatry. There are significant practical issues when accessing and citing audiovisual sources, and Joice takes us through these problems without losing sight of the incredible potential of moving, speaking images. Films made by psychologists and psychiatrists are clearly extremely relevant here, and covered in detail, but anthropological films and commercial films about asylums and psychiatric treatment are also rich and valuable, as Joice shows. Scandal and other adverse publicity are crucial aspects of psychiatry's modern history, and films loom large here after the Second World War, but as well as exposés, there are also films that produce new professional knowledge for psychiatrists, psychologists, and a host of other professionals. Finally, Joice makes clear that there are serious ethical questions around patient consent to being filmed, and powerful empathetic and emotional reactions that audiovisual sources can both capture in the subject and provoke in the viewer, both of which must be accounted for by any researcher who uses these materials.

Finally, Victoria Hoyle navigates the practicalities of interviews and the power of oral histories in Chapter 14. Oral histories have often been focused upon marginalised groups, whose documentary traces might be more sparse than dominant groupings. This is especially important in the history of psychiatry, a discipline strafed by power relations and inequalities. The ethics of interviewing (both practical and theoretical) are covered in depth, and this is especially pertinent considering that the content of interviews about the history of psychiatry can contain sensitive and potentially traumatic material. Hoyle also deftly explicates the methodological issues in using this kind of testimony, which is a rich resource, but with many pitfalls for the unsuspecting historian. Rarely are accounts so rich, useful, unreliable, and conflicting as when they are charged memories.

In each of these chapters, care has been taken to combine the intellectual and theoretical possibilities of particular source types with practical advice as to their use. All chapters contain worked-through examples of how to read, analyse, and use these sources. Where appropriate any administrative, archival, or ethical difficulties associated with sources have been flagged, even if some of these issues are thorny and largely insoluble. The history of psychiatry has much to contribute to any assessment of human society, human frailty, and human marginalisation. It can only do this in a responsible and properly historical manner if the sources of the accounts are well-understood and adequately contextualised. This book is our attempt at providing such tools and examples, whether for students embarking upon primary source work for the first time, or for seasoned researchers new to the sub-discipline of psychiatric history, who need signposts for the ethical, practical, and theoretical problems that these sources present.

Notes

1 One of the more prominent examples here is Professor Sir Simon Wessely, a former President of the Royal College of Psychiatrists, and keen contributor to varied historical scholarship on psychiatry. For example: Richard A.A. Kanaan and Simon C. Wessely, 'The Origins of Factitious Disorder', *History of the Human Sciences*, 23, 2 (2010), pp. 68–85; Edgar Jones and Simon Wessely, *Shell Shock to PTSD: Military Psychiatry from 1900 to the Gulf War* (London: Psychology Press, 2005).
2 Tom Burns, *Our Necessary Shadow: The Nature and Meaning of Psychiatry* (London: Penguin, 2013), p. xxiv.

3 Brian Cooper, 'British Psychiatry and Its Discontents', *Journal of the Royal Society of Medicine*, 103, 10 (2010), pp. 397–402: p. 398.
4 Just three examples from a huge, sprawling literature: Charlotte MacKenzie, *Psychiatry for the Rich: A History of Ticehurst Private Asylum 1792–1917* (London: Routledge, 1992); Edward B. Renvoize and Allan W. Beveridge, 'Mental Illness and the Late Victorians: A Study of Patients Admitted to Three Asylums in York, 1880–1884', *Psychological Medicine*, 19, 1 (1989), pp. 19–28; Cathy Smith, 'Family, Community and the Victorian Asylum: A Case Study of the Northampton General Lunatic Asylum and Its Pauper Lunatics', *Family & Community History*, 9, 2 (2006), pp. 109–24.
5 Roy Porter, 'The Patient's View: Doing Medical History from Below', *Theory and Society*, 14, 2 (1985), pp. 175–98.
6 A small number of examples from a huge variety of works: Peter Bartlett and David Wright (eds), *Outside the Walls of the Asylum: The History of Care in the Community 1750–2000* (London: The Athlone Press, 1999); Vicky Long, 'Rethinking Post-War Mental Health Care: Industrial Therapy and the Chronic Mental Patient in Britain', *Social History of Medicine*, 26, 4 (2013), pp. 738–58; Andrew Smith, *Victorian Demons: Medicine, Masculinity and the Gothic at the fin de siècle* (Manchester: Manchester University Press, 2004); Akihito Suzuki, *Madness at Home: The Psychiatrist, the Patient, and the Family in England, 1820–1860* (Oakland, CA: University of California Press, 2006); Mathew Thomson, *Psychological Subjects: Identity, Culture, and Health in Twentieth-Century Britain* (Oxford: Oxford University Press, 2006); Jonathan Toms, *Mental Hygiene and Psychiatry in Modern Britain* (Basingstoke: Palgrave Macmillan, 2013).
7 Russell Barton, *Institutional Neurosis* (Bristol: Wright, 1959); J.K. Wing and G.W. Brown, *Institutionalism and Schizophrenia: A Comparative Study of Three Mental Hospitals, 1960–1968* (Cambridge: Cambridge University Press, 1970); G.W. Brown, E.M. Monck, G.M. Carstairs, and J.K. Wing, 'Influence of Family Life on the Course of Schizophrenic Illness', *British Journal of Preventive & Social Medicine*, 16, 2 (1962), pp. 55–68.
8 Available at Andrew Roberts' Home Page, http://studymore.org.uk/xpowell.htm, accessed 24 Mar. 2021.
9 Barbara Taylor, 'The Demise of the Asylum in Late Twentieth-Century Britain: A Personal History', *Transactions of the Royal Historical Society*, 21 (2011), pp. 193–215; Barbara Taylor, *The Last Asylum: A Memoir of Madness in Our Times* (London: Penguin, 2014).
10 See for example Deborah Doroshow, Matthew Gambino, and Mical Raz, 'New Directions in the Historiography of Psychiatry', *Journal of the History of Medicine and the Allied Sciences*, 74, 1 (2019): pp. 15–33.
11 Greg Eghigian, 'Deinstitutionalizing the History of Contemporary Psychiatry', *History of Psychiatry*, 22, 2 (2011): pp. 201–14.
12 See https://wellcomecollection.org/pages/YA64vRMAACAAgRjZ#online-collections, accessed 24 Mar. 2021.
13 US National Library of Medicine/National Institutes of Health, PubMed Central, https://www.ncbi.nlm.nih.gov/pmc/ and Europe PMC Consortium, http://europepmc.org/.
14 Sally Swartz, 'Asylum Case Records: Fact and Fiction', *Rethinking History*, 22, 3 (2018): pp. 289–301.
15 Catharine Coleborne, *Why Talk About Madness? Bringing History into the Conversation* (Cham, Switzerland: Palgrave Macmillan/Springer Nature, 2020), p. 41, citing David Wright 'Getting Out of the Asylum: Understanding the Confinement of the Insane in the Nineteenth Century', *Social History of Medicine*, 10, 1 (1997), pp. 137–55: p. 155.
16 Matthew M. Heaton, *Black Skin, White Coats: Nigerian Psychiatrists, Decolonization, and the Globalization of Psychiatry* (Athens, OH: Ohio University Press, 2013); Richard C. Keller, 'Madness and Colonization: Psychiatry in the British and French Empires, 1800–1962', *Journal of Social History*, 35, 2 (2001), pp. 295–326; Erik Linstrum, *Ruling Minds: Psychology in the British Empire* (Cambridge, MA: Harvard University Press,

2016); Katie Kilroy-Marac, *Postcolonial Psychiatry and the Work of Memory in a West African Clinic* (Oakland, CA: University of California Press, 2019); Yolana Pringle, 'Neurasthenia at Mengo Hospital, Uganda: A Case Study in Psychiatry and a Diagnosis, 1906–50', *Journal of Imperial and Commonwealth History*, 44, 2 (2016), pp. 241–62.

17 See for example Caroline Bressey, 'The City of Others: Photographs from the City of London Asylum Archive', *19: Interdisciplinary Studies in the Long Nineteenth Century*, 13 (2011); Katherine D.B. Rawling, "She Sits All Day in the Attitude Depicted in the Photo': Photography and the Psychiatric Patient in the Late Nineteenth Century', *Medical Humanities*, 43 (2017): pp. 99–100; Susan Sidlauskas, 'Inventing the Medical Portrait: Photography at the 'Benevolent Asylum' of Holloway, c.1885–1889', *Medical Humanities*, 39, 1 (2013): pp. 29–37.

18 See for example Hayden V. White, *The Content of the Form: Narrative Discourse and Historical Representation* (Baltimore, MD: Johns Hopkins University Press, 1987).

19 For example Karen Harvey (ed.), *History and Material Culture: A Student's Guide to Approaching Alternative Sources* (London: Routledge, 2009); Lorraine Daston (ed.), *Things that Talk: Object Lessons from Art and Science* (New York: Zone Books, 2004).

20 Joan Wallach Scott, *Gender and the Politics of History* (New York: Columbia University Press, 1988).

21 Excellent examples of this literature include: Chiara Beccalossi, *Female Sexual Inversion: Same-Sex Desires in Italian and British Sexology, c.1870–1920* (Basingstoke: Palgrave Macmillan, 2012); Gilbert Herdt (ed.), *Third Sex, Third Gender: Beyond Sexual Dimorphism in Culture and History* (New York: Zone Books, 1994); Kate Fisher and Sarah Toulalan (eds), *Bodies, Sex and Desire from the Renaissance to the Present* (Basingstoke: Palgrave Macmillan, 2011); Matt Houlbrook, *Queer London: Perils and Pleasures in the Sexual Metropolis, 1918–1957* (Chicago, IL: University of Chicago Press, 2005); Julie Peakman (ed.), *A Cultural History of Sexuality* (Oxford: Berg, 2011).

22 Michel Foucault, *Histoire de la sexualité*, 4 vols (Paris: Éditions Gallimard, 1976–2018).

23 Two classic examples are: Andrew Cunningham and Perry Williams (eds), *The Laboratory Revolution in Medicine* (Cambridge: Cambridge University Press, 1992) and John Harley Warner, 'The History of Science and the Sciences of Medicine', *Osiris*, 10 (1995), pp. 164–93. For a more recent example, see Andreas Mayer, 'Why Does Psychoanalysis Matter to History and Philosophy of Science? On the Ramifications of Forrester's Axiom', *Psychoanalysis and History*, 19, 2 (2017), pp. 151–66.

24 Nikolas Rose, *The Psychological Complex: Social Regulation and the Psychology of the Individual* (London: Routledge & Kegan Paul, 1985) and *Governing the Soul: The Shaping of the Private Self* (London: Free Association Books, 1999).

1

ASYLUM RECORDS: FILES, NOTES, CASEBOOKS, AND PATIENT REGISTERS

Cris Sarg, Cheryl McGeachan, and Chris Philo

Asylum archives

In Tom Pow's poem 'The Great Asylums of Scotland' he considers the moul-
dering archives forgotten in the attics of these historic institutions, most now
standing empty or converted to other uses:

> In attic rooms the sky's light pours over
> …
> a tide-wrack of maps, plans, records – a grid
> to lay over a waste of rage, grief, anger
> and pain.[1]

In a few cases such words are literally true, as Kim Ross found when seeking the
'lost archive' of the Lanark District Asylum, Hartwood, one of Scotland's lesser-
known lunatic asylums.[2] In some cases these archives have been saved and to an
extent organised and even catalogued on site, as Emily Donoho was relieved to
find at the Argyll and Bute District Asylum, Lochgilphead.[3] In other cases what
survives of these archives has been transferred to the safe keeping of local health
board collections, themselves now stored in county record offices or city libraries
with historic records sections. Donoho was able to consult the archives of the
other Highlands public asylum, the Inverness District Asylum, at the Highlands
Archives Centre in the same city, while Ross lists and discusses the range of
'resource centres' visited in the course of tracing Scottish district asylum records.[4]
What Pow suggests about Scotland's asylum archives is applicable more generally,
of course, and during their research on several different asylums in Nottingham,
England, Hester Parr and Chris Philo veered from stumbling on the remaining
records of the Nottingham Borough Asylum, Mapperley, in a higgledy-piggledy

DOI: 10.4324/9781003087694-2

over-spilling glass-fronted cabinet in the corner of the 'hospital library', to rooting through materials helpfully catalogued in Nottinghamshire County Archives and the Nottinghamshire County Library Local History Department.[5] Useful guides exist for searching and locating British asylum records, providing an invaluable platform for anyone commencing their own research into the histories (and geographies) of 'madness, asylums, and psychiatry' (what we fondly term MAP).[6]

The latter part of the extract from Pow's poem, above, is worth underlining at the outset. Clearly, the 'official' or institutional documents comprising an asylum's archive – Pow gestures to 'maps, plans, records' – can only open a relatively narrow window on to what really occurred behind the high walls and bolted gates of an asylum. They indeed comprise 'a grid to lay over a waste of rage, grief, anger and pain'. This phrase does two things. On the one hand, it hints at an 'official' approach to ordering and controlling an asylum: a pre-set 'grid' of ideas and practices, often enacted with the best of intentions but now sometimes seen as wrong-headed and even brutal.[7] Much contained within an asylum's records tells a 'top-down' story, testifying to the entanglement of culture, knowledge, and power within a given society, time, and place, as we will show in this chapter. On the other hand, Pow's phrase betrays all that cannot but escape the 'grid': the broiling emotional landscapes of an asylum in its everyday workings, the 'rage, grief, anger and pain' often felt by those confined within, many against their wishes, whose own mental traumas and demons – irrespective of how they were labelled – were doubtless exacerbated by their immuration in a strange home surrounded by strangers. The daily grind of an asylum, its conflicted encounters and relations, as well as the immediacy of what patients felt, hoped, and feared – even what doctors, nurses, attendants, and other asylum workers similarly felt – all remain opaque from the standard asylum records. Insofar as it is possible, such feelings have to be recovered from other kinds of sources, some of which are examined in other contributions to this collection.

It now seems completely 'natural' that an institution such as an asylum should create its own 'official' documents either to facilitate its workaday operations, chiefly for internal use, or to encapsulate and maybe justify its own performance for external audiences or audit purposes. Nonetheless, such 'documenting' should itself be seen as an invention and a process, reflecting growing accountability demands from the eighteenth century, when charitable 'lunatic hospitals' began to report back to, and seek more, subscribers. Such demands then became more insistent in the lurch towards governmental inspection and regulation, at national and local levels, during the nineteenth century. We are particularly referencing the British context here, unevenly played out between different parts of the British 'nation', but similar developments unfolded elsewhere across western Europe, North America, and beyond over the last two centuries, not least, and not always happily, under the impress of colonialism. The documents created have varied greatly in character and coverage, often a reflection of whether the asylums in question have been private, charitable, or public in their constitution, and much energy was expended by nineteenth-century lunacy experts in agitating for 'uniformity' in how asylums reported on – and deployed written information in managing – their occupants and activities.[8] It is these documents, however, that now survive – if not rotting in the attic, consumed by fire, or otherwise lost – and which can be consulted by the asylum researcher.

There are perhaps three most obvious types of such documents, each typically combining printed headings with handwritten or, later, typed entries. Their precise form and content can vary considerably by institution and time period, but certain root principles remain broadly stable. The first type is the admission documentation, sometimes called the case files but not to be confused with case notes, containing basic reception and certification papers for an individual patient. In many asylum archives, these may be listed as 'reception orders'. These papers include personal data such as name, sex, age, next of kin, and address, alongside varying levels of detail about the circumstances of admission, the patient's health history, and preliminary medical judgements about the patient's apparent mental disorder. The second is the patient register, a full tabular listing of all patients admitted to the asylum, usually organised by date of admission, including the most skeletal demographic and medical 'facts' of each case, followed by dates of discharge or death. The third is patient case notes or casebooks, providing descriptions of the health, conduct, and progress of each patient, including diagnoses and prognoses of their 'mental affliction', spread over the weeks, months, or years during which the patient was an asylum resident. In what follows we provide a case study of how such sources can be utilised, based on the doctoral research of the first author, Cris Sarg, on Jewish patients in two Scottish 'royal' asylums from the 1870s to the 1930s.[9]

There are other kinds of documents worth mentioning, notably asylum annual reports, increasingly produced by all types of British asylums during the nineteenth century, which combined often-lengthy textual passages – usually penned by the medical superintendent, sometimes revealing their own understandings of and approaches to 'madness' – with statistical summaries of the changing patient cohorts from one year to the next. It was once objected that '[n]o one who has not … examined year after year the whole series of [annual reports] can have any idea of the sameness of their contents',[10] and their sheer proliferation – too much to be sensibly appraised – led them to be left 'lying in a heap of confusion at the bottom of some cupboard specially reserved for the reception of the "dead dogs," as they have been called'.[11] For the researcher, though, these reports can be a treasure trove, yielding insights into the peculiarities of particular asylum regimes, and they certainly helped us to appreciate why our two different Scottish asylums had seemingly dissimilar experiences with respect to their Jewish inmates. There are other documents – meeting minutes, staff records, financial transactions and balance sheets, and the 'maps and plans' mentioned by Pow – which can all be invaluable depending on the exact focus of a researcher's inquiries, but we do not have space to consider them all in this chapter. In what follows, therefore, we will first introduce case files and patient registers, noting the quantitative insights into asylum worlds that they can offer. Next, we will explore case notes through the example of one asylum patient, Fanny Finestein, to demonstrate in miniature what can be excavated of asylum experiences through such qualitative sources.

Case files and patient registers

'We want, in fact, a scientific statistical record of the entrance, life and death of every inmate,' wrote Charles Lockhart Robertson in 1861, 'which, at the end of each year may then, from the several reports, be massed and grouped into figures, uniform and accurate, and pregnant with information on the history of mental disease.'[12] That was the ideal, though, and Robertson called for greater standardisation in combining the facts of a patient's 'career', from admission through to discharge or death, with information on 'the influences of age, sex, occupation, social relations on the incubation, progress and result of the disease'.[13] Individual entries in case files and subsequent notes appended to them – ideally including information about bodily changes, diet, exercise, and the like – were crucial, certainly for the management of individual cases, but also for what might be possible when aggregating these details into the larger datasets that Robertson envisaged. 'The reams of statistical tables continued to appear as if this were a ritual process that would one day mysteriously lay bare the facts of insanity',[14] muses historian Richard Russell, but this 'ritual process' is a boon for the asylum re-searcher, especially for one with demographic or socio-economic interests asking questions such as: who was turning up in the asylum? Why were they arriving? And with what consequences (personally and societally)?

In the work of the lead author here, use is made of case files and patient registers to investigate the relationship between asylums and the Anglo-Jewry (Jewish people living in Britain). Specifically, she investigates the cohorts of Jewish patients – or, rather, of patients convincingly identified as 'Jewish'[15] – admitted to, and then either discharged from or dying in, the two most prominent 'chartered' lunatic asylums in Scotland between 1870 and 1939. Predominantly taking patients with kith and kin able to pay fees, but with some poorer inmates cross-subsidised from these fees, the Royal Edinburgh Asylum (REA) and the Glasgow (or Gartnavel) Royal Asylum (GRA) took, respectively, 20,123 and 10,181 patients in total and 49 (0.24%) and 46 (0.45%) Jewish patients over this period. For comparison, in the middle of the nineteenth century the Jewish communities of Edinburgh and Glasgow were of about equal size, but gradually, with Glasgow's increasingly heavy industrial and commercial dominance, there was more opportunity for both established community members and recent immigrants to find employment, particularly low-status work that could lead to 'pauperisation' if this work was lost. The Jewish population of Glasgow soon far exceeded that of Edinburgh: c.12,000 in Glasgow compared with c.1,500 in Edinburgh by 1914, but overall Scotland's Jewish population re-mained less than 1% of its overall population.[16]

A database has been created that examines the Jewish patient cohorts of REA and GRA in several different ways. Specialist software for database development and associated statistical analysis may make this task easier, but databases can be created using readily available software that enables the manipulation of spreadsheets. Case files provide researchers with a wealth of information from which to build a database, such as the institution (when working with records from multiple institutions), as well as individual patient details: name; sex; age; class or occupation; religious affiliation; address prior to admission; admission date; numbers of previous admissions; initial diagnoses, and discharge or death dates – among other variables for potential comparison. Examination of these data points can reveal patterns such as an older or younger than expected patient population, or patients enduring extended stays within the asylum who were all diagnosed with a particular condition. These patterns can then be used in combination with medical journals or textbooks of the period to explore the practical implications of prevailing medical ideas.

The database created in this case matched Jewish with 'Control' (non-Jewish) patients, the latter simply being the next non-Jewish patient listed in the patient register, as a sampling strategy allowing a four-way comparison to be made: between Jewish and non-Jewish patients and between the two asylums. Table 1.1 carries some basic demographic information extracted from the database, providing headcounts and percentages (the latter relative to the host asylum). It reveals intriguing inter-asylum contrasts such as Jewish male admission rates to REA appearing to be proportionally greater than to GRA, and female admissions correspondingly less, perhaps reflecting the fact that many Glaswegian male Jews becoming mentally afflicted may have been truly 'paupers' – linked to the city's industrial and commercial dominance – and hence without family means to gain admission to GRA. Indeed, no Jewish 'pauper' males were admitted to GRA (and only two 'pauper' females), reflecting an explicit policy from the 1870s to restrict GRA to private patients, meaning that we must look elsewhere than GRA to locate them (to the state-run pauper district asylums opening around Glasgow).[17]

More intriguing still are contrasts revealed between average ages at first admission and average lengths of stay, with the former being noticeably lower for the Jewish than the Control cohorts and the latter noticeably longer. There are many complications to consider, not all shown in the table, including what appear to be overall gendered variations (males being first-admitted younger; all women staying longer) and classed ones (paupers tending to be first-admitted earlier [although maybe not for Jews]; private patients definitely staying longer). Then there are further inter-asylum differences, notably GRA Jewish pauper males being first-admitted younger and all GRA Jewish pauper patients staying less time than occurred at REA. The exact reasons behind these patterns cannot be discerned from the bald figures, but what the figures do prompt – and why they can be so useful for the researcher – are profound questions. What dynamics or pressures within, and pressing upon, the Jewish communities of Edinburgh and Glasgow led them to 'yield' their mentally unwell members to the asylum so much earlier, within individual lifespans, than was true of non-Jewish society? What happened in the asylum that led Jewish patients to continue being 'detained' for so much longer than their non-Jewish counterparts?

TABLE 1.1 Basic Jewish and Control demographics (combining and contrasting REA and GRA)

	REA	GRA	Total or average
Jewish headcount (%)	49	46	95
Control headcount (%)	49	46	95
Jewish male headcount (%)	32 (65.31%)	17 (36.96%)	49
Control male headcount (%)	18 (36.73%)	17 (36.96%)	35
Jewish female headcount (%)	17 (34.69%)	29 (63.04%)	46
Control female headcount (%)	31 (63.27%)	29 (63.04%)	60
Jewish average age at first admission	39.43 yrs	35.13 yrs	37.28 yrs
Control average age at first admission	46.33 yrs	45.24 yrs	45.79 yrs
Jewish male average age at first admission	40.09 yrs	27.82 yrs	33.96 yrs
Control male average age at first admission	44.61 yrs	39.06 yrs	41.84 yrs
Jewish female average age at first admission	38.18 yrs	39.41 yrs	38.80 yrs
Control female average age at first admission	47.33 yrs	48.86 yrs	48.10 yrs
Jewish average length of stay	1,617 days	1,361 days	1,489 days
Control average length of stay	1,107 days	337 days	722 days

The point here is not to offer answers, merely to note, in a substantive example, what possibilities can be opened up by case files and patient registers. That said, we can show some additional data derived from the registers of REA and GRA concerning mental disorders that were attributed to patients, whether as a description of symptomology (REA) or explicitly as a diagnosis (GRA), the different emphases here probably reflecting different clinical cultures established under the various medical superintendents of the two asylums.[18] Records of diagnoses can indeed be used to illustrate differences in asylum cultures, particularly when combined with other sources such as annual reports. Did different institutions and superintendents tend to favour particular diagnoses, perhaps reflecting a preference for more holistic engagements with patients – such as 'case conferences' (see under 'Case Notes' below) – over the straight 'factual' reporting of histories and symptoms? How do such variations fit within the wider trajectory and milieu of psychiatric history? These types of question can also shed light on how differences in clinical cultures impacted patients' lived experience in terms of diagnostic and prognostic trends, as we will show.

An attempt has nonetheless been made here to bridge these differences in clinical cultures by grouping together broadly similar terms deployed at both REA and GRA, such as dementia praecox, paraphenia, and schizophrenia (arguably describing the same 'disease' process over the period) or persecution, paranoia, psychosis, and delusions (meaning similar things and commonly used in conjunction). This grouping procedure produced 11 categories, on the basis of which it was possible to detect whether Jewish patients were disproportionately assigned to particular categories. Table 1.2 picks out the two composite classifications just referenced as ones where such a disproportionality appears to arise.

In qualitative chapters of the first author's doctoral thesis, chapters using case notes, she charts the prevalence of 'persecution complexes' in a number of individual cases, thinking more broadly about the historical-cultural circumstances that have arguably led to Jews as a people – translated into individuals – feeling persecuted. Elements of persecution mixed with delusion also feature, moreover, in the case study of Fanny presented below. With respect to dementia praecox, meanwhile, there is evidence to suggest a contemporary assumption that this condition was especially prevalent among Jews, perhaps predisposing clinicians to recording dementia praecox in asylum records pertaining to Jewish patients. An example is seen in D.K. Henderson and R.D. Gillespie's *A Text-Book of Psychiatry for Students and Practitioners*: 'With the Italians, [Jews] have the highest proportional incidence of dementia praecox among the Massachusetts admissions for 1917–19.'[19] The edition quoted here was dated 1940, at the close of the period under investigation, but it was the fifth edition of a textbook widely used in the Anglo-speaking world. Tellingly, Henderson held the post of Medical Superintendent at both REA and GRA at different times during the period under investigation; his learning about the Jewry and dementia praecox would have been familiar to, and an influence upon, clinicians at both establishments. The section of the textbook containing this quote addressed how race and ethnicity supposedly impacted the incidence of psychiatric disorders, a perspective within which certain mental disorders – under the umbrella of 'scientific racism' – became particularly associated with Jews, cast as inherently less robust and more prone to disease (particularly 'excitable' mental diseases) than other European populations.[20]

Case notes

'A book containing within the compass of a single volume, or of one for each sex, complete records of all the cases actually under treatment, is probably a *desideratum* in most asylums,' remarked 'T.B.B.' in the *Journal of Mental Science* in 1865. Typically, though, the reality was simply one of

> filling up successive books with more or less fragmentary accounts … and if a patient live many years in an asylum, the history of his case may ultimately have to be sought in detached notes, scattered through ten or twenty books.

'T.B.B.' continued: 'A striking illustration … recently occurred in one large asylum where, on the occasion of an official visit, a view of the Case Book being requested, a small cartload of bulky volumes was placed before the dismayed visitors.'[21] To be sure, patient case notes, dispersed chaotically across bound

TABLE 1.2 'Attributions' of diagnoses/symptomologies (combining REA and GRA)

	Jewish patients with this 'attribution': headcount	Jewish patients with this 'attribution': %	Control patients with this 'attribution': headcount	Control patients with this 'attribution': %
1. Alcohol (i.e. alcohol-induced mental disorders)	0	0	2	2.11%
2. Confusional Insanity or Mental Confusion	5	5.26%	5	5.26%
3. Congenital Imbecility, Mental Defect, or Mental Unsoundness	5	5.26%	3	3.16%
4. Dementia or Senile Dementia	5	5.26%	10	10.53%
5. Dementia Praecox, Paraphenia, or Schizophrenia	18	18.95%	9	9.47%
6. Epilepsy	3	3.16%	3	3.16%
7. General Paralysis or Syphilis	5	5.26%	7	7.37%
8. Manic, Mania, Manic Depression, Melancholia, Melia, Excitement, or Exhaustion	39	41.05%	38	40.00%
9. Moral Insanity	1	1.05%	0	0
10. Persecution, Paranoia, Psychosis, or Delusions	9	9.47%	5	5.26%
11. Not Answered or Illegible	5	5.26%	13	13.68%
Totals	95	100%	95	100%

casebooks and interleaved with 'detached' ephemera, were notoriously difficult to access, process, and act upon. Even when converted into singular books for each patient, they remained – and remain – weirdly inconsistent documents, at one moment full of detail, texture, touches of humanity and speculation, but at the next terse and uninformative ('Discharged, unimproved'; 'Transferred to London asylum').

Nonetheless, case notes are arguably the closest that we can get through the official institutional records to the intimacies of asylum lives, as well as to the thought processes, professional judgements, and treatment-related decision-making of the clinicians (and sometimes nurses) responsible for individual cases. There is now a sizeable secondary literature on case notes.[22] A good example is Hazel Morrison's attention to the clinical practice of Henderson, mentioned above, and his emphasis on recovering substantive case histories of patients, their families, and present illnesses through what became known as the patient 'case conference', which he championed and believed could greatly illuminate a patient's current actions and reactions. Morrison remarks that, for Henderson, describing a patient's symptoms was of little value 'unless information is collected elsewhere regarding the setting in which the symptoms have occurred and the causes that have been instrumental in producing them'.[23]

In Sarg's work use is made of case notes – supplemented by admission information in case files – to probe the individual stories of numerous Jewish patients who passed through REA and GRA, locating the human scale of experiences, sadnesses, clinical interpretations, and related treatments lying behind the tables and numbers discussed in the previous section. In what follows, we will briefly consider one particular 'case', that of Fanny Finestein.[24] A key point to note is how we weave case notes from the archive together with other primary sources, such as marriage resisters, as well as existing studies in the academic literature.[25] The aim is to illustrate something of how a researcher might deploy and tackle case note evidence. Fanny's case was selected because it comprises 83 unbound and unnumbered pages, giving us much to work with, while her narrative as disclosed within the case notes touches upon several themes illustrative of the Jewish patient experience within both REA and GRA. Stripped of the thicker interpretative context given in the doctoral examination of Fanny's case – alert to the complex entanglings of ethnic, religious, class, and gender identities, representations and politics bound up in the paired histories of the Anglo-Jewry and the historical asylum system – our account below is unavoidably partial, but in introducing Fanny's story we can still highlight the potential for excavating patient experience from the archive. We begin by tracing a brief biography of Fanny's 'life-path', situating her asylum story within the larger context of her various familial worlds before moving to chart her admission to REA in January 1934.

Fanny Finestein's story

Fanny Josephart was born on 26 December 1879 in Latvia, the sixth of eight children. Her father was a merchant in Latvia who had studied veterinary science but never practised, most likely due to his Jewish origins and the restrictions placed on Jews in the Russian Empire.[26] Fanny's mother died when she was very young and her father remarried when she was seven in 1886. One sister, who became, when married, a Mrs Rifkins, living in Mount Florida, Glasgow, had a son who ended up in a home/hospital with 'loss of all his senses' as a result of a blow to the head from a cricket bat.[27] The link with Fanny's nephew was important in the eyes of clinicians because it suggested evidence of a hereditary predisposition towards 'madness' within Fanny's family, notwithstanding his initial injury being physical, not 'psychiatric', in nature. Fanny went to school until the age of 14, implying a sufficiently well-to-do family background, before leaving Latvia to come to Glasgow to live with one of her sisters, possibly Mrs Rifkins, who had recently married. Between 1894 and 1899, while living with her sister, she took in dressmaking to earn money. In 1899 she met Isaac, and Fanny and Isaac Finestein were married on 30 August 1899 in Glasgow.[28]

Isaac worked as a traveller or itinerant pedlar, primarily in jewellery, and Fanny and Isaac moved to Inverness in about 1901, where they purchased a business, a jewellery store, which was successful. In 1903 Fanny gave birth to her first child, a boy who died at birth, which could be seen as one cause of her later mental distress, while at the time so-called puerperal insanity was linked to traumatic or prolonged labour, or stillbirth.[29] In 1906 she gave birth to her second child, Morris, who was one of the 'informants' to the asylum when she was admitted, as will be elaborated below. In 1908 she gave birth to her third child, Lily, and before 1912 to her fourth child, a boy, who died six hours after his birth, surely a further factor in her later mental ill health. Finally, in 1912 she gave birth to her fifth child, Daisy, suffering from a prolapsed uterus after this delivery. Daisy was interviewed by Henderson regarding the history of her mother's illness when Fanny was admitted to REA. Sometime in 1915, Daisy related, Fanny had undergone an operation, described on several occasions in the sources as an 'ovariectomy', the complete surgical removal of the uterus and ovaries, perhaps following complications from the prolapsed uterus or as a form of birth control, there being few options for women to control their fertility during this period. In 1917, Fanny and Isaac expanded their business to include an antique store. They were again successful, sufficiently so that they were able to send all their children away to boarding schools. Morris completed the undergraduate qualification in medicine at Edinburgh University, while Daisy and Lily were able to pursue music to a high level, studying for and completing a musical qualification, Licentiate of the Royal Academy of Music or LRAM. All three of Fanny's surviving children were successful, an important aspiration of Jewish motherhood and a possible dimension in Fanny's unwellness.

On admission to REA, three accounts of Fanny's illness were given and recorded in the case notes, one by herself and two from her children, Morris and
Daisy. It is unclear why no account from Isaac exists in the case notes, since legally
he was the person who had to petition for Fanny to be admitted. The three
accounts held different levels of importance for the clinicians. Morris's was the
longest and arguably carried the most weight for the clinicians because he was a
fellow medical practitioner or researcher, based at the Lister Institute for
Preventative Medicine in London,[30] while Fanny's own words seemingly held the
least weight with the clinicians and was the shortest of the three. According to
Morris:

> ... following a scene with my father, we decide to call in the services of Dr
> McAlister, who decided that she suffered from paranoia and recommended
> her removal to hospital. This the father was loath to do, more particularly as
> my sisters were still at school. I may emphasize that during all this time, my
> father's affection for my mother remained remarkably stable. He seemed
> unable to realise the change which had come over her, and frequently
> presented her with valuable gifts, which she received without even an
> expression of thanks, and which she regarded as a form of bribery.[31]

Morris later stated that '[a]s it was obvious that Lily could no longer live at home
and it did not appear advisable to leave my sister Daisy alone with my mother, we
took steps to have her examined and certified'.[32]

It was related that in mid September 1933 Lily had travelled to London 'to
escape her mother's persecution',[33] after which Fanny became more antagonistic
and violent towards Daisy. Lily had returned to Edinburgh in late December 1933,
but Fanny began to be hostile towards Lily and told her 'to return to her immoral
life in London'.[34] During a particularly heated exchange, Fanny threatened Lily
with a fire poker, after which Isaac, her three children, and Mr Furst, together
with a Dr McAlister and a Mr Ingram KC, took action to have Fanny certified.
Fanny was duly admitted to REA on 4 January 1934 due to her alleged 'paranoid
delusions' about murder plots directed towards her by her husband and children.
Over the course of her seven-month stay in the institution, however, she successfully litigated her way out of the asylum – showing remarkably proactive
agency for a patient, itself possibly colouring how her condition was interpreted by
the asylum authorities – and was discharged 'relieved' by 'order of the sheriff' on
30 July 1934.

Abuse, Jewish motherhood, and stereotypical pathologies

Fanny herself spoke of being in an abusive relationship, distorted, it seems, by
lying, avarice, and sexual perversion, thereby ensnaring herself in problematic
tropes with which Jews were often represented:

The rest of it all is money; it's money from the family's part and from the husband's part, he doesn't care what happens. The family all want a share of my money and the husband has put them up to it. I wouldn't have grudged giving them the money, and Lily wanted £2000 to get married and I wouldn't give it to her and therefore she turned against me. And Furst [Isaac's lawyer and mentor to the children] drew her away from her first boy and spoilt her. She says that Furst made love to Lily at the instigation of Mr Finestein with the intent to hurt Mrs Finestein's feelings.

...

Of her husband she says, "He has been cruel in every way; he did all he could to spoil my life; he tells lies and rumours, wicked lies about me to everyone. He is a manufacturer of lies. He does it to affect my health." Pressed to give an example of the lies, Mrs Finestein said it was a long story, and that they were wicked lies. She appeared somewhat at a loss to remember any of the lies.[35]

With the statement about Mr Furst, Fanny invoked the image of the lustful Jew, and compounded matters with allusions to stereotypes of the Jewish prostitute and pimp embodied in her daughter and husband. The impression from the wordings here, recorded verbatim together with some limited interpretation from a 'case conference' interview with the patient conducted by Henderson and colleagues, is that the clinicians were sceptical about Fanny's claims, seeing here evidence of her 'paranoid delusions'.

Moreover, subtly woven through the case notes are hints at how the clinicians were 'reading' this particular Jewish-mother-body. A general point is that such notes often fuse specialist medical language with 'non-medical' terms, the latter serving to smuggle contemporary norms, values, and prejudices into the apparently objective professional judgements being passed. Joyce Antler, in her history of 'the Jewish mother', reconstructs (from Biblical sources onwards) 'the image of the Jewish mother in song and story … as strong, determined, family-bound, and loyal matriarch, raising her children, helping to sustain the family economically, and keeping the domestic flame of Judaism alive'.[36] As Antler implies, the upshot was something almost pathological, a distinctive constellation of 'mad Jewish mother':

the portrayal of the [Jewish] mother as overbearing and manipulative has [over time led to] the depiction of the father as ineffectual, weak, and passive. … Strong, indomitable, and dangerous, the developing Jewish mother icon was fashioned as a warning against the usurpation of patriarchal authority.[37]

Arguably, such a proactive matriarchal figure sat uneasily with a more acquiescent Victorian and Edwardian understanding of quiet 'Anglo' feminine domesticity, counterposed to the restricted, less active, less authority-wielding expectations of a respectable British woman in relation to her family and household.

These claims intersect with other attributed dimensions of Jewish motherhood:

> [a]chievement is a great theme in a Jewish mother's relationship with her children. A child's failure in getting ahead educationally, financially, or in marrying and having children is experienced by the Jewish mother as her failure and thus the source of her own personal pain.[38]

Linked to Antler's account, the implication is that the Jewish mother will be vocal and proactive with regards to her children, possibly in a manner counter to what would have been expected of a respectable British, even 'properly assimilated' Anglo-Jewish, mother. The way Fanny was portrayed by herself, clinicians, and her family, for good or ill, was hence that of the stereotypical

> … Jewish mother [who] does not sacrifice stoically or silently, as does the Irish mother. She suffers and sacrifices "in public" – talking about it to her husband, her children and of course her fellow Jewish mothers. The active expression of her suffering is to ensure that her children appreciate what she has done.[39]

Some of the more negative interpretations of the Jewish mother – from an Anglo perspective – were read through Fanny's disease history, as related to Henderson by Fanny's daughter Daisy. Fanny was painted as highly involved – over-involved perhaps – in her children's lives, intervening in matters such as who they interacted with and what they did in their time away from the family home in Edinburgh:

> [Fanny] would never believe a word that her daughters told her. If they went out to the pictures in the evening, on their return she would accuse them of not having been at the pictures, but of having visited some friend from whom [Fanny] was at the moment estranged, and of having told lies about her to this friend. The daughters had to be very careful not to speak of anyone of whom their mother did not approve, otherwise [Fanny] was sure to conclude that they were in league with this person against her.[40]

Henderson concluded that Fanny had a high opinion of herself and was very proud, whereas Fanny thought herself very virtuous, that she had never told a lie, and that no one could be her equal. She was undoubtedly ambitious for her children, determined that they would be successful to the point that she spared no expense to give them the best education. The consequences for the children were revealing and were clearly central to how the clinicians interpreted Fanny's case, with residual intimations throughout of them harbouring negative responses to the interventionist Jewish mother-figure (albeit one, in this instance, who almost certainly did prove counterproductive for her children's welfare).

Fanny's case can therefore be seen as indicative of prevailing attitudes towards 'pathological' Jewish female bodies, biology, and gender in general. Based on Fanny's case notes – albeit ideally we would compare her case with those of several other Jewish patients identified in the Scottish asylum records – we can see the relevance of what Antler conjectures:

> Excessive, overprotective, neurotically anxious, and ever present, the Jewish mother became a scapegoat for ambivalent and hostile sentiments regarding assimilation in a new society, changing family dynamics, and shifting gender roles. ... This combination of diverse and malleable characteristics allowed each generation to manipulate the Jewish mother image to suit its particular needs.[41]

As can be seen from Fanny's experience, the 'diverse and malleable characteristics' of Jewish motherhood could likely instil psychic tensions in an individual, perhaps leading Fanny to extreme internal distress – self-delusion and passing blame to others – at not being able to live up to an extremely demanding ideal. At the same time, the pursuit of such an ideal – itself geographically 'out of place' when shifted from Latvia to Britain, from the Eastern European Jewry to the Anglo-Jewry – could lead to, or at least become tangled up with, attributions of mental pathology on the part of otherwise well-meaning lunacy experts.

Concluding remarks

In this chapter we have discussed and illustrated how a variety of asylum records, such as case files (admission papers or reception orders), patient registers, and case notes (or casebooks), can both quantitatively and qualitatively be analysed to explore asylum worlds and patients' lived experiences. The merging of quantitative and qualitative materials allows a diverse picture to emerge, highlighting the contrasts between different asylum systems and regional settings – in which regard the quantitative database discloses broader patterns and prompts fresh questions – as well as qualitatively scissoring into the intricacies of patient lives. Drawing on Fanny's case study, we have highlighted in miniature how patient stories are deeply connected to wider political, social, and cultural stories of family, identity, and place. More particularly, the range of 'voices' captured in Fanny's case demonstrates the importance of using such sources to listen more intently to the patient's own words and ways of expressing their own asylum stories.[42] As demonstrated in this example, key to Fanny's asylum narrative are her family networks and the various ways in which the words and experiences of close relatives collide, challenge, and often collude with medical discourse. Catharine Coleborne's work shows how engaged families have often been with the asylum, at once 'outside' and 'inside' of the institution, simultaneously everywhere and nowhere in histories of psychiatry.[43] Using case files, patient registers, and case notes in the ways outlined above helps to reconfigure the family and diverse family voices as an integral part of the asylum system, and in doing so aids in opening up patient experience beyond the institution itself.

As historians of psychiatry continue to diversify their methodological approaches to tracing asylum histories, particularly in relation to the lives of its various inhabitants, the more complex and entangled the stories become. As highlighted in the case study above, the variety of sources required to tell a partial account of Fanny's experience point to the limitations present in such an undertaking. However, this chapter has centred on showcasing the possibilities that such sources – rescued from the attics, wrestled with in the records office – can offer the researcher in their own studies. In demonstrating how we have given attention to 'the grid' of asylum histories, we have begun to reveal the possibilities for learning more about the variety of experiences of 'rage, grief, anger and pain' that have existed within their confines.

Notes

1 Tom Pow, 'The Great Asylums of Scotland [Poems by Doctors]', *British Journal of Psychiatry*, 198 (2011), p. 427. This poem originally appeared in Tom Pow, *Dear Alice – Narratives of Madness* (Cambridge: Salt Publishing, 2008) and we gratefully acknowledge Tom Pow for granting us permission to quote from it in our chapter.

2 Kim A. Ross, 'The Locational History of Scotland's District Lunatic Asylums, 1857–1913'. Doctoral thesis, University of Glasgow, 2014, esp. pp. 114–5 (on 'the lost archive'). Available online at http://theses.gla.ac.uk/5320/.

3 Emily S. Donoho, 'Appeasing the Saint in the Loch and the Physician in the Asylum: The Historical Geography of Insanity in the Scottish Highlands and Islands, from the Early Modern to Victorian Eras'. Doctoral thesis, University of Glasgow, 2012. Available online at http://theses.gla.ac.uk/3315/.

4 Ross, 'Locational History', Appendix A.

5 Hester Parr and Chris Philo, *'A Forbidding Fortress of Locks, Bars and Padded Cells': The Locational History of Mental Health Care in Nottingham* (Glasgow: Historical Geography Research Group [HGRG], 1996).

6 'How to look for records of asylums, psychiatric hospitals and mental health', https://www.nationalarchives.gov.uk/help-with-your-research/research-guides/mental-health/, accessed 3 Feb. 2021; 'The GenGuide [to] Lunatic Asylum Records', www.genguide.co.uk/source/lunatic-asylum-records/125/, accessed 3 Feb. 2021.

7 This statement hints at a highly contested historiographic landscape, ranging from straightforwardly laudatory accounts of progressive improvements through time in how 'madness' has been understood (perhaps as 'mental illness') and treated, to more critical accounts condemnatory of how 'madness' has been progressively captured, silenced, and subjected to corrective measures by the apparatuses of medicine, psychiatry, and other 'psy' disciplines. In these orbits, the asylum appears as either humane site of respite, care, and cure or as carceral site of removal, detention, and disciplining. A recent overview giving some sense of this complex landscape is Andrew Scull, *Madness in Civilization: From the Bible to Freud, from the Madhouse to Modern Medicine* (London: Thames & Hudson, 2015).

8 C. Lockhart Robertson, 'Suggestions Towards an Uniform System of Asylum Statistics (with Tabular Forms)', *Journal of Mental Science*, 7, 36 (1861), pp. 195–211; J.A.

Campbell and J. Todd, 'Uniformity in Public Asylum Reports', *Journal of Mental Science*, 19, 85 (1873), pp. 67–78.

9 Cristin M. Sarg, 'Scottish-Jewish 'Madness'? An Examination of Jewish Admissions to the Royal Asylums of Edinburgh and Glasgow, c.1870–1939'. Doctoral thesis, University of Glasgow, 2017. Available online at http://theses.gla.ac.uk/8496/.

10 Anon., 'Asylum Reports', *Journal of Mental Science*, 8, 42 (1862), p. 276.

11 Anon., 'Asylum Reports for 1872', *Journal of Mental Science*, 19, 86 (1873), p. 266.

12 Robertson, 'Suggestions', pp. 197–8.

13 Ibid., p. 197.

14 Richard Russell, 'The Lunacy Profession and its Staff in the Second Half of the Nineteenth Century, with Special Reference to the West Riding Lunatic Asylum', in W.F. Bynum, Roy Porter, and Michael Shepherd (eds), *The Anatomy of Madness: Essays in the History of Psychiatry, Vol. III: The Asylum and its Psychiatry* (London: Routledge, 1988), pp. 297–315: p. 298.

15 'Jewishness' was determined by answers supplied to question No. 5 of the Admission Warrants/Certification Papers, which asked about religious affiliation. This information was confirmed by what was sometimes mentioned in case notes regarding religious affiliation. Information about a patient's religious affiliation was not routinely recorded in the Patient Registers. Making Jewish-ethnic determination only using patient surname is imprecise because there had been a fair amount of Anglicisation: Schwartz might become Black and Cohen, Cowen.

16 Kenneth E. Collins, *Scotland's Jews: A Guide to the History and Community of the Jews in Scotland* (Glasgow: Scottish Council of Jewish Communities, 2008), p. 16.

17 On the district asylums, see Ross, 'Locational History'. The first author is now collecting data on Jewish admissions to Glasgow and region's district asylums.

18 Sarg, 'Scottish-Jewish 'Madness'?', esp. Ch. 4.

19 D.K. Henderson and R.D. Gillespie, *A Text-Book of Psychiatry for Students and Practitioners*, 5th edn (London: Oxford Medical Publications, 1940), p. 69.

20 Sarg, 'Scottish-Jewish 'Madness'?', Ch. 7. For some of the foundational works of 'scientific racism' as regards mental disorders, see Samuel Cartwright, 'Diseases and Peculiarities of the Negro Race' (originally published in 1851), in Arthur L. Caplan, James J. McCartney, and Dominic A. Sisti (eds), *Health, Disease, and Illness: Concepts in Medicine* (Washington, DC: Georgetown University Press, 2004), pp. 28–39.

21 T.B.B., 'The Asylum Case Book', *Journal of Mental Science*, 11, 53 (1865), p. 144.

22 See Jonathan Andrews, 'Case Notes, Case Histories, and the Patient's Experience of Insanity at Gartnavel Royal Asylum, Glasgow, in the Nineteenth Century', *Social History of Medicine*, 11, 2 (1998), pp. 255–81; Carol Berkenkotter, *Patient Tales: Case Histories and the Uses of Narrative in Psychiatry* (Columbia, SC: University of South Carolina Press, 2008).

23 Hazel Morrison, 'Unearthing the 'Clinical Encounter': Gartnavel Mental Hospital, 1921–1932. Exploring the Intersection of Scientific and Social Discourses which Negotiated the Boundaries of Psychiatric Diagnosis.' Doctoral thesis, University of Glasgow, 2014, p. 14. Available online at http://theses.gla.ac.uk/5766/; also Hazel Morrison, 'Conversing with the Psychiatrist: Patient Narratives within Glasgow's Royal Asylum 1921–1929', *Journal of Literature & Science*, 6, 1 (2013), pp. 18–37.

24 Fanny's name has been altered to comply with the UK Data Protection Act and out of consideration for her family. It is easier to write this sort of analysis by using proper names, even made-up ones, as opposed to the somewhat flat 'Patient A' designation.

25 Specialist works informing this endeavour include: Sander Gilman, 'Jews and Mental Illness: Medical Metaphors, Anti-Semitism and the Jewish Response', *Journal of the History of the Behavioural Sciences*, 20, 2 (1984), pp. 150–9; Ann Goldberg, 'The Limits of Medicalization: Jewish Lunatics and Nineteenth-Century Germany', *History of Psychiatry*, 7, 26 (1996), pp. 265–85; Jan Goldstein, 'The Wandering Jew and the Problem of Psychiatric Anti-Semitism in Fin-de-Siècle France', *Journal of Contemporary*

History, 20, 4 (1985), pp. 521–52; Carole Anne Reeves, 'Insanity and Nervous Diseases Amongst Jewish Immigrants to the East End 1880–1920.' Doctoral thesis, University of London, 2001; Leonard D. Smith, 'Insanity and Ethnicity: Jews in the Mid-Victorian Lunatic Asylum', *Jewish Culture and History*, 1, 1 (1998), pp. 27–40. A contribution containing materials specifically about the treatment/care of 'insanity' in/by Victorian Glasgow's Jewish community is Kenneth Collins, *Be Well!: Jewish Immigrant Health and Welfare in Glasgow, 1860–1914* (East Linton, East Lothian: Tuckwell Press, 2001), esp. pp. 115–30.

26 Lothian Health Board (LHB) 7/1/Craighouse Box 4, Royal Edinburgh Hospital Case Notes (loose).

27 LHB 7/1/Craighouse Box 4.

28 1899 Statutory Marriages (Glasgow/Gorbals) 644/12 0520, 1899 Marriage Register for Finestein, Isaac L. and Josephart, Fanny (http://www.scotlandspeople.gov.uk, accessed Aug. 2015).

29 Morag Allan Campbell, '"Noisy, restless and incoherent": Puerperal Insanity at Dundee Lunatic Asylum', *History of Psychiatry*, 28, 1 (2017), pp. 44–57.

30 Lister Institute of Preventive Medicine was founded in 1891 and is one of the UK's oldest medical charities.

31 LHB 7/1/Craighouse Box 4, Dr Finestein's Letter to Dr Munro – 04-03-1934.

32 Ibid.

33 LHB 7/1/Craighouse Box 4, Daisy's History of Illness.

34 Ibid.

35 LHB 7/1/Craighouse Box 4, Fanny Finestein Mental Status 04-03-1934.

36 Joyce Antler, *You Never Call! You Never Write!: A History of the Jewish Mother* (Oxford: Oxford University Press, 2007), p. 16.

37 Ibid., p. 9.

38 Lois Braverman, 'Jewish Mothers', *Journal of Feminist Family Therapy*, 2, 2 (1990), pp. 9–14: p. 9.

39 Ibid., p. 10.

40 LHB 7/1/Craighouse Box 4, Daisy's History of Illness.

41 Antler, *You Never Call!*, pp. 2–3.

42 Brendan D. Kelly, 'Searching for the Patient's Voice in the Irish Asylums', *Medical Humanities*, 42, 2 (2016), pp. 87–91.

43 Catharine Coleborne, *Madness in the Family: Insanity and Institutions in the Australasian Colonial World, 1860–1914* (Basingstoke: Palgrave Macmillan, 2009).

Select bibliography

Andrews, J., 'Case Notes, Case Histories, and the Patient's Experience of Insanity at Gartnavel Royal Asylum, Glasgow, in the Nineteenth Century', *Social History of Medicine* 11, 1998, pp. 255–281.

Berkenkotter, C., *Patient Tales: Case Histories and the Uses of Narrative in Psychiatry*, Columbia, SC: University of South Carolina Press, 2008.

Gen Guide, 'The GenGuide [to] Lunatic Asylum Records', www.genguide.co.uk/source/lunatic-asylum-records/125/.

Kelly, B.D., 'Searching for the Patient's Voice in the Irish Asylums', *Medical Humanities* 42, 2016, pp. 87–91.

Morrison, H., 'Conversing with the Psychiatrist: Patient Narratives within Glasgow's Royal Asylum 1921–1929', *Journal of Literature & Science* 6, 2013, pp. 18–37.

The National Archives, 'How to Look for Records of Asylums, Psychiatric Hospitals and Mental Health', https://www.nationalarchives.gov.uk/help-with-your-research/research-guides/mental-health/.

2

PHOTOGRAPHIC SOURCES IN THE HISTORY OF PSYCHIATRY

Beatriz Pichel

Ever since the public announcement of the first photographic processes in 1839, cameras have captured the world around us, shaping how we see it. The rapid expansion of photographic studios, the creation of photographic societies, and the development of photographic technologies such as printing techniques and portable cameras meant that, by the early twentieth century, photographs were everywhere. The great number of photographic materials preserved in libraries, museums, and archives around the world attests to this fact. Yet, photographic collections are not always easy to identify. When we talk about nineteenth-century photography, we usually think about prints such as Figure 2.1: an image printed on cardboard or paper, which normally belongs to a larger group of prints or an album. However, photographs often appear as illustrations in books, journals, and magazines, are pasted in the pages of other documents, or take other forms such as glass plates, lantern slides, or stereoscopic cards. The diversity of photographic materials is particularly relevant when researching the history of psychiatry. Psychiatrists, doctors, and alienists in the late nineteenth and early twentieth centuries used photography extensively to keep records of patients, to communicate with one another, as a diagnostic tool, and as an aid for research. Some of these photographs have been lost, others (usually the most famous ones) are carefully preserved in archives. Most of them, however, are spread among publications and casebooks, often with no indication whatsoever of their presence. Historical psychiatric photographs are ambivalent objects, rare and ubiquitous at the same time.

This chapter will help students and researchers to integrate photographs into their work on the history of psychiatry, even when photographs are not the main focus of the research. While identifying photographic collections in archives can be a difficult task, finding textbooks and journals illustrated with photographs is fairly common. The question is what to do with the photographs. Images have

DOI: 10.4324/9781003087694-3

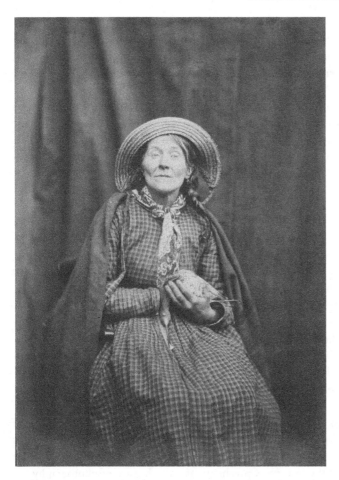

FIGURE 2.1 Hugh Welch Diamond, Seated Woman with a Bird. Surrey, c.1855. Albumen silver print, 84.XP.927.3. The J. Paul Getty Museum, Los Angeles. Digital image courtesy of the Getty's Open Content Program

often been relegated to a secondary role, becoming illustrations that are simply descriptive, reinforcing what has already been said rather than making contributions of their own.[1] The text might refer to them, but the main argument is not drawn from the analysis of photographic materials. This happens, for instance, when photographs are bundled together in the central pages of a book. The fact that they are presented detached from the text suggests that one could, potentially, read the text without looking at the images. Against this, scholarship in photographic history and the history of medicine has shown different ways in which we can treat photographs as historical evidence, placing them at the centre of the historical inquiry. Using photographic sources poses its own challenges, different from those raised by textual sources, but it also opens up new questions that are worth exploring.

Contrary to popular belief, photographs in the history of psychiatry are quite diverse.[2] Beyond the full frontal 'mugshot' focused on the face of the patient, we can find images of bodies in movement, post-mortem examinations of the brain, and pictures of asylum facilities and personnel. More importantly, photographs are more than images. A doctor or a photographer took the photograph with particular equipment, in a certain space (usually a dedicated studio, a ward, or a garden), with a specific purpose in mind. Afterwards, they developed the photograph and stored it in a drawer, pasted it in a casebook, sent it to a colleague, or used it for teaching or publication. All of these actions are integral to the making of photographic meaning and reveal as much about the history of photography as about the history of psychiatry. Examining photographic practices, as well as representations, is key to using photographic sources in a productive way.

The first section of this chapter examines several case studies in the history of psychiatric photography, from the renowned photographs taken by Hugh Welch Diamond and Jean-Martin Charcot, to lesser-known material. This section is not an exhaustive catalogue of all the photographic sources one can find in the history of psychiatry, but introduces the main types of photographs, highlighting the importance not only of their visual style (how they represent their content) but also their materiality and the purpose of the images at the time. The aim is to offer enough variety so the analysis can be applied to other sources. The second section examines the main methodological and historiographical approaches to medical photography, from Marxist and Foucauldian-inspired analyses of power and the medical gaze, to the influence of material culture studies. A final section on archives examines the main issues involved in collecting and locating photographic medical collections, as well as the need to consider the ethical repercussions of using medical photographs in research and publication. Overall, this chapter aims to provide the tools for students and researchers to contextualise psychiatric photography within the history of psychiatry and the history of photography.

Histories of photography

Many histories of medical photography start with Hugh Welch Diamond's speech before the Royal Society on 23 April 1856.[3] Diamond, Resident Superintendent of the Surrey County Lunatic Asylum and an avid amateur photographer, defended the benefits of photographing female patients with mental disorders. The photographs, circulated among the audience during the presentation, were later disseminated by renowned British psychiatrist John Connolly, who included them as engravings in his work on mental disorders.[4] While the use of photography in the asylum was a novelty, Diamond's photographs followed the nineteenth-century tradition of visual representation of mental disorders for diagnostic purposes. Prominent examples of this tradition include Alexander Morison's *The Physiognomy of Mental Diseases* (1839) and J.E.D. Esquirol's sketches of patients.[5] Diamond's photographs did not represent a complete break with tradition, rather an innovative use of technology that integrated artistic conventions and new medical theories of the physiognomy of the insane.

All the photographs Diamond took at the Surrey Lunatic Asylum adopt a similar style. They portray a single female patient, usually sitting on a chair against a draped background. Some images show the floor covered with a patterned carpet. The women in the pictures sometimes look directly into the camera, but more often than not their gaze is directed outside the frame, looking down or to one side. They wear nice dresses made of different fabrics and hold accessories like bags, hats, and books. One of the patients is even holding a bird on her lap (Figure 2.1). None of this would be remarkable if these were studio portraits, which displayed similar props and poses. The fact that Diamond appropriated these conventional codes of representation to portray his patients demonstrates the blurry boundaries between science and art and the need to situate these images within broader cultural and artistic contexts.

Simultaneously invented in 1839 by Louis-Jacques-Mandé Daguerre in France and Henry Fox Talbot in England, photography expanded around the world in the 1840s and 1850s.[6] Photographic societies played a key role in the development of photographic technologies and connected photographers with one another. This is important to note because professional and amateur photographers were not just image-makers; they often built their own equipment and experimented with chemicals and photographic processes. In Britain, Diamond founded, together with other photography pioneers, the Photographic Society in 1853. He wrote several articles on photographic techniques and participated in exhibitions showcasing his photographs of patients as well as portraits and landscapes.[7] Technological advances in photography, therefore, went hand in hand with the making of photographic visual languages. In the midst of the debate on whether photography was art or science, Diamond used his camera both to record patients' mental states and to represent people and objects in artistic ways.[8] Thus, it is not surprising that Diamond photographed patients in similar ways as he photographed his other sitters.[9]

Diamond's ideas on photography also reflected the views of his contemporaries. He wrote that photographs produced a 'perfect and faithful record', unlike drawings, which depended on the artist's skills and judgement, and language, which was always a mediated form of communication.[10] This idea of photographic cameras and plates as devices that recorded nature *as it was* was widespread at the time. As historians Lorraine Daston and Peter Galison have argued, nineteenth-century science aspired to let nature 'speak for itself', without the interference of the scientist's judgement or values, in order to achieve the scientific ideal of objectivity.[11] While this ideal was never attained, and contemporary critics challenged the camera's power to directly reproduce nature, Diamond mobilised the ideal of scientific objectivity to defend the benefits of photographing patients.

Diamond proposed three main uses of portraits of the insane: to diagnose patients; as a form of treatment; and to serve as institutional records. At the core of Diamond's confidence in the power of photography to document mental illness was his belief in physiognomy. As Sharrona Pearl has argued, Diamond's photographs and writings echoed Johann Kaspar Lavater's physiognomic ideas at the same time that they challenged them. Lavater's physiognomy ascribed moral characteristics to the face, associating certain features such as a large nose or a prominent forehead with personality types.[12] Against this static model, which implied the existence of permanent qualities, Diamond transformed physiognomy into a dynamic study of mental illness and health. In Pearl's words, 'Diamond's photographic analyses were tracing behaviour rather than personality, based on the assumption that a mind gone wrong could be righted.'[13] As a result, facial and bodily aspects that were excluded in traditional physiognomic studies, such as hair and clothing, became meaningful features that could express the patient's state of mind. In his communication to the Royal Society, Diamond illustrated the case of a patient who had recovered with four photographs that showed a progression from dishevelled hair and absent gaze to the 'perfect calm' of a nice dress, a nice hat, and a nice shawl.[14] The womanly accessories mentioned in the previous paragraph acquire, therefore, further meaning. The hat or the way in which patients sat on the chair were not only bourgeois photographic conventions but also key elements that communicated the mental illness or health of patients. Diamond's photographs, therefore, exemplify how the photographic medium contributed to shaping medical theories of insanity.

Throughout the second half of the nineteenth century, a growing number of doctors and alienists around the world started to incorporate photography into their medical practice. Photography became a useful tool in asylums, keeping a record of patients and their mental disorders. One of the earliest examples is the Romanian *Photographic Atlas of the Main Types of Mental Alienation*, published by Nicolae G. Chernbach in 1870.[15] Illustrated with 12 photographic plates taken by a commercial photographer, this atlas followed some of Diamond's conventions while introducing new elements. Influenced by Connolly's physiognomy of insanity, the photographs helped the reader to visualise how a diverse range of mental disorders such as pellagra mania (caused by a vitamin deficit and prominent in rural areas), congenital idiocy (understood as a mental deficiency rather than a disease) and general paralysis (characterised by loss of memory, dementia, delusion, and neurological symptoms) manifested in patients.[16] The images show individual patients sitting on a chair looking at the camera, but, unlike Diamond's portraits, Chernbach's photographs are standardised: the background is a blank sheet, which helps the viewer focus on the sitter's face and body, and most patients wear similar white clothes. Patients' hands are on their lap or their knees, so they are visible, and only in one case are the patient's feet visible, indicating that they might be relevant to the diagnosis. The disposition of the photographs in the atlas and their standardisation suggests that they helped alienists to examine patients and to compare them to one another. While this atlas represents one of the earliest works in psychiatric photography in Eastern Europe, it presents many features that characterised psychiatric photography in Europe and America.

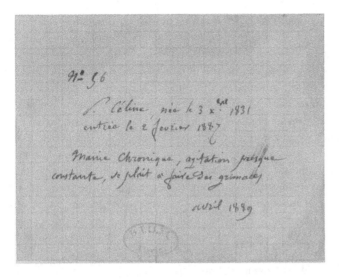

FIGURE 2.2 Henri Dagonet, N. 56. Manie chronique, agitation presque constante, se plaît à faire des grimaces, Album de 26 photographies d'aliénés annotés par Henri Dagonet. CISA 911. BIU Santé/Bibliothèque numérique Medica

From the 1880s onwards, many medical institutions started to paste pictures of patients into the casebook pages or to compile them into albums. For instance, the French psychiatrist Henri Dagonet collected photographs of patients in two small albums.[17] Unlike Chernbach's *Atlas*, the albums were not intended for public dissemination. In fact, they were commercial photographic albums that, instead of containing personal images, were repurposed for medical use. As Figure 2.2 shows, each photograph was accompanied by a short description of the disorder and, sometimes, brief notes about the progress of the patient. Interestingly, the albums included images taken by doctors from other institutions, suggesting not only that photography was widespread in French asylums by the 1880s, but also that photographs circulated extensively within medical circles. For instance, the photograph of a patient suffering from hydrocephalia taken by A. Malfilâtre was included in Dagonet's album, reproduced in Dagonet's *Treatise of Mental Diseases* (1894), and used by the physiologist Charles-Émile François-Franck in his course on emotions (1900/1901) at the Collège de France.[18] This circulation is important because it demonstrates the key role of photographs in the history of medicine. Photographs were not simply illustrations but medical evidence, documents that had the same authority as textual accounts.

One of the main sources in the study of asylum photography are casebooks, which historians of psychiatry have extensively used to examine the daily life of patients in the asylum (on casebooks, see Sarg et al.'s chapter in this volume). Photographs kept in casebooks complement the written sources, revealing key aspects of the relationship between alienists, nurses, and patients. For instance, the Holloway Sanatorium casebooks present a remarkable variety of photographs, as scholars have recently noted.[19] While the images are hardly interesting examined individually, collectively they bring to light the diverse practices of photography in the asylum. Some patients pose with elegant clothes imitating the bourgeois portrait, others hide their faces by looking downwards or upwards, and others are pictured in the garden, unaware of the presence of the camera. Most of the patients were photographed once, some were photographed twice or more, while others were never portrayed. The photographs are sometimes placed on the margins of the casebook, while others are pasted in the middle of the page. These details help us to understand the specific ways in which photography was incorporated into the asylum. As historian Katherine Rawling has suggested, the lack of standardisation suggests that doctors were inventive, adapting their practice to the particular situation of each patient. It also hints at a more complex use of the camera, which was not reduced to an identification or diagnostic tool. Rawling has argued that 'patient photographs can help provide insight into the relationships and interactions that occurred in the everyday life of the asylum'.[20] In the case of the Holloway Sanatorium, the casebook photographs show that photography was a co-creation between doctors and patients.[21] Some patients complied and posed for the camera, while others rebelled, looking down or making gestures. This is important because it allows for a subtler understanding of photography in the asylum. Instead of reducing photographic encounters to a coercive or controlling act, Rawling emphasises the agency and subjectivity of the patient, who, in their vulnerable state, could still find ways to present their individuality in front of the camera.

Patient agency in the context of asylum photography is even more important to examine in relation to race. As anthropological and ethnographic studies of race gained prominence in the nineteenth century, the representation of Black mental patients acquired further meanings. Historian Rory du Plessis has argued that the photography of Black patients at the Grahamstown Lunatic Asylum in South Africa between 1890 and 1907 shows the contrast between the public image of the asylum as a healing institution and the reality of patients' lived experience.[22] These photographs reveal the inequalities in access to treatment between white and Black patients. Following theories of 'moral therapy', according to which physical activity helped to treat mental disorders, Black patients were forced into labour, while white (paying) patients played sports, exercised, or danced.[23] Moreover, while the photographs that reached the public depicted 'domesticated' Black bodies that had been successfully reintegrated into the workforce, casebook photographs show patients 'confronting, refusing and resisting the asylum administration'.[24] Photographs, therefore, became tools of the colonial project that both represented and reinforced imperial hierarchies and ideologies.

It is important to remember that psychiatry was a nascent discipline in the nineteenth century that shared questions and methods with other medical and scientific fields such as physiology, neurology, and pathology, as well as areas such as criminology. The history of psychiatric photography, therefore, cannot be reduced to asylum photography. Medical photographs often entered into dialogue with other types of images such as the photographs of criminals made by Cesare

Lombroso (Italy), Alphonse Bertillon (France), and Francis Galton (Britain). Borrowing from physiognomic ideas, they defended the existence of a 'criminal type'. For them, criminals had particular facial and bodily features, which could be identified with the proper photographic method. Bertillon established an extensive protocol for the photography of criminals, which integrated images and anthropometric data such as head measurements on filing cards, and a system to classify and retrieve images from the police archive.[25] In contrast, Galton's 'composite portraits' aimed to provide the general features of a type by superimposing images of individuals one on top of the other. In line with his eugenic beliefs, Galton also produced composite portraits of other social types such as 'the Jew'. While he also made a composite portrait of asylum patients, he concluded that there were no specific facial features that could predict insanity.[26] Lombroso, who popularised the idea of the 'born criminal' in his 1870 book *Criminal Man*, collected hundreds of photographs between 1850 and 1909, including photographs of psychiatric patients from Italian asylums.[27] While the criminals and the insane were not necessarily or always the same, both psychiatry and criminology embraced a similar project, using photography to identify individuals, determine the general features of insanity and criminality respectively, and predict who would become insane or a criminal.

One of the best examples of the interdisciplinary nature of nineteenth-century medical photography is the production related to Jean-Martin Charcot, a French pathologist, neurologist, and psychiatrist working at the Parisian Hospital La Salpêtrière between 1862 and 1893. During Charcot's tenure, the Salpêtrière consolidated itself as a modern teaching institution, with students coming from all around the world to attend Charcot's lectures (Freud was among them).[28] Thanks to public funding, between 1875 and 1900 the Salpêtrière built anatomical and pathological laboratories, an amphitheatre with a capacity for 500 people, a pathological museum, and up to 3 photographic studios.[29] Photography at the Salpêtrière was not the personal initiative of a doctor, but a centralised system unparalleled at the time. Albert Londe, head of the Photography Laboratory since 1884, designed a protocol for the photography of patients, organised the construction of an archive of the photographs, and their public dissemination through books and journals, including *Nouvelle Iconographie de la Salpêtrière* (*New Iconography of the Salpêtrière*, 1880–1918).[30] The analysis of Salpêtrière's most famous photographs, the images of hysteric patients (1875–1880), reveals the complexity of photographic practices in medical institutions as well as the intimate relationship between photographs, textual accounts, and other visual sources.

Between 1875 and 1880 Charcot, together with Desiré Magloire Bourneville and Paul Regnard, published five issues of *Iconographie photographique de la Salpêtrière* (*Photographic Iconography of the Salpêtrière*), first as a compilation of photographs and later as a combination of photographs and clinical histories of women suffering from hysteria. *Iconographie* followed in the footsteps of the *Photographic Journal of Parisian Hospitals* (1869–1872), the first medical journal to publish photographic plates, not simply drawings or engravings after photographs.[31] The photographs in *Iconographie*

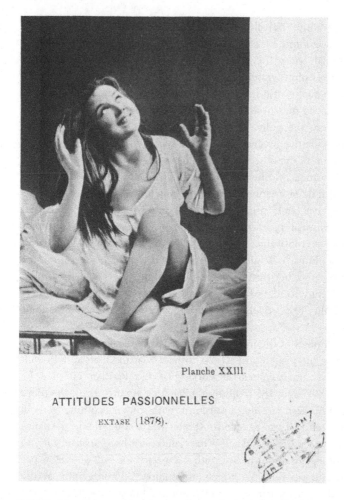

Planche XXIII.

ATTITUDES PASSIONNELLES

EXTASE (1878).

FIGURE 2.3 *Iconographie photographique de la Salpêtrière: service de M. Charcot,* par Bourneville et P. Regnard (1878), Planche XXIII, Attitudes Passionnelles, 'Extase'. Wellcome Collection. Attribution 4.0 International (CC BY 4.0)

showed patients in the middle of a hysterical attack, making exaggerated gestures such as 'amorous supplication', 'ecstasy' (Figure 2.3), or even 'crucifixion'. Some of these patients were photographed in bed, others were in the garden. This lack of visual consistency was intentional. Charcot's aim was to identify and define the stages of the hysterical attack in order to better understand its nervous origins. While the photographic studio was equipped with a bed, and many photographs were taken there, the camera had to chase the patients, wherever the attack happened, in the studio, the wards, or outdoors. This was possible thanks to the use of dry gelatine plates, which, unlike the older wet collodion process, allowed photographers to load the glass plates in advance and did not require the development of the plate immediately after taking the photograph. The Salpêtrière's team took advantage of the new possibilities afforded by technological innovations to advance a new way to visualise mental disorders. Unlike the portraits of the insane previously explored, hysteria was not attached to any particular facial features, but to a series of movements. Visualising hysteria as a dynamic flow was key to Charcot's new conceptualisation of the disease.

Despite the long history of hysteria, it still persisted as a cluster of symptoms that was easier to diagnose than to explain.[32] The so-called 'grand hysteria' often manifested in crises where women suffered from convulsions, the paralysis of limbs, and fits such as the famous 'arch of hysteria', where the patient's body formed an arch supported by the head and feet. These symptoms, however, were shared with other disorders such as epilepsy and tetanus.[33] Charcot studied hysterical attacks by combining the visual observation of the body of patients with post-mortem studies of the brain that would confirm neurological and nervous disorders (on post-mortem investigation, see Jennifer Wallis's chapter in this volume). Photographs became essential tools to identify hysteria's specific symptoms and its four phases: 'epileptoid', 'clownism', 'passionate attitudes', and 'delirium', characterised by particular movements.[34] For instance, Figure 2.3 shows a patient in the stage of passionate attitudes, while Figure 2.4 shows the same woman with a contracture in her leg, belonging to the first stage of the attack. These movements were captured thanks to instantaneous photography, but it was the publication of the photographs in *Iconographie* that helped to make sense of the attacks by putting together images and text. Each issue focused on a few patients, noting the cause of their admission, their daily routines, and their symptoms. Some patients suffered multiple attacks in a day, and hysterical stages lasted for only a brief time, barely 10 or 20 seconds. The speed with which patients went from one phase to the next reveals the utility of photography, which captured moments that the naked eye did not fully register. The references to the images in the clinical histories also confirm that the photographs documented different attacks over several days. However, by serialising the photographs, *Iconographie* presented them to the reader as the images of 'grand hysteria', rather than as pictures of the particular attack suffered by a specific patient. Therefore, while clinical histories described individual cases, photographs presented general conclusions. This generalisation was possible thanks to the interaction between text and image.

Photographs also acquired meaning through their relation with other visual media. At the Salpêtrière, doctor Paul Richer often drew sketches from photographs and modelled wax sculptures of patients presenting bodily pathologies.[35] Unlike photographs, which were sometimes blurred and showed both the patient and her surroundings, the simplicity of the handwritten lines helped viewers to focus on the essential details. In 1885, Richer compiled all the drawings of the different stages of the hysterical attack into one synoptic table (Figure 2.5).[36] By presenting all the variations of movement in each stage, Richer's table visualised the hysterical attack as a whole. Photographs, which had provided the raw data, were absent from the table, but formed the basis of it. This combination of photographs and drawings was common in medical publications. Journals and

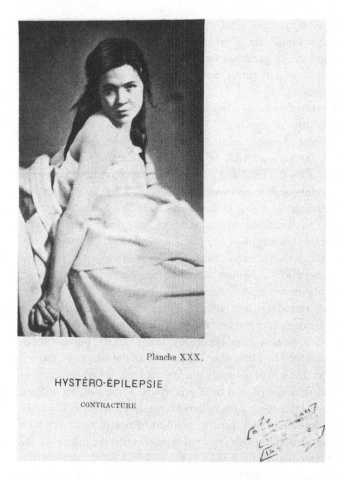

FIGURE 2.4 *Iconographie photographique de la Salpêtrière: service de M. Charcot*, par Bourneville et P. Regnard (1878), Planche XXX, 'Hystero-epilepsie, contracture'. Wellcome Collection. Attribution 4.0 International (CC BY 4.0)

textbooks often included photographic images, drawings, or engravings after photographs and other data visualisation objects such as diagrams and graphic inscriptions of the pulse, breath, etc. Reading photographs alongside other visual media shows the particular role of photographs in psychiatric research. As mental disorders were understood as nervous disorders, and therefore as something having an organic origin, photographs and graphic inscriptions showed the relationship between external and internal changes.

Historiographies and methods

Historians of photography, psychiatry, and medicine routinely use photographs like those examined in this chapter. However, it has not always been like this.

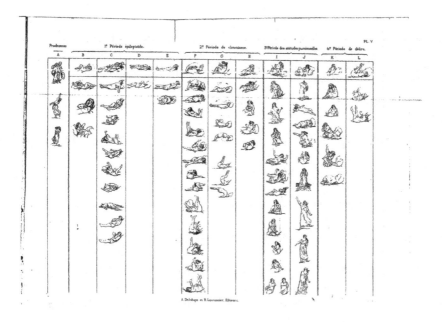

FIGURE 2.5   Paul Richer, *Etudes cliniques sur l'hystéro-épilepsie ou grande hystérie*, 2nd edn (Paris: Delahaye et Lecrosnier, 1885), Planche V, 'Tableau synoptique de la grande attaque hystérique'. Gallica/Bibliothèque nationale de France

Only a handful of publications referred to nineteenth-century medical photographs up until the 1960s.[37] Sander Gilman's *The Face of Madness*, published in 1976, was the first time that Diamond's photographs and speech were published. It was not until the late 1980s, with the work of John Tagg and Allan Sekula, that medical photography became a mainstream topic in the history of photography. Gilman's books in the 1980s also contributed to the popularisation of photographs in the history of medicine.[38] While these works focused on medical photography as a topic, recent scholarship seeks to fully integrate photographs into the history of medicine, using photographic materials alongside other sources to explore topics such as the body in nineteenth-century asylum research, the history of 'incurables' in the Victorian asylum, or the AIDS epidemic.[39]

John Tagg's *The Burden of Representation* (1988) and Allan Sekula's 'The Body and the Archive' (1986) have been tremendously influential, defining the main approach to medical photography for generations. In line with Marxist and Foucauldian analyses of power, Tagg and Sekula explore the social and political processes by which photographs became evidence in courtrooms, police quarters, and hospitals in the nineteenth century. Tagg's work focuses on the 'power effects' of photographic representations such as the criminal mugshot and the medical image, which did not simply record reality like a mirror but produced social realities.[40] Examining medical photography alongside criminal and police photography, Tagg emphasises their regulatory and surveillance role. Similarly, Sekula explores medical photography in relation to Galton and Bertillon and the emergence of the modern archive, which he defines as the 'dominant institutional basis for photographic meaning'.[41] For Sekula, photography, and particularly the photographic archive, contributed to regulating society by means of defining what constituted deviation from the norm, such as the criminal or the insane. Both Tagg and Sekula, therefore, understand medical photographic representations as institutional tools for social control.

Chris Amirault has written about the parallels between Foucault's concept of the medical gaze and nineteenth-century ideas of photographs as objective representations.[42] Focusing on the differences between photographic and artistic images, Amirault argues that 'in its fantasy of objectivity, medical photography instituted the enforcement of the objective subject called the patient'.[43] The analysis of early medical photographs also reveals, according to Amirault, that the medical gaze was a male gaze.[44] The sexualisation of female patients by male photographers and doctors is a prominent topic in the literature. Charcot's photographs of hysterical women, only dressed in their nightgowns, showing their bare shoulders and legs and unaware of the camera, have often raised these criticisms.[45] In the same line, Erin O'Connor has argued that the use of photography in the consolidation of anorexia nervosa as a diagnostic category reinforced traditional ideas about the female body, its appearance, and its sexuality.[46] When doctors started to identify anorexia nervosa with a thin body, according to O'Connor, 'it was not necessary to understand why the fasting girl had made her body so thin in order to treat her thinness effectively'.[47] Photography reinforced this process by documenting patients' bodily changes, staging 'the reconfiguration of the female body as the restoration of health, fusing questions of personal appearance and physical well-being so thoroughly that the management of starvation became indistinguishible from the management of sexuality'.[48] For O'Connor, photographic representations of the female body became evidence of a new medical discourse for which 'the restoration of female health' became 'the restoration of gender'.[49]

Shifting the focus away from representations, recent work has examined photographic practices from a material point of view. Inspired by material culture studies, photographic historians such as Elizabeth Edwards have argued that just as important as the content of the image is the material format of the photograph (paper, cardboard, glass, film), as well as any traces or inscriptions on the surface.[50] This perspective examines photographs as cultural and social objects, asking not what photographs represent, but what photographs *do*. Applied to medical photography, focusing on material practices helps to recognise cameras and other photographic equipment such as backdrops, props, and artificial lighting as medical tools. In relation to the Salpêtrière, for instance, I have argued that the use of different photographic cameras, rather than different images, contributed to the conceptualisation of facial expressions and bodily gestures as organic signs of emotions.[51]

Historians have also used medical photographs to explore questions not necessarily related to medicine. Caroline Bressey, for instance, has used medical photographic records to reconstruct the social history of Black Londoners in a multicultural city.[52] More broadly, Suzannah Biernoff has examined the ethical implications of digital uses of historical medical photographs, particularly in the context of video games.[53] Medical photographs are, therefore, versatile sources that can be examined in myriad ways. As an emerging subfield, sitting between the history of medicine, the history of photography, and social and cultural history, the history of medical photography offers innovative ways to use visual and material evidence.

Archives and ethics

Photographs can be found everywhere. However, as Elizabeth Edwards and Christopher Morton warn, 'their very ubiquity counts against them, for beyond those photographs categorized as "art" or as "masterpieces of early photography" and the like, photographs sit low in the hierarchy of museum values'.[54] With the exception of photographs that are firmly established in the canonical history of photography, the masses of 'anonymous, unregistered' photographs do not feature prominently in museums or archival collections.[55] The fact that photographs are not always preserved in the more recognisable forms of prints and albums, often attached to or printed on other types of documents, only complicates the situation. Within the history of psychiatry, and medicine in general, there is an increasing recognition of the value of photographic materials as historical documents. However, the history of medical photography collecting in archives and museums presents the same characteristics described by Edwards and Morton. The production of 'early masters' such as Diamond and Charcot is relatively easy to locate. A quick Google search shows that Diamond's prints are currently preserved at the J. Paul Getty Museum in Los Angeles, the Metropolitan Museum of Art in New York, and the Victoria & Albert Museum (V&A) in London, all major art institutions (which, incidentally, might indicate that Diamond's photographs are now considered part of the history of art). Charcot's production at the Salpêtrière is a different case, as the photographic prints have mostly been lost.[56] However, copies of *Iconographie* and *Nouvelle* can be easily accessed in medical libraries. More difficult to uncover are the thousands of photographs taken in hospitals and asylums around the world.

Digitisation projects carried out by heritage institutions such as the Wellcome Library in the UK or the BIU-Santé in France, as well as online repositories such as The Medical Heritage Library, have broadened access to medical collections.[57] Browsing digital collections also makes the identification of illustrated books, journals, and casebooks easier. This is clearly a positive development, as digital projects have widened access to archive collections.

As ever with medical history collections, the Wellcome Library is the best starting point in the UK. Among its holdings, the Wellcome preserves the photographs made by James Crichton-Browne at the West Riding Pauper Lunatic Asylum, Wakefield, in the early 1870s. Crichton-Browne sent copies of his photographs to Charles Darwin for his study on the expression of the emotions in man and animals, which are now preserved at the University of Cambridge.[58] Other interesting photographic collections are the photographs from the Royal Albert Asylum in Lancaster, which include documents such as Figure 2.6, a plate combining photographs of a brain from different perspectives.[59] While a good number of these photographs are available through the Wellcome Images catalogue, many are not. The richly-illustrated Holloway Sanatorium casebooks, for instance, need to be accessed through the main catalogue in spite of being richly illustrated.[60] The fact that a particular casebook or book is not identified as being illustrated or does not come up in image results does not mean that it does not include pictures.

Medical photographs are not only preserved in medical libraries. For example, the V&A currently holds several of Diamond's prints because they are part of the Royal Photographic Society collection that the Museum recently acquired, and which also includes other medical photographs.[61] Local archives, and record offices in particular, are especially helpful. For instance, the Leicester Records Office preserves the casebooks of the former Leicester Borough Lunatic Asylum, and the Tyne and Wear Archives Service holds the Newcastle City Lunatic Asylum casebooks.[62] Sometimes, medical photographs are not identified as specific collections and lay around in boxes and drawers, labelled as 'ephemera'. This is the case with the late 1800s album that the medical photographer Anni Skilton found at the Bristol Royal Infirmary in 2012. Containing around 250 photographs arranged over 100 pages, the images in this album are not unusual for their time, but throw light on the relationships between photography, medical specimens, surgery, and medical museums in the late nineteenth century.[63] Now safely stored at the Bristol Records Office and digitally available via the Wellcome catalogue, the story of this album illustrates the multiple trajectories of medical photographs.

However, researchers need to be aware of the risks attached to medical images. Medical photographs are sensitive sources. Nowadays, medical photographers need to abide by ethical protocols, making sure that they have the informed consent of the patient for the taking and circulation of the photographs, anonymise the images, and store them privately and securely.[64] However, no such codes exist for medical photographs that are over 100 years old. Some institutions are reviewing their ethical guidelines in relation to the access and dissemination of their archival collections, but no standard or universal conventions exist.[65] In spite of this, as researchers, we need to be aware of our responsibility towards the people we study. Nineteenth- and early twentieth-century medical photographs often show patients, sometimes children, naked, in distress, and in vulnerable situations. Moreover, these images can trigger all sorts of responses from viewers, from sympathy and shock to disgust and trauma. Therefore, we need to think twice

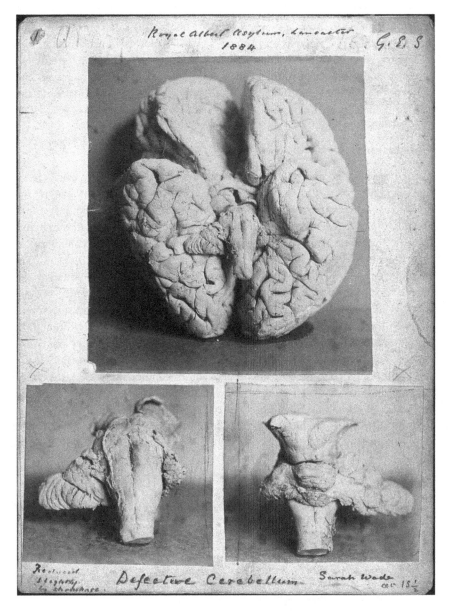

FIGURE 2.6   Royal Albert Asylum, Lancaster: brain with a defective cerebellum, seen from different angles. Three photographs, 1884. Wellcome Collection. Attribution 4.0 International (CC BY 4.0)

about why we want to use a particular image and whether we need to use it at all. For instance, we might need to publish the photographs as part of the argument, but what would be the effect of naming the patient? Would that contribute to further stigmatisation or acknowledge the individual lives of patients? Similarly, we need to discuss how and when to share medical images on social media. Posting medical photographs on platforms with limited space for discussion, such as Twitter, runs the risk of decontextualising the images, turning them into objects of shock and a means to prompt quick emotional reactions. There are no easy answers, but it is our responsibility to thoroughly consider the potential harm that sharing medical images can cause viewers and historical subjects.

Conclusions

Using photographic materials as sources in the history of psychiatry can be challenging, but it can also open up new research questions. Photography was common practice in many institutions in the nineteenth century, and doctors and alienists routinely used photographs to identify patients, diagnose, research, and communicate with their peers. Photographs were more than passive illustrations and, therefore, we should examine them as the active agents they were. The multiplicity of images and the various uses of photographs examined in this chapter demonstrate that photography was a fluid, often experimental, practice that was adapted to the circumstances of each institution. This is not, therefore, a linear history, as several practices often overlapped in the same institution. The historiography section has shown that photographs are versatile sources that can be interpreted in different ways. Photographic meaning is inherently unstable, as it is the product of a continuous dialogue between the author's intention, the image content, and the viewer's reading. This chapter has provided some historical and methodological tools for using photographs as sources in the history of psychiatry, locating them in the archives, and considering the ethical issues involved in disseminating them.

Notes

1 Peter Burke, *Eyewitnessing: The Uses of Images as Historical Evidence* (Ithaca, NY: Cornell University Press, 2001), p. 10.
2 See Katherine D.B. Rawling, '"The Annexed Photos Were Taken Today": Photographing Patients in the Late Nineteenth-Century Asylum', *Social History of Medicine*, hkz060 (2020). https://doi.org/10.1093/shm/hkz060, accessed 15 Mar. 2021.
3 Hugh Welch Diamond, 'On the Application of Photography to the Physiognomic and Mental Phenomena of Insanity', in Sander Gilman (ed.), *The Face of Madness. Hugh Welch Diamond and the Origins of Psychiatric Photography* (New York: Brunner/Mazel, 1976), pp. 17–24. Pearl, 'Through a Mediated Mirror'.
4 John Conolly, 'Case Studies from the Physiognomy of Insanity', *The Medical Times and Gazette* (1858). Reproduced in Gilman, *Face of Madness*, pp. 25–72.
5 Gilman, *Face of Madness*, p. 7.
6 See Tanya Sheehan and Andres Mario Zervigón (eds), *Photography and its Origins* (New York and London: Routledge, 2015).
7 Sharrona Pearl, 'Through a Mediated Mirror: The Photographic Physiognomy of Dr Hugh Welch Diamond', *History of Photography*, 33, 3 (2009), pp. 288–305: p. 291; Laurie Dahlberg, 'Dr Diamond's Day Off', *History of Photography*, 39, 1 (2015), pp. 3–17: p. 7.

8 For this debate, see Joan Schwartz, 'Records of Simple Truth and Precision': Photography, Archives and the Illusion of Control', *Archivaria*, 50 (2000), pp. 1–40.
9 Dahlberg, 'Dr Diamond's Day Off'.
10 Diamond, 'On the Application of Photography'.
11 Lorraine Daston and Peter Galison, *Objectivity* (New York: Zone Books, 2007). See also Jennifer Tucker, *Nature Exposed. Photography as Eyewitness in Victorian Science* (Baltimore and London: John Hopkins University, 2005).
12 Johann Kaspar Lavater, *Essays on Physiognomy; for the Promotion of the Knowledge and the Love of Mankind*, trans. Thomas Holcroft (London: G.G.J. and J. Robinson, 1789).
13 Pearl, 'Through a Mediated Mirror', p. 290.
14 Diamond, 'On the Application of Photography'.
15 N.G. Chernbach, *Atlas Photographic de Cateva Typuri Principale de Alienati* (Bucharest: Noua Tipografie a Laboratorilor Romani, 1870).
16 Octavian Buda, 'The Face of Madness in Romania: The Origin of Psychiatric Photography in Eastern Europe', *History of Psychiatry*, 21, 3 (2010), pp. 278–93.
17 Henri Dagonet, Album de 26 photographies d'aliénés annotés par Henri Dagonet. CISA 911. Album de 49 planches rassemblant 76 photographies d'aliénés annotés par Henri Dagonet. CISA 911. BIU Santé, Paris. The albums have been digitised and are available online: https://www.biusante.parisdescartes.fr/histoire/medica/resultats/index.php?fille=o&cotemere=CISA0911, accessed 15 Oct. 2020.
18 N. 22, 'Hydrocephalia', CISA 911, BIU Santé; Dagonet, *Traité des maladies mentales*, 3rd edn (Paris: J.-B. Baillière, 1894), p. 672; Sarah Rey, 'Les Fonds François-Franck – Janet – Dumas. L'invention de la psychologie moderne' Salamandre. Fonds de plaques de verre photographiques François-Franck, Collège de France.
19 Rawling, "Annexed Photos"; Susan Sidlauskas, 'Inventing the Medical Portrait. Photography at the 'Benevolent Asylum' of Holloway, ca. 1885–1889', *Medical Humanities*, 39, 1 (2013), pp. 29–37.
20 Rawling, "Annexed Photos", p. 6.
21 Ibid., p. 3.
22 Rory du Plessis, 'Photographs from the Grahamstown Lunatic Asylum, South Africa, 1890–1907', *Social Dynamics*, 40, 1 (2014), pp. 12–42.
23 Ibid., pp. 15–6.
24 Ibid., p. 13.
25 Alphonse Bertillon, *La photographie judiciare: avec un appendice sur la classification et identification anthropométrique* (Paris: Gauthier-Villars, 1900).
26 Fae Brauer, 'Framing Darwin. A Portrait of Eugenics', in Fae Brauer and Barbara Larson (eds), *The Art of Evolution: Darwin, Darwinisms and Visual Culture* (Hanover and London: University Press of New England, 2009), pp. 124–54: p. 137.
27 Nicoletta Leonardi, 'It metodo lombrosiano e la fotografia come oggetti sociale', in Silvano Montaldo and Cristina Cilli (eds), *Il Museo di Antropologia Criminale "Cesare Lombroso" dell'Universita di Torino* (Cinisello Balsamo, MI: Silvana Editore, 2015), pp. 36–51.
28 Mark S. Micale, 'The Salpêtrière in the Age of Charcot. An Institutional Perspective on Medical History in the Late Nineteenth Century', *Journal of Contemporary History*, 20, 4 (1985), pp. 703–31.
29 Ibid., p. 709.
30 Albert Londe, *La photographie médicale. Application des sciences médicales et physiologiques* (Paris: Gauthier-Villars et Fils, 1893).
31 *Revue photographique des hôpitaux de Paris* (Paris: A. Delahaye, 1869–1872), 4 vols.
32 Sabine Arnaud, *On Hysteria: The Invention of a Medical Category between 1670 and 1820* (Chicago, IL: Chicago University Press, 2015).
33 Diana P. Faber, 'Charcot and the Epilepsy/Hysteria Relationship', *Journal of the History of the Neurosciences*, 6, 3 (1997), pp. 275–90.

34 Georges Didi-Huberman, *Invention of Hysteria. Charcot and the Photographic Iconography of the Salpêtrière*, trans. Alisa Hartz (Cambridge, MA and London: MIT Press, 2003), p. 115.

35 Natasha Gomez Ruiz, 'The 'Scientific Artworks' of Doctor Paul Richer', *Medical Humanities*, 39, 1 (2013), pp. 4–10.

36 Paul Richer, *Etudes cliniques sur l'hystéro-épilepsie ou grande hystérie*, 2nd edn (Paris: Delahaye et Lecrosnier, 1885).

37 Alison Gernsheim, 'Medical Photography in the Nineteenth Century', *Medical and Biological Illustration*, 11 (1961), pp. 85–92; Robert Ollerenshaw, 'Medical Illustration: The Impact of Photography on Its History', *Journal of the Biological Photographic Association*, 36 (1968), pp. 6–13.

38 Sander L. Gilman, *Seeing the Insane* (Lincoln, NE and London: University of Nebraska Press, 1982); Sander L. Gilman, *Disease and Representation: Images of Illness from Madness to AIDS* (Ithaca, NY and London: Cornell University Press, 1988).

39 Jennifer Wallis, *Investigating the Body in the Victorian Asylum: Doctors, Patients, and Practices* (Cham, Switzerland: Palgrave Macmillan, 2017); Stef Eastoe, *Idiocy, Imbecility and Insanity in Victorian Society: Caterham Asylum, 1867–1911* (Cham, Switzerland: Palgrave Macmillan, 2020); Lukas Engelmann, *Mapping AIDS. Visual Histories of an Enduring Epidemic* (Cambridge: Cambridge University Press, 2018).

40 John Tagg, *The Burden of Representation: Essays on Photographies and Histories* (The Macmillan Press, 1988), p. 21.

41 Allan Sekula, 'The Body and the Archive', *October*, 39 (1986), pp. 3–64.

42 Chris Amirault, 'Posing the Subject of Early Medical Photography', *Discourse*, 16, 2 (1993/1994), pp. 51–76.

43 Amirault, 'Posing the Subject', p. 70. See also Erin O'Connor, 'Camera Medica: Towards a Morbid History of Photography', *History of Photography*, 23, 3 (1999), pp. 232–44.

44 Amirault, 'Posing the Subject', p. 69.

45 See Didi-Huberman, *Invention of Hysteria*; Asti Hustvedt, *Medical Muses: Hysteria in Nineteenth-Century Paris* (London: Bloomsbury, 2011).

46 Erin O'Connor, 'Pictures of Health: Medical Photography and the Emergence of Anorexia Nervosa', *Journal of the History of Sexuality*, 5, 4 (1995), pp. 535–72.

47 Ibid., p. 541.

48 Ibid.

49 Ibid. p. 543.

50 Elizabeth Edwards and Janice Hart (eds), *Photographs, Objects, Histories: On the Materiality of Photography* (London: Routledge, 2004).

51 Beatriz Pichel, 'From Facial Expressions to Bodily Gestures. Passions, Photography and Movement in French 19th Century Sciences', *History of the Human Sciences*, 29, 1 (2016), pp. 27–48; Beatriz Pichel, 'Photographing the Emotional Body. Performing Expressions in the Theatre and Psychological Sciences', in Dolores Martin-Moruno and Beatriz Pichel (eds), *Emotional Bodies. The Historical Performativity of Emotions* (Urbana, IL: University of Illinois Press, 2019), pp. 97–119.

52 Caroline Bressey, 'The City of Others. Photographs from the City of London Asylum Archive', *19: Interdisciplinary Studies in the Long Nineteenth Century*, 13 (2011), https://19.bbk.ac.uk/article/id/1661/, accessed 15 Mar. 2021.

53 Suzannah Biernoff, 'Medical Archives and Digital Culture: From WWI to BioShock', *Medical History*, 55, 3 (2011), pp. 325–30.

54 Elizabeth Edwards and Chris Morton (eds), *Museums, Photographs, Collections: Between Art and Information* (London and New York: Bloomsbury, 2015), p. 3.

55 Ibid.

56 The photochronographic plates taken by Albert Londe, director of the photography laboratory at the Salpêtrière in the 1890s, are currently preserved at the Paris École Nationale Supérieur des Beaux Arts. The Bibliothèque Charcot also preserves some

photographic prints. The Centre for the History of Medicine at the Countway Library (Harvard University) preserves thousands of glass plates of the Salpêtrière and related hospitals.

57 Wellcome Images: https://wellcomecollection.org/works; BIU Santé, Medica: https://www.biusante.parisdescartes.fr/histoire/medica/index.php, Medical Heritage Library: http://www.medicalheritage.org/. All links last accessed 15 Sept. 2020.

58 See University of Cambridge Library, Darwin Papers, particularly DAR.51.1.

59 Wellcome Library no. 39152i. Royal Albert Asylum, Lancaster, 1884. G.E.S. Reduced slightly by shrinkage. Defective cerebellum. Sarah Wade at 151/2.

60 https://wellcomelibrary.org/search-the-catalogues/, accessed 25 Mar. 2021.

61 See V&A Collections, https://collections.vam.ac.uk/search/?id_person=C6869, accessed 29 Mar. 2021.

62 Rawling has examined the Newcastle casebooks in "Annexed Photos". The Leicester case books have only been the object of an undergraduate dissertation by Deimena Daugelaite at De Montfort University.

63 Anni Skilton, 'Recording the Diseased and the Deceased. A Historical Look at Medical Illustration in 19th-Century Bristol', *Journal of Visual Communication in Medicine*, 38, 1/2 (2015), pp. 85–94.

64 Tiana Kazemi, Kachiu C. Lee, and Lionel Bercovitch, 'Just a Quick Pic: Ethics of Medical Photography', *Journal of the American Academy of Dermatology*, 80, 4 (2019), pp. 1172–4.

65 Mineke te Hiennepe, 'Private Portraits or Suffering on Stage: Curating Clinical Photographic Collections in the Museum Context', *Science Museum Group Journal*, 5, 5 (2019), http://dx.doi.org/10.15180/160503, accessed 15 Mar. 2021; Beatriz Pichel, Katherine Rawling, and Jennifer Wallis, 'Historical Photographs as Sensitive Sources: Questions and Challenges', Royal Historical Society blog (2020), http://blog.royalhistsoc.org/2020/09/07/photographs-sensitive-sources/, accessed 15 Sept. 2020.

Select bibliography

Burke, P., *Eyewitnessing: The Uses of Images as Historical Evidence*, Ithaca, NY: Cornell University Press, 2001.

Edwards, E. and Hart, J. (eds), *Photographs, Objects, Histories. On the Materiality of Photography*, London: Routledge, 2004.

Gilman, S., *Disease and Representation. Images of Illness from Madness to AIDS*, Ithaca, NY: Cornell University Press, 1988.

Gilman, S. (ed.), *The Face of Madness: Hugh W. Diamond and the Origins of Psychiatric Photography*, New York: Brunner/Mazel, 1976.

O'Connor, E., 'Camera Medica. Towards a Morbid History of Photography', *History of Photography* 23, 1999, pp. 232–244.

Sekula, A., 'The Body and the Archive', *October* 39, 1986, pp. 3–64.

Tagg, J., *The Burden of Representation. Essays on Photographies and Histories*, Basingstoke: The Macmillan Press, 1988.

Tucker, J., *Nature Exposed: Photography as Eyewitness in Victorian Science*, Baltimore, MD: Johns Hopkins University Press, 2005.

3

USING ASYLUM POST-MORTEM RECORDS IN THE HISTORY OF PSYCHIATRY

Jennifer Wallis

For many years, the history of psychiatry was primarily a social history, concerned with the experiences of patients and families, the everyday life of institutions, and the operation of power within the psychiatric encounter. The impetus to place patient experience at the heart of the analysis, while productive in so many ways, has, however, often had the unintended effect of effacing much of the *scientific* work of psychiatry. Historical interest in these scientific practices has grown in recent years.[1] This renewed interest in the scientific side of psychiatry is not intended to replace or to overwrite socially-oriented histories, rather to acknowledge the diversity of past psychiatric practice. After all, many of the laboratory spaces and experimental practices described in this body of work underpinned patient experiences and treatments.

In melding the scientific and social aspects of psychiatry's history, several historians have focused on death in the asylum, most notably in the 2012 special issue of *History of Psychiatry*, 'Lunacy's Last Rites: Dying Insane in Britain, c.1629–1939'. The authors explore, among other issues, the role of asylums within nineteenth-century networks for supplying bodies for anatomical teaching, and the provision of asylum cemeteries.[2] Jonathan Andrews notes in his article in that issue that post-mortem data is an often-overlooked source in the history of psychiatry.[3] There are exceptions, of course: post-mortem records have been used by Eric Engstrom in his study of imperial German psychiatry, by Gayle Davis on Scotland, by Dolly MacKinnon on Australia, and by Lynsey Cullen and myself on Britain.[4] In each of these examples, post-mortem records are used to enhance our understanding of institutional preoccupations as well as broader contemporary psychiatric landscapes, from changing diagnostic criteria throughout a patient's stay to debates surrounding bodily injury. The authors combine post-mortem records with information from casebooks and other sources. If we are to better understand the scientific aspects of the history of psychiatry, including the ways in which this

DOI: 10.4324/9781003087694-4

influenced patient care, post-mortem records are important documents. This is particularly the case when looking at the late nineteenth and early twentieth century, a period when psychiatry strived to prove itself to be a 'natural science with its own rigorous techniques and modes of observation'.[5]

Throughout this chapter I use the term 'post-mortem' and 'post-mortem records'. The applicability of this term to the procedure in asylums is discussed in more detail in Cullen's work.[6] Strictly speaking, 'post-mortem' refers to an examination that takes place by order of a coroner; in Britain for instance, under the terms of the 1862 Lunacy Amendment Act, the local coroner was to be informed of every death within an asylum.[7] In most institutional records, however, the term 'post-mortem' was used to refer to the examination of the body after death whether or not the examination was taking place under coroners' orders.[8] Most surviving 'post-mortem books' contain the records of *all* deaths within an institution, not just coroners' cases, and so this chapter uses 'post-mortem' to refer to the procedure in this broad sense as used by many asylum doctors at the time.[9]

This chapter begins with a brief overview of post-mortems within psychiatry, including some of the legislative developments that affected practices in the second half of the nineteenth century in Britain. Although the bulk of my examples come from the nineteenth-century British context (thus, I use the term 'asylum' rather than 'institution' or 'mental hospital'), the questions raised are directly applicable to other contexts. The chapter considers how to find and interpret post-mortem records, offering guidance for understanding their layout and content as well as highlighting the challenges the historian faces in using them – such as dealing with unfamiliar and outdated medical terminology. Strategies for dealing with these challenges are considered, including how post-mortem records might be better contextualised and understood with the help of other sources such as textbooks. Finally, the chapter offers some examples of how historians have used post-mortem records in their work, arguing that these are sources with much to offer the historian of psychiatry.

Post-mortems and pathology in psychiatry

Although the second half of the nineteenth century was the period when the post-mortem became more firmly entrenched in psychiatry, there was already a long-standing interest in the pathology of insanity. Eighteenth-century Italian anatomist Giovanni Battista Morgagni examined the bodies of several insane patients, and rudimentary observations of the brains and viscera of insane patients were made by Herman Boerhaave (Dutch Republic) and Jean-Étienne Dominique Esquirol (France), among others. In France, the Inspector-General of Asylums Jean-Baptiste-Maximiem Parchappe de Vinay was writing about his pathological investigations of the brain in the late 1830s. Achille-Louis Foville was undertaking anatomical investigations of the brain and spinal cord during the same period, and France's Charenton Asylum (where Foville was located for part of his career) was notable for its connection to Antoine Laurent Jessé Bayle and Louis-Florentin

Calmeil, both of whom researched the anatomical features of General Paralysis of the Insane (GPI) early in the nineteenth century.[10]

Much of this early work relied upon animals as experimental material, but human bodies were preferable. During the nineteenth century, the use of human bodies for anatomical teaching and experimentation – a fate previously reserved for executed criminals – expanded with the introduction of new legislation. The 1832 Anatomy Act in Britain stipulated that the unclaimed bodies of paupers dying in public institutions were legitimate subjects for anatomical examination; the Act was followed by similar legislation in other countries. The implications of such legislation, with asylums joining workhouses and prisons as sources of 'unwanted' bodies for anatomical teaching and research, have been explored by a number of historians.[11] Elizabeth Hurren, for instance, highlights Cambridge Professor Alexander Macalister's reliance upon bodies from the local asylum for his research into heredity and evolution.[12]

As interest in the pathology of insanity grew, the bodies of asylum patients were increasingly viewed as valuable material for research into psychiatric illness, prized by asylum superintendents for the insights they might offer into complex conditions like GPI. As well as admiration for the earlier work of figures like Bayle, Calmeil, and Foville in France, psychiatrists the world over were looking to Germany, where pathological research and post-mortem investigation was becoming more systematised. The so-called German model, in which psychiatric provision was divided between chronic asylums and acute units attached to teaching hospitals (and where, in most states, doctors did not need a family's explicit consent to perform an examination[13]), was an aspirational one that would be carried out in a modified form by several institutions in Britain and America.[14] During the 1870s there were attempts to embed pathological work more firmly in psychiatric practice; there was an unsuccessful call to make post-mortems compulsory in British asylums, for example.[15]

The specific legislation governing post-mortem procedure will vary according to your own region of study, and general works on the history of dissection will be a helpful starting point in getting to grips with this.[16] At some institutions, carrying out a post-mortem was further dependent on gaining the consent of the patient's family or friends. When seeking this consent, the post-mortem was often cast as being for the greater good. At the same time, bodies were viewed as the 'property' of institutions.[17] The opportunity to register an objection to a post-mortem could depend on the way in which the intention to conduct one was communicated, as well as the literacy level of the patient and/or their family. Determining an institution's procedures for obtaining consent can be tricky for the historian, but annual reports and meeting minutes can be useful here, as well as any collections of ephemera containing documents such as letters sent to patients' families at the point of admission or death. The Medical Superintendent's report for Manchester's Prestwich Asylum in 1874, for instance, noted that post-mortem examinations would have been made in all deaths were it not for the fact that 'in numerous instances the friends could not be prevailed upon to grant the necessary permissions'.[18] Glimpses of permissions given or withheld can occasionally be seen in notes within post-mortem records, with the refusal or partial refusal of families entered into the record, such as 'Thorax only permitted to be examined'.[19] Here, post-mortem records may also be revealing of local religious communities, mourning traditions, and burial customs.[20]

Asylums and their staff were accountable to government-appointed bodies as well as patients' families. In Britain the Commissioners in Lunacy, a public body established in 1845 to oversee the operation of asylums, viewed post-mortem records as important documents supplementing other data (on recovery rates, for instance), as well as providing evidence of any incidences of injury or assault. Individual pieces of legislation, like the 1885 Lunacy Acts Amendment Act in Britain, encouraged meticulous record-keeping that aimed to protect doctors from accusations of negligent treatment.[21] The Commissioners believed in the merits of the post-mortem as a knowledge-making exercise, too. In their report on the West Riding Asylum in Yorkshire in 1891, the Commissioners noted with regret that 'the Pathologist is not directing his attention to the relation of the cerebellum to the cerebrum, and to that part of the brain which is concerned with vision'.[22]

By this time, some asylums – in Britain and elsewhere – had appointed pathologists to their staff, also supplementing mortuaries with pathological laboratories and museums. One early adopter of this approach was the Royal Edinburgh Asylum in Scotland, which renovated its mortuary facilities in the 1850s.[23] In Canada in the 1880s, Kingston Asylum constructed an anatomy theatre to seat 70 people, testament to the importance of asylums as sites of teaching as well as sites of care.[24] By 1899 one contributor to the British *Journal of Mental Science* declared:

> It is probably not an exaggeration to say that no physicians have so many favourable opportunities for pathological observations as those connected with asylums. Post-mortem examinations are generally expected to be made in all patients who die in asylums. There are in most, if not in all the asylums, well-appointed mortuaries for conducting these examinations, and every facility is available for preparing and preserving morbid specimens and making microscopical and other observations.[25]

It is important to recognise that this increasing focus on pathology was not universally welcomed. William P. Phillimore, Superintendent of Nottingham County Asylum, wrote in the *British Medical Journal* that he believed his time better spent in the observation of insanity during life rather than after death.[26] Although high rates of post-mortem examination impressed the Commissioners, critics like Phillimore pointed to unclear consent procedures, a competitive spirit between asylums as to the numbers performed, and disparities in practice between pauper and private asylums. The spread of new practices and techniques was uneven: some asylums could not boast a microscope, let alone a full suite of laboratories.[27]

Nevertheless, by the turn of the century psychiatry could be more confident in presenting itself as a discipline based on empirical observation and experiment; the work of researchers like neurologist David Ferrier, who utilised the spaces and resources of asylums, was testament to this. In the preface to *The Microscopical Examination of the Human Brain* (1894), pathologist Edwin Goodall wrote with pride of the great increase of workers in 'cerebral pathology' in asylums.[28] By the beginning of the twentieth century, then, post-mortem examinations in asylums were by no means unusual, with objections to the procedure steadily diminishing even if professional enthusiasm for pathological investigation waxed and waned. By 1913, post-mortems were said to be performed in three out of four deaths in British asylums.[29] With many asylum archives containing reports of these procedures, where should the historical researcher start?

Finding post-mortem records

Before beginning your search for post-mortem records, it is worth considering what you might see in them, and if these are sources that you wish to engage with as part of your research. Detailed descriptions of procedures, and the presence of photographs and other visual materials, can be upsetting. Photographs may be stuck between the pages of books with no prior indication of their presence, and the physical effects of incidents such as sexual assault or suicide described in graphic detail. Post-mortem records were often present in the rooms where procedures were carried out, whether completed during or immediately after an examination. Their pages sometimes carry visible traces of pathological work, making them unusually resonant objects: pages may be stained with blood, or damaged by chemicals used in the preservation of specimens. If you decide to work with such sources, archivists will be well-placed to advise you about the content and state of an institution's records. When considering a timetable for your research, you might build in regular breaks, or identify supervisors and peers with whom you can share experiences and coping strategies when working with these materials.[30]

With these issues considered, how should you begin your search? Not all post-mortem records will be catalogued as such; when searching archival catalogues, it is advisable to also search for keywords such as 'pathology' or 'pathological'. Annual reports and meeting minutes are additional sources that often yield information about the pathological work done at an institution, the number of post-mortem examinations carried out, the instruments and equipment bought, and the research endeavours of individual staff members. Many asylums published their annual reports, and physical copies of these can often be found in medical libraries such as the Wellcome Library in London. Sometimes, doctors' notebooks will contain records of post-mortem observations and practices. The source you are most likely to encounter, though, is the chronological post-mortem record, often in the form of a large bound book.

The most extensive post-mortem records tend to be from those institutions that had a particular interest in, or reputation for, scientific research. During the late nineteenth and early twentieth centuries, notable institutions in this regard included the Claybury and West Riding Asylums in England, the Royal Edinburgh Asylum under W. Ford Robertson in Scotland (he went on to become the head of the Scottish Asylums' Pathological Scheme begun in 1896–7), Cardiff City Mental Hospital in Wales, and Massachusetts' McLean Asylum and the short-lived New York State Pathological Laboratory (later Institute) in the United States. These were institutions that carried out significant numbers of post-mortems. A Commissioners' Report for the West Riding in 1901 recorded that post-mortems had been made in 90 per cent of deaths that year,[31] and by the end of the nineteenth century all deaths at Claybury were said to be subject to post-mortem exam.[32] Post-mortems were carried out regularly enough at Washington D.C.'s Government Hospital for the Insane in the early 1900s that pathologist I.W. Blackburn's volume on brain anatomy could be based upon the results of 2,350 examinations.[33] At many – but by no means all – asylums, then, the post-mortem was becoming a standard part of institutional practice.

In many of these asylums, post-mortems and other pathological investigations were undertaken not by a dedicated member of staff but by superintendents and medical officers alongside their other work, a 'professional polymorphism' that critics worried was not conducive to rapid progress in psychiatric research.[34] Blackburn, above, was one of several dedicated pathologists working in asylums at the turn of the century, as research-focused asylums began to appoint pathologists to their staff. There were also pathologists who – although the asylum they worked for may not have had the reputation of Claybury or McLean – were active investigators in their own right, such as Hubert Bond (who worked at Morningside, West Riding, and Bexley asylums, among others). In cases like this, it is worthwhile searching library and archival catalogues for work by a named individual, as well as journal repositories such as *Brain, Journal of Mental Science* (*British Journal of Psychiatry*) and *American Journal of Insanity* (later *American Journal of Psychiatry*). In the absence of detailed archival records about pathological work, journal articles can prove useful in shedding light on an institution's practices. Researchers engaged in a particular course of research often pursued their work across several different institutions as they moved from place to place. Harvey Baird, for example, drew upon post-mortem data collected during his time at the West Riding Asylum and London County Asylum at Horton in his published work on GPI.[35] Such movement between institutions also transferred personal research materials across institutional archives. Thus, if the work of a particular pathologist proves helpful to your study, it is worth tracking down any records connected to them at other institutions (if they published regularly, journals can again be helpful in building a timeline of institutional affiliations).

Individual pathologists, however, would generally not be permitted to take an institution's post-mortem records with them upon their departure. Thus, extensive runs of post-mortem records can be found in almost all asylum archives, regardless of whether the institution demonstrated a particular commitment to pathological research. Working with these records can be daunting. Books are frequently chaotic, added to in different hands over a long period of time. It can take time to become accustomed to each writer's personal style of recording, as well as their handwriting, but after viewing a number of records it becomes easier to pick out specific sections of interest.

Interpreting post-mortem records

Let us consider what a typical post-mortem record might look like. The layout of post-mortem records depends upon the period being studied. In the first half of the nineteenth century, post-mortem observations tended to appear as short additions to a patient's casebook entry. As the century progressed, dedicated volumes were introduced containing pre-printed forms. Some asylums, such as the Royal Edinburgh and Brookwood in Surrey, introduced separate post-mortem books as early as the 1850s,[36] but most asylums would implement these in the last quarter of the century. Mid to late nineteenth-century records tend to be carefully delineated, with staff organising their observations in sections – typically head, thorax, and other organs.[37] Some records – especially those of smaller institutions – might consist of one continuous stream of text, making it harder to quickly identify relevant information.[38] Claybury's post-mortem books dedicated four pages to each patient: 'two for the results of the naked-eye examination, one for the results of the microscopic examination, and one for the clinical history'.[39] New sections might be added to books over time according to what was considered most worthy of record, or which body parts were feasible objects of study as techniques and technologies developed.[40]

Post-mortem records are complex and ever-changing documents, then. When I took my seat at a table in an archive search room and first looked down at an 1880 post-mortem record from the West Riding Asylum, I was overwhelmed by the variety of information contained within it.[41] At the head of the page was the patient's name, date and time of death, and a note of when the examination was performed ('23 hours after death'). This was followed by a short description of the condition of the body: 'Body much emaciated. Post mortem rigidity present in lower extremities. ... Abdomen greenish from decomposition.' This section also noted any injuries or scars on the body, in this case 'a bed sore'. The record went on to describe the condition of the head, brain, and (in less detail) major organs including heart and lungs. Many records from this period include a list of the weights of these organs and – especially at the end of the century as interest in brain anatomy and cerebral localisation burgeoned – the constituent parts of the brain: 'Whole brain weighs 1270 grammes. Right hemisphere weighs 518. ... Cerebellum weighs 170.' The record was methodical in its layout, but as it was not arranged in pre-printed sections staff were granted a degree of freedom in the amount of detail they chose to include.

Exchanging the bulky volume for another from the same institution from 1899, and resettling in my seat, I could immediately see that some changes had been introduced.[42] Now, the book was made up of pre-printed forms. At the top of each entry were spaces for the usual particulars of name and time of death, but also

'Form of Mental Disorder on Admission' and 'Form of Mental Disorder at Death'. Each record was split into clearly marked sections to be filled in: 'External appearances' ('State of nutrition', 'P.M. Rigidity', 'External marks, Bruises, Bed Sores, Injuries or Signs of Disease'), 'HEAD', 'NECK', 'THORAX', 'ABDOMEN', 'JOINTS', and finally a space for 'Macroscopic appearances, microscopical notes, special notes'. The form acted as a prompt for the pathologist, sometimes with hints about appearances to look for, such as 'HEAD, Pia-arachnoid. – Opacity, Thickening, Adhesions', or reminders to check the ribs for signs of fracture. Standardised forms recommended by the Commissioners were also in widespread use at the end of the century in Britain; they left little space for elaborate detail, with just one page per patient.[43] Lisa Gitelman, in *Paper Knowledge* (2014), notes that pre-printed forms '[work] to structure knowledge' within bureaucracies and institutions.[44] Such structuring work, however, can also be a process of exclusion: the detailed observations and rich language of earlier free-form documents is lost with the introduction of pre-printed forms. Chicago pathologist Ludvig Hektoen wrote that forms were 'useful as a general guide to the beginner and the non-expert physician', but allowed for little 'individuality of description'.[45] In many pre-printed forms, pathologists completed the record with one- or two-word responses such as 'Liver: Small. Otherwise normal'.[46] Forms are helpful, though, for the researcher who is interested in a particular body part or condition, as they can be skimmed at speed for pertinent information.

The West Riding records described above are just two examples; the length and detail of records will vary according to individual doctors' available time and inclination, as well as institutional guidelines. A book from The Retreat in York, England contains entries of varying length, with some examinations meriting only a few lines while others expand to fill two pages.[47] In general, though, the post-mortem record becomes more standardised as the century goes on, as institutions were expected to account for both the clinical treatment of their patients and the rigour of their pathological practice. That such records were monitored and checked can be seen in comments such as 'Space out more. Double [page] for each', or signatures in books from visiting Commissioners.[48]

The historian might take comfort in the fact that the challenge of using such idiosyncratic records was also recognised by contemporary researchers. 'Anyone who has attempted to work up statistical facts from a Pathological Record,' wrote Montrose Asylum (Scotland)'s James Howden in 1871, 'must have felt how much time and trouble were wasted in wading through case after case which had no connection whatever with the subject in hand.'[49] Even within the most research-oriented institution, lackadaisical record-keeping could be frustrating: records kept by previous pathologists were taken with them upon their departure, thrown away, or were simply unintelligible.[50] There were some attempts to make the comparison of post-mortem data across institutions easier by adopting identical classification systems, as well as sharing information between colleagues.[51] Meaningful comparison was often hindered by different institutional conventions, however, or 'too much individualism' on the part of staff.[52] The use of different, and constantly evolving, classification systems was also a stumbling block. As a published collection of 458 post-mortems at Norristown State Hospital for the Insane (Pennsylvania) noted: 'During the past several years, all clinical mental diagnoses have been gradually revised by the Resident Physicians to conform with the classification of Kraepelin. It will therefore be noticed that the older cases in this volume retain the older form of mental diagnosis.'[53] In Britain, classification systems were a constant thorn in the side of the Medico-Psychological Association, whose introduction of a set of statistical tables in the 1860s led to as much debate as clarification; the following years would see competing systems regularly discussed in medical journals. As well as a contemporary bone of contention, changing classification systems can lead to confusion for the historian. Asylum staff sometimes added retrospective data to records (both post-mortem and other types such as casebooks) – including coding nineteenth-century records with later classification schemes such as the 'Schedule of causes' introduced by the Commissioners in 1907.[54] Such amendments tend to be written in a different hand or ink and can be confusing at first glance.

Some asylums attempted to make the work of comparison easier by adding brief overviews of each case to the header or footer of records, such as 'Case of Idiocy. Small & light brain, but without convolutionary or structural peculiarity to naked eye. Death from Phthisis'.[55] These are helpful when consulting large numbers of records at once. Howden's response to the growing mountain of data was to introduce indexes to post-mortem records. Where they exist, indexes can be a helpful device for the researcher with limited time, or who is looking for a specific condition or pathological feature. One should bear in mind, however, that indexes were constructed by medical officers and pathologists with the preoccupations of their day in mind. They might display a particular interest in one condition and its pathological appearances (this is often the case with GPI), or simply chart anomalous appearances and 'abnormalities'.

Rather than relying on indexes alone, it is advisable to browse complete volumes of records or – if time is short – to adopt a sampling method. Whether dealing with indexes or individual records, terminology can pose a challenge: the historian is faced with a large amount of technical medical terms, many of which are no longer in use. Records discussing 'pia mater' and 'dura mater', or 'lateral ventricles' and 'lepto-meninges', can be overwhelming to the reader without a medical background. To clarify these terms, contemporary textbooks are of particular use: volumes such as Emil Kraepelin's *Compendium der Psychiatrie* (1883), William Bevan Lewis's *Text-book of Mental Diseases* (1889), Daniel Hack Tuke's *Dictionary of Psychological Medicine* (1892), or Jelliffe and White's *Diseases of the Nervous System* (1915).[56] Contemporary guides for medical students are also helpful for clarifying any Latin terms used, such as W.T. St. Clair's *Medical Latin* (1897).[57] In accessing such works, the Wellcome Library and online repositories the Internet Archive and Hathi Trust are invaluable, as they collect together a lot of nineteenth- and early twentieth-century textbooks in easily searchable databases.[58] Modern textbooks and encyclopaedia entries can be helpful, but as the meaning and application of a term may change over time, it is profitable to combine older and newer sources. Astrocytes, for instance, a type of cell specific to the nervous system, have been referred to as 'phagocytes', 'scavenger cells', and 'spider cells' as terminology has changed over time and according to individual writers.[59] Language can also be revealing as regards contemporary psychiatric thought, pointing to the influence of phrenology within an institution, for example.[60] Indeed, when consulting post-mortem records, it is crucial to bear in mind that anatomical evidence often played a part in supporting scientific racism and eugenically-inflected conceptions of disability.[61] At the same time that they use specialist or loaded terminology, however, post-mortem records often contain the everyday language used by many medical staff to describe their findings: tumours 'the size of a thrush's egg' or 'as large as an orange'.[62] Thus, post-mortem records (in psychiatry and elsewhere) can be valuable sources for the historian interested in medical language and analogy.

As is the case with other source types covered in this volume, the post-mortem record can rarely be used alone. The information within it has been used by historians in conjunction with casebooks, coroners' records, newspaper reports, and other sources. Here, I wish to highlight just one source type that can usefully supplement post-mortem records: the published book or journal article. In the introduction to *Index of 458 Post-Mortems of the Insane* (1915) Norristown pathologist Allen J. Smith suggested that publishing post-mortem data was a duty of the committed psychiatric researcher:

> I know of no better disposition... of such records, otherwise so hopelessly buried in the dusty record book of an isolated institution, than that they should be printed and distributed, making them available as the bases for correlative study and the evolution of principles which eventually will react upon psychiatric practice.[63]

Many textbooks, too, derived a significant degree of their intellectual weight from their basis in large amounts of post-mortem data. Bevan Lewis's *Text-book*, for instance, drew heavily upon post-mortem findings, especially in relation to alcoholism, epilepsy, and GPI. Similarly, journal articles contain a wealth of material based on post-mortem findings. Asylums with a strong research focus might produce their own medical journals. In Britain, the most notable are Claybury's *Archives of Neurology* (not to be confused with the journal of the same name produced by the American Medical Association) and the West Riding's *West Riding Medical Reports*. Much of the content of these journals had a strong pathological bent, connected to prominent asylum laboratories and drawing upon extensive post-mortem records. Many articles addressed topics of contemporary interest (such as alcoholism) or anomalous cases (brains of 'excessive weight' or post-mortem appearances that were 'difficult to explain').[64] Crucially, published materials like this may provide information that does not survive in the archive; an article by Goodall about a case of 'spastic hemiplegia', for example, contains extensive detail about microscopical examination.[65] This detail no longer exists in the archive as it was contained within a separate volume dedicated to microscopical work, possibly one that Goodall took with him upon his departure, or which was damaged in storage. Published work is, of course, highly mediated (as highlighted by Chris Millard's chapter in this volume), but where archival records are sparse or incomplete it can be immensely helpful in building up a more detailed picture of an institution's or a pathologist's practices. This junction between archive and publication may also be a site where the work of 'invisible technicians' comes into view: the administrative labour of compiling indexes, taking photographs, and producing illustrations.[66]

The importance of post-mortem records in the history of psychiatry

The value of post-mortem records was clearly recognised by asylum staff and inspectors, and contemporary researchers in other fields. Statisticians, for instance, considered large asylum populations as providing useful insights into disease and mortality rates, forming a kind of microcosm of society as well as a highly regulated experimental population.[67] Post-mortems held out the promise of understanding complex conditions like GPI but also issues with broader relevance to society, such as the effect of alcohol on the brain or the spread of dysentery within institutional populations.[68]

Although post-mortem records have been relatively under-used within the history of psychiatry compared to medical casebooks, these are records that can add much to asylum historiography. To end this chapter, I wish to briefly highlight some specific examples of how historians have used post-mortem records, and whose work you should therefore find useful and encouraging. Davis, in her book '*The Cruel Madness of Love': Sex, Syphilis, and Psychiatry in Scotland, 1880–1930* (2008), draws upon post-mortem records to build a more complete picture of one condition's aetiology and classification from asylum admission to death. By charting a patient's journey through the asylum, Davis demonstrates how the post-mortem could cement tentative diagnoses of GPI made during a patient's lifetime.[69] GPI is also the subject of my own book-length study, *Investigating the Body in the Victorian Asylum: Doctors, Patients, and Practices* (2017), which draws upon post-mortem data to highlight how the bodies of GPI patients were investigated in life and after death. Here, we see that post-mortem findings sometimes informed clinical treatment: the presence of large amounts of cerebrospinal fluid in the skulls of deceased GPI patients, for instance, led more than one doctor to experiment with trepanation as a potential solution to the symptoms during life. Pathological findings were also incorporated into contemporary debates surrounding fractures in asylums during the 1870s.[70] Looking beyond studies of particular conditions or injuries, Cullen's 2017 article, 'Post-mortem in the Victorian Asylum', uses post-mortem records to explore the multiple motivations for examination, but also discusses the specific points to be borne in mind when studying post-mortems in the asylum, such as the surveying role of the Commissioners. Her work is an important addition to more general histories of post-mortem and dissection, which do not often analyse the practices of psychiatric institutions in detail. Cullen also demonstrates how post-mortem records can provide information about the local prevalence of endemic conditions such as tuberculosis.

These are just three examples; the notes within this chapter will yield further references. Besides this, there are many other areas in which post-mortem records might be profitably used. For the researcher interested in histories of scientific practice, medical museums, or the history of the body, these are records that offer a great deal. They document a wide range of practices: the importance of the pathologist's sense of touch in examining a brain; the way in which a cast of the skull was taken; a record of the specimens preserved for museum and teaching collections, and descriptions of the equipment used to perform pathological investigations and bacteriological tests. Besides their written content, post-mortem records may also include materials that illuminate visual and print culture within psychiatry: pre-printed illustrations of organs upon which staff could indicate areas of softening or lesion; diagrams of the body to record tattoos, scars, or fractures, and photographs of the body and its parts.

Post-mortem records pose interpretive challenges, from their changing layout and language to the ad hoc annotations made by asylum staff and Commissioners. Yet, the same features that make post-mortem records challenging to work with, testify to their importance. They are sources that provide an insight into myriad issues beyond the simple mechanics of pathological practice: changes in record-keeping and administration; contemporary theoretical and taxonomical debates; relationships between institutions, families, and local communities. As we seek to deepen our knowledge of the social *and* scientific aspects of the history of psychiatry, post-mortem records remind us that the two cannot, in any case, be neatly separated. In capturing the minutiae of death, they also capture something of lives lived, both inside and outside the asylum. They are dynamic, rich, and vital documents.

Notes

1 For example Tatjana Buklijas, 'The Laboratory and the Asylum: Francis Walker Mott and the Pathological Laboratory at London County Council Lunatic Asylum, Claybury, Essex (1895–1916)', *History of Psychiatry*, 28, 3 (2017), pp. 311–25; Eric J. Engstrom, *Clinical Psychiatry in Imperial Germany: A History of Psychiatric Practice* (Ithaca, NY: Cornell University Press, 2003); L. Stephen Jacyna and Stephen T. Casper, *The Neurological Patient in History* (Rochester, NY: University of Rochester Press, 2012); Tom Quick, 'From Phrenology to the Laboratory: Physiological Psychology and the Institution of Science in Britain (c. 1830–80)', *History of the Human Sciences*, 27, 5 (2014), pp. 54–73; Jennifer Wallis, *Investigating the Body in the Victorian Asylum: Doctors, Patients, and Practices* (Cham, Switzerland: Palgrave Macmillan, 2017).

2 Elizabeth T. Hurren, "Abnormalities and Deformities': The Dissection and Interment of the Insane Poor, 1832–1929', *History of Psychiatry*, 23, 1 (2012), pp. 65–77; Chris

Philo, 'Troubled Proximities: Asylums and Cemeteries in Nineteenth-Century England', *History of Psychiatry*, 23, 1 (2012), pp. 91–103.

3 Jonathan Andrews, 'Death and the Dead-House in Victorian Asylums: Necroscopy versus Mourning at the Royal Edinburgh Asylum, c. 1832–1901', *History of Psychiatry*, 23, 1 (2012), pp. 6–26: p. 7.

4 Engstrom, *Clinical Psychiatry in Imperial Germany*; Gayle Davis, '*The Cruel Madness of Love': Sex, Syphilis and Psychiatry in Scotland, 1880–1930* (Amsterdam: Rodopi, 2008); Dolly MacKinnon, 'Bodies of Evidence: Dissecting Madness in Colonial Victoria (Australia)', in Sarah Ferber and Sally Wilde (eds), *The Body Divided: Human Beings and Medical 'Material' in Modern Medical History* (Farnham: Ashgate Publishing, 2011), pp. 75–107; Lynsey T. Cullen, 'Post-mortem in the Victorian Asylum: Practice, Purpose, and Findings at the Littlemore County Lunatic Asylum, 1886–7', *History of Psychiatry*, 28, 3 (2017), pp. 280–96; Wallis, *Investigating the Body*.

5 Engstrom, *Clinical Psychiatry in Imperial Germany*, p. 89.

6 Cullen, 'Post-mortem in the Victorian Asylum'.

7 Practices and legislation varied. In Australia, for instance, the 1865 Coroners Act stipulated that coroners were to conduct an inquest in cases of death in prisons, but not asylums. MacKinnon, 'Bodies of Evidence', p. 81.

8 Cullen, 'Post-mortem in the Victorian Asylum'.

9 I am very grateful to Nicol Ferrier for helping me to clarify my thoughts on this problem of definition.

10 John Charles Bucknill, 'The Pathology of Insanity', *The Asylum Journal of Mental Science*, 4, 23 (1857), pp. 42–93.

11 See for example Hurren, 'Abnormalities and Deformities' (on Britain); Helen MacDonald, *Human Remains: Dissection and its Histories* (New Haven, CT: Yale University Press, 2005) (on Australia); Ruth Richardson, *Death, Dissection and the Destitute: The Politics of the Corpse in Pre-Victorian Britain* (London: Routledge & Kegan Paul, 1987) (on Britain); Michael Sappol, *A Traffic of Dead Bodies: Anatomy and Embodied Social Identity in Nineteenth-Century America* (Princeton, NJ: Princeton University Press, 2002) (on America); David Wright, Laurie Jacklin and Tom Themeles, 'Dying to Get Out of the Asylum: Mortality and Madness in Four Mental Hospitals in Victorian Canada, c. 1841–1891', *Bulletin of the History of Medicine*, 87, 4 (2013), pp. 591–621 (on Canada). There is a useful short overview of legislation in D. Gareth Jones and Maja I. Whitaker, *Speaking for the Dead: The Human Body in Biology and Medicine* (Farnham: Ashgate, 2009), pp. 25–34.

12 Hurren, 'Abnormalities and Deformities', p. 71.

13 Engstrom, *Clinical Psychiatry in Imperial Germany*, p. 95.

14 Buklijas, 'Laboratory and the Asylum', p. 311.

15 Andrews, 'Death and the Dead-House', p. 15.

16 For example, MacDonald's *Human Remains*, Richardson's *Death, Dissection and the Destitute*, Sappol's *Traffic of Dead Bodies*.

17 An excellent recent work providing an in-depth overview of these issues is Tinne Claes, *Corpses in Belgian Anatomy, 1860–1914. Nobody's Dead* (Cham, Switzerland: Palgrave Macmillan, 2019), esp. pp. 77–152.

18 Lancaster County Lunatic Asylum, *Reports of the County Lunatic Asylums at Lancaster, Prestwich, Rainhill and Whittingham: with the accounts of the receipts and payments of the respective treasurers of the said asylums* (Lancaster: T. Snape and Co., 1875), p. 72.

19 West Yorkshire Archive Service (WYAS), Wakefield. C85/1124 Post-mortem reports vol. 7 (1881–1884), p. 439. Also see Anon., 'The Attitude of the Public Towards Post-Mortem Examinations', *The Lancet*, 167, 4298 (13 Jan. 1906), p. 109.

20 See for example Andrews, 'Death and the Dead-House'.

21 Cullen, 'Post-mortem in the Victorian Asylum', p. 282.

22 WYAS C85/1/12/10 *Report of the Sub-Committee and of the Medical Superintendent of the West Riding Pauper Lunatic Asylum, Wakefield, for the year 1891* (Wakefield: West Yorkshire Printing Co Limited, 1892), p. 36.

23 Andrews, 'Death and the Dead-House', p. 11.

24 Wright et al., 'Dying to Get Out', p. 615.

25 A.H. Newth, 'The Necessity for a Museum and Laboratory of Cerebral Pathology and Physiology', *Journal of Mental Science [JMS]*, 45, 189 (1899), pp. 321–5: p. 321.

26 Wm. P. Phillimore, '*Post Mortem* Examinations in Lunatic Asylums', *British Medical Journal [BMJ]*, 2, 886 (22 Dec. 1877), pp. 908–9.

27 Richard Noll, *American Madness: The Rise and Fall of Dementia Praecox* (Cambridge, MA: Harvard University Press, 2011), pp. 32–3.

28 Edwin Goodall, *The Microscopical Examination of the Human Brain: Methods; with an Appendix of Methods for the Preparation of the Brain for Museum Purposes* (London: Baillière, Tindall & Cox, 1894), unnumbered page.

29 Sidney Coupland, 'Remarks on Death Certification and Registration', *JMS*, 59, 244 (1913), pp. 27–53: p. 28.

30 University of Sheffield, 'Specialist Research Ethics Guidance Papers: Emotionally Demanding Research: Risks to the Researcher', https://www.sheffield.ac.uk/polopoly_fs/1.834056!/file/SREGP-EmotionallyDemandingResearch.pdf, accessed 23 Mar. 2021.

31 WYAS C85/1/12/6 Annual Reports of the Medical Superintendent (1894–1904). *Report of the Sub-Committee and of the Medical Superintendent of the West Riding Pauper Lunatic Asylum, Wakefield, for the year 1901* (Wakefield: West Yorkshire Printing Co., 1902). Copy of Commissioner's Report.

32 Anon., 'The Pathology of Insanity', *BMJ*, 1, 1990 (1899), pp. 420–2: p. 421.

33 I.W. Blackburn, *Illustrations of the Gross Morbid Anatomy of the Brain in the Insane* (Washington: Government Printing Office, 1908), p. 2.

34 Anon., 'Pathology in Asylums', *JMS*, 43, 180 (1897), pp. 106–9: p. 106.

35 Harvey Baird, 'Statistical Observations on General Paralysis', *JMS*, 51, 214 (1905), pp. 581–5.

36 Andrews, 'Death and the Dead-House', pp. 10, 22 (n. 9).

37 For example Wellcome Library, George Edward Shuttleworth Archives MS4566/4568 Notes of post-mortem examinations at Earlswood Asylum, 1869, 1870 (1869–1870). Available online here: https://wellcomelibrary.org/item/b18274924#?c=0&m=0&s=0&cv=0&z=-0.5169%2C-0.064%2C2.0338%2C1.2792, accessed 27 Mar. 2021.

38 For example Wellcome Library/Borthwick Institute for Archives, University of York, The Retreat Archive RET/6/17/1/1 Notes on a post mortem examination, name of patient not given (1870s). Available online here: https://wellcomelibrary.org/item/b2494581x#?c=0&m=0&s=0&cv=0&z=-0.6056%2C0.1871%2C1.8282%2C1.1499, accessed 27 Mar. 2021.

39 Anon., 'Pathology of Insanity', p. 421.

40 Cullen, 'Post-Mortem in the Victorian Asylum', p. 283.

41 WYAS C85/1123 Post-mortem reports vol. 6 (1879–1881), p. 177.

42 WYAS C85/1132 Post-mortem reports vol. 15 (1899–1901).

43 This can be seen for example in Wellcome Library, Ticehurst House Hospital Papers MS6245/6317/6325 Post-mortem book (1896–1929). Available online here: https://wellcomelibrary.org/item/b18423644#?c=0&m=0&s=0&cv=0, accessed 27 Mar. 2021.

44 Lisa Gitelman, *Paper Knowledge: Towards a Media History of Documents* (Durham and London: Duke University Press, 2014), p. 24. Also see Volker Hess and Andrew Mendelsohn, 'Case and Series: Medical Knowledge and Paper Technology, 1600–1900', *History of Science*, 48, 3/4 (2010), pp. 287–314.

45 Ludvig Hektoen, *The Technique of Post-Mortem Examination* (Chicago, IL: The W.T. Keener Company, 1894), p. 12.

46 WYAS C85/1132, Post-mortem reports vol. 15, p. 20.

47 Wellcome Library, The Retreat archives RET/6/17/2/1 Post-mortem book (Apr. 1892–Oct. 1916).

48 Ibid., p. 11.

49 James C. Howden, 'An Analysis of the Post-Mortem Appearances in 235 Insane Persons', *JMS*, 17, 77 (1871), pp. 83–93: p. 83.

50 Francis O. Simpson, *The Pathological Statistics of Insanity* (London: Baillière, Tindall and Cox, 1900), p. 7.

51 For example W.G. Balfour, 'Pathological Appearances Observed in the Brains of the Insane', *JMS*, 20, 89 (1874), pp. 49–60. MacKinnon writes that reports from an asylum in Victoria, Australia, made their way to the library of the Royal Edinburgh Asylum in Scotland (MacKinnon, 'Bodies of Evidence', pp. 80–1).

52 Newth, 'Necessity for a Museum', p. 321.

53 Chas. J. Swalm, Abraham L. Mann, and Allen J. Smith, *Index of 458 Post-Mortems of the Insane. State Hospital for the Insane, Norristown, P.A.*, Vol. II (Pennsylvania: Norristown State Hospital for the Insane Board of Trustees, 1915), Preface.

54 This can be seen, for example, in WYAS C85/3/6 Male medical casebook M54 (1889–1890).

55 WYAS C85/1123 Post-mortem records vol. 6 (1879–1881), p. 342.

56 Emil Kraepelin, *Compendium der Psychiatrie* (Leipzig: Abel, 1883); William Bevan Lewis, *A Text-book of Mental Diseases: With Special Reference to the Pathological Aspects of Insanity* (London: Charles Griffin, 1889); Daniel Hack Tuke, *A Dictionary of Psychological Medicine: Giving the Definition, Etymology and Synonyms of the Terms Used in Medical Psychology with the Symptoms, Treatment, and Pathology of Insanity and the Law of Lunacy in Great Britain and Ireland*, 2 vols (London: J. & A. Churchill, 1892); Smith Ely Jelliffe and William A. White, *Diseases of the Nervous System: A Text-book of Neurology and Psychiatry* (Philadelphia, PA: Lea & Febiger, 1915).

57 W.T. St. Clair, *Medical Latin Designed Expressly for Elementary Training of Medical Students* (Philadelphia, PA: P. Blakiston, Son & Co., 1897).

58 Wellcome Library, https://wellcomelibrary.org/; Internet Archive, https://archive.org/; Hathi Trust Digital Library, https://www.hathitrust.org/.

59 Wallis, *Investigating the Body*, p. 167.

60 Cullen, 'Post-Mortem in the Victorian Asylum', p. 288.

61 See for example Simon Jarrett, 'Consciousness Reduced: The Role of the 'Idiot' in Early Evolutionary Psychology', *History of the Human Sciences*, 33, 5 (2020), pp. 110–37.

62 William T. Benham, 'The Result of a Post-Mortem Examination on a Hydrocephalic Idiot (Congenital),' *JMS*, 20, 90 (1874), pp. 259–62: p. 261; Frederick W. Mott, 'Frontal Tumour Simulating General Paralysis', *Archives of Neurology from the Pathological Laboratory of the London Co. Asylums*, 3 (1907), pp. 364–8.

63 Swalm et al., *Index of 458 Post-Mortems of the Insane*, Introductory Note.

64 John Sutcliffe and Sheridan Delepine, 'An Abnormal Brain of Excessive Weight', *JMS*, 48, 201 (1902), pp. 323–7; Edwin Goodall, 'Post-Mortem Appearances (some of which were difficult to explain) of Certain Parts of the Nervous System in a Case of Spastic Hemiplegia', *JMS*, 37, 157 (1891), pp. 248–57.

65 Goodall, 'Post-Mortem Appearances'.

66 Steven Shapin, 'The Invisible Technician', *American Scientist*, 77, 6 (1989), pp. 554–63.

67 Wright et al., 'Dying to Get Out', pp. 598–9.

68 Frederick W. Mott, 'Alcohol and Insanity. – The Effects of Alcohol on the Body and Mind as Shown by Asylum and Hospital Experience in the Wards and Post-Mortem Room', *JMS*, 52, 219 (1906), pp. 673–711; Anon., 'Report of Drs. Mott and Durham on Colitis or Asylum Dysentery', *BMJ*, 1, 2101 (6 Apr. 1901), pp. 838–9.

69 Davis, *'Cruel Madness of Love'*, p. 113.

70 Jennifer Wallis, 'The Bones of the Insane', *History of Psychiatry*, 24, 2 (2013), pp. 196–211. Also see Kai Sammet, 'Controlling Space, Transforming Visibility: Psychiatrists, Nursing Staff, Violence, and the Case of Haematoma Auris in German

Psychiatry, c.1830 to 1870', in Jonathan Andrews, James E. Moran, and Leslie Topp (eds), *Madness, Architecture, and the Built Environment: Psychiatric Spaces in Historical Context* (London: Routledge, 2007), pp. 287–304.

Select bibliography

Andrews, J. (ed.), 'Lunacy's Last Rites: Dying Insane in Britain, c.1629–1939 (special issue)', *History of Psychiatry* 23, 2012.

Buklijas, T., 'The Laboratory and the Asylum: Francis Walker Mott and the Pathological Laboratory at London County Council Lunatic Asylum, Claybury, Essex (1895–1916)', *History of Psychiatry* 28, 2017, pp. 311–325.

Cullen, L.T., 'Post-mortem in the Victorian Asylum: Practice, Purpose, and Findings at the Littlemore County Lunatic Asylum, 1886–7', *History of Psychiatry* 28, 2017, pp. 280–296.

Davis, G., '*The Cruel Madness of Love': Sex, Syphilis and Psychiatry in Scotland, 1880–1930*, Amsterdam: Rodopi, 2008.

Engstrom, E.J., *Clinical Psychiatry in Imperial Germany: A History of Psychiatric Practice*, Ithaca, NY: Cornell University Press, 2003.

Quick, T., 'From Phrenology to the Laboratory: Physiological Psychology and the Institution of Science in Britain (c.1830–80)', *History of the Human Sciences* 27, 2014, pp. 54–73.

Wallis, J., *Investigating the Body in the Victorian Asylum: Doctors, Patients, and Practices*, Cham, Switzerland: Palgrave Macmillan, 2017.

4

PSYCHIATRY'S MATERIAL CULTURE: THE SYMBOLIC POWER OF THE STRAITJACKET

Sarah Chaney

Close your eyes and imagine an early Victorian psychiatric hospital. Picture the beamed ceilings, high windows, and long galleried corridors; the bird cages, framed prints, books, and domestic trappings. Such a scene is filled with material things (Figure 4.1). Fast forward a century and consider the same setting in the 1950s. The battered tables and chairs in a tobacco-stained day room; a well-used pack of playing cards, perhaps even a black and white television set high on the wall. These objects and settings are not sources that historians have traditionally used. Yet, by exploring the material world of psychiatry we can uncover detail about institutional life that may not be present in written sources, in particular, the experiences of those who left few other records. Because of this, the goods that people own, use, or make have begun to feature more heavily in historical analysis, from the early modern period to modern ethnography. As Tara Hamling and Catherine Richardson note in a recent sourcebook on material culture in the early modern period, seemingly mundane items can help us to access the daily lives of people in parts of society previously neglected by historians. Through their material goods, we can gain 'a more textured and nuanced understanding of past beliefs and practices'.[1] In psychiatry in particular, as Monika Ankele and Benoit Majerus explain in the introduction to *Material Cultures of Psychiatry* (2020), approaching history through material culture makes it possible to encompass the critical histories of the 1970s while moving beyond a 'narrative that reduces psychiatry to a tool of social domination and control'.[2]

No element of material culture has perhaps proved more iconic in psychiatry than the straitjacket. Invented in France in around 1770, the straitjacket (at first known as a camisole or strait-waistcoat) is a garment with extremely long sleeves, usually crossed over the chest and tied or buckled behind the back. It was used in most western countries – with some exceptions – throughout much of the nineteenth and twentieth centuries. It was not until 1994, according to *The New*

DOI: 10.4324/9781003087694-5

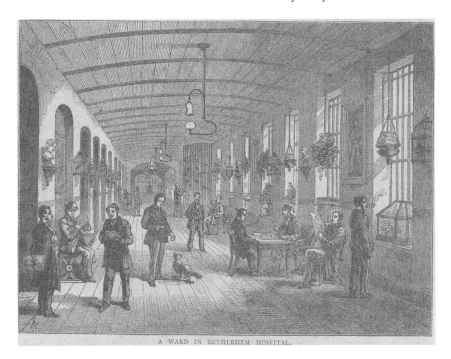

A WARD IN BETHLEHEM HOSPITAL.

FIGURE 4.1 'The Gallery for Men at Bethlem Royal Hospital' from Edward Walford's *Old and New London: Vol. VI* (1878). Birdcages, plants, pictures, sculptures, and lamps are all very prominent in appearance. Author's collection

York Times, that hospitals in New York State abandoned the use of straitjackets.[3] And, while mechanical restraints are now 'not acceptable' in the UK, a Royal College of Nursing report of 2008 indicated that vest, belt, or cuff devices that restrain movement by preventing patients from getting out of bed or chairs remain 'in relatively common use in hospital and care home settings in many countries outside the UK, including in Europe, the USA and Australia'.[4]

Despite its disappearance from hospitals, the straitjacket remained a staple feature of mental health depictions in popular culture in the second half of the twentieth century. In the 1960s and 1970s criticism of restraint – of all kinds – dominated the 'anti-psychiatry' agenda in films as diverse as Frederick Wiseman's 1967 documentary *Titicut Follies* and Miloš Forman's 1975 adaptation of Ken Kesey's *One Flew Over the Cuckoo's Nest*. Even today, despite the rarity of its actual use, the straitjacket remains a quick shorthand for insanity. In the 1997 *Buffy the Vampire Slayer* episode 'Helpless' we instantly know that vampire Zachary Kralik is mad because he's in a straitjacket, as are the inhabitants of the fictional Arkham Asylum in feature film (*Batman Begins*, 2005; *The Dark Knight*, 2008) and the TV series *Gotham* (2014–2019).[5] In some representations, restraint is also a visual shorthand for psychiatric cruelty. In the 1948 film of Mary Jane Ward's semi-autobiographical novel, *The Snake Pit*, Virginia Cunningham is restrained after abusive treatment by the jealous Nurse Davis, while *One Flew Over the Cuckoo's Nest* is famously dominated by the cruel Nurse Ratched. Yet the straitjacket is just as often used to indicate the dangerousness of the wearer. In the BBC *Sherlock* episode 'His Last Vow' (2014), Sherlock imagines his arch-enemy Moriarty in a padded cell, writhing in a straitjacket. Moriarty, as every episode of *Sherlock* emphasises, is criminally insane. So too is Hannibal Lecter, the cannibal psychiatrist who invariably appears bound in a straitjacket, the lower half of his face covered by a mask. Moriarty and Hannibal, this imagery quickly tells the viewer, are too dangerous to others to be allowed their freedom.

This complex symbolism, in which the straitjacket functions as a metaphor for both the perceived violence of psychiatric practice *and* the supposed danger of the person identified as mad, indicates some of the challenges and opportunities for the historian of psychiatry in interpreting material culture. Many psychiatric objects function as both object and metaphor: from the bird cage common in the Victorian institution to the head attendant's bunch of keys, which both speak to wider themes of freedom and constraint. Yet, despite the important role that material culture holds in the history of psychiatry, 'remarkably little has been written about psychiatric collections and their display', Dolly MacKinnon and Catharine Coleborne noted in 2011.[6] Their edited volume, *Exhibiting Madness in Museums*, attempts to provide a framework for addressing this gap in the scholarship, bringing together approaches from the material turn in history with contemporary museum studies on 'making history'.[7] This approach addresses both the ways in which objects can be used and interpreted in history – analysed or contextualised with or without the support of other sources – as well as understanding and appreciating the power relations inherent in the way psychiatric collections have been created. Objects – including clothing, furniture, and keys – served to construct specific identities for patients and staff within an institutional dynamic.[8] These items thus demonstrate 'layers of meaning', as Elizabeth Willis puts it, for a single object may have meant very different things to different people in an institution.[9] More recently, Ankele and Majerus have described this as the 'transformation' of everyday objects within a psychiatric setting.[10] Ankele explores the way that beds, textiles, and baths become transformed within hospitals, while Marianna Scarfone's detailed examination of patients' 'lives in storage' describes the 'disconcerting banality' of the toothbrushes, lipsticks, cigarettes, and shoes in a forgotten hospital storage room.[11] The complexity of these layers means that psychiatry's material culture cannot speak for itself.

Histories of material culture tend to set objects within context. Hamling and Richardson indicate two main strands of writing on material culture in history. The first approach begins with the object or group of objects, moving out from it to 'wider questions of social and cultural value'.[12] The second uses objects as one among a range of forms of evidence to generate new research questions. In either case, however, the term 'material culture' within history 'encapsulates not just the physical attributes of an object, but the myriad and shifting contexts through which it acquires meaning'.[13] Ankele and Majerus, meanwhile, take an even broader view of material culture to include the asylum space, its inhabitants, and their actions: sounds, images, and shades of light and darkness as well as objects themselves.[14] Within the history of psychiatry, material culture can help us to uncover the experiences of people who left no written records. It allows historians to 'illuminate the gap between the public rhetoric and the actual practice in the institution', while prompting new questions and unexpected answers.[15] Here, focusing on the straitjacket and other restraint devices as a primary example throughout, I look at these opportunities alongside some of the key questions surrounding the use of material culture as a source in the history of psychiatry. Where do we find psychiatric objects? How can the historian use them as a source? What do these sources offer us that might not be found elsewhere? And, finally, what can these objects and the ways and places in which they have been collected tell us about how we, as historians, approach psychiatry past and present?

Where do we find psychiatry's material culture?

The vast majority of psychiatric object collections are attached to former or current institutions: examples include Bethlem Museum of the Mind, Glenside Hospital Museum, and Wakefield Mental Health Museum in the UK; Museum het Dolhuys in the Netherlands; Museum Dr Guislain in Belgium, and Uppsala Museum of Medical History in Sweden.[16] Coleborne and MacKinnon's *Exhibiting Madness in Museums* outlines similar collections in Australia and New Zealand.[17] You might find items on permanent display or in storage. Some collections have online catalogues; at other institutions you will need to contact curatorial staff to find out more details about what they hold. Collections are often large, so be as specific as possible about what you are looking for. Depending on the size and procedures of the institution, you should be able to undertake a research visit to investigate items more closely, just as you would archival material. You may be able to handle the objects (wearing gloves), or a member of staff might display them for you. Find out about the provenance of each item you examine. Does the museum have a record of when it was made, and when and why it was added to the collection? Was there a particular person or group of people instrumental in retaining these objects?

Across the western world, most psychiatric collections emerged from the closure of large institutions in the late twentieth century, an important factor to consider when we approach them for analysis.[18] These are by no means the only items that could have been retained, but have been selected for a variety of reasons, including available storage space, the condition of the item, and the elements of institutional history that the collectors wished to preserve. Within psychiatric institutions, this practice of collecting has almost invariably been driven by staff, in some cases by psychiatrists, in others by nurses or administrators. A shared sense of nostalgia for life in these disappearing institutions formed a major drive in their collecting practice.[19] This has affected what items are retained, as well as the stories that they are used to tell. Bronwyn Labrum describes the way psychiatric collections have tended to focus on 'hard' items – medical instruments, tools of treatment, and architectural remnants – rather than on everyday clothing or decorative items, even though the latter held more significance in the daily lives of most patients.[20] These 'hard' objects were used by their collectors to support an evolutionary history of psychiatry, presenting a 'clear and coherent narrative of the progressive nature of institutional care' – as the founders of the Stanley Royd Museum in Wakefield aimed to do in the 1970s.[21] As Coleborne and MacKinnon conclude, while psychiatric collections do include 'evidence of past practices', their use as display items means they are often 'as much about constructing the present and the future of psychiatry'.[22]

As far as restraint is concerned, this process of construction is by no means new. In 1892, British psychiatrist and author Daniel Hack Tuke described a display of iron fetters in London's Guildhall Museum. The Treasurer and Governors of Bethlem Hospital – Tuke among them – had, Tuke said, presented specimens of 'the heavy chains formerly in use' alongside 'the celebrated figures by [sculptor Caius Gabriel] Cibber of raving madness and melancholy, bound in fetters' to the museum. These objects were intentionally displayed to the public 'as the outward and visible sign of the blessed change which has taken place in asylum treatment'.[23] They thus represented not only the brutal past, but a newly enlightened present. At Hanwell Asylum – one of the earliest institutions to adopt a policy of 'non-restraint' in 1840 – replicas of formerly used chains and straps were created, presumably to display the same idea of progressive change to patients and staff.[24] Other objects were adapted for new purposes. When restraint reduction began at Bethlem Hospital in the 1840s, the annual report commented that 'it was highly interesting to see the iron circlets, which had formerly been used as manacles, converted into stands for the irons employed in ironing the linen'.[25]

Restraints have thus long been on display – to the public, staff, and patients – in a variety of ways. The aim of these exhibitions was similar to what Coleborne and MacKinnon see as the 'unifying quality' in modern psychiatric collections: the presentation of an 'evolutionary history of psychiatry, where the past represents a "horror" that contrasts with the more enlightened practices of the present'.[26] In 1911, when the Wellcome Historical Medical Museum in Wigmore Street, London, decided to display 'appliances for the restraint of the insane', these were placed alongside historic 'instruments of torture', suggesting that the two things were synonymous (Figure 4.2). This was by no means a given before the 1840s, when restraint was still considered an occasionally necessary medical practice. By the twentieth century, however, the idea that psychiatry's benevolent future could be understood by comparison to a cruel past was widespread.

How do we interpret psychiatric objects?

The first challenge for the historian, then, is to move beyond the intentions of those who collected and displayed psychiatry's material culture and explore individual items or groups of items in depth. One curatorial technique that can help

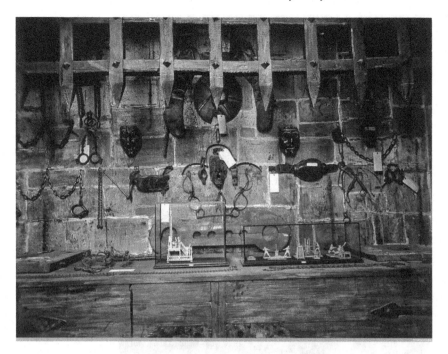

FIGURE 4.2   Wellcome Historical Medical Museum, Wigmore Street, London: a display of instruments of torture and appliances for restraint of the insane. Photograph. Wellcome Collection. Attribution 4.0 International (CC BY 4.0).

the historian of material culture here is the practice of deep observation. The curator approaches the object directly – before reading any background information – recording first what he or she sees, feels, or smells, avoiding interpretation wherever possible. We might look at the shape, size, and colour of the item; the techniques or materials of production, or any defects, damage, or signs of use and repair. Taking this approach can offer new insight into items with emotive resonance, such as a straitjacket. Elizabeth Willis expressed surprise that a worn and much mended straitjacket in the Charles Brothers Collection in Australia features 'a roll of stockingette around the collar', sewn onto the garment by some anonymous person 'to prevent the rough canvas chafing the neck of the wearer'.[27] Garments in the Bethlem Museum of the Mind include similar embellishments, such as an incongruous frilled collar on a padded grown.

Looking closely at these garments reveals that they were made as clothing, as well as for restraint. The dress with the frilled collar in the Bethlem collection is quilted in a style common in the second half of the nineteenth century: a diamond pattern that formed a decorative feature in many women's petticoats.[28] It features snap fasteners instead of buttons, dating the garment to after 1885 when fasteners became a new and much sought-after addition to clothing. The quilting served to keep a person warm – an important feature in a large and poorly-heated institution – though in a

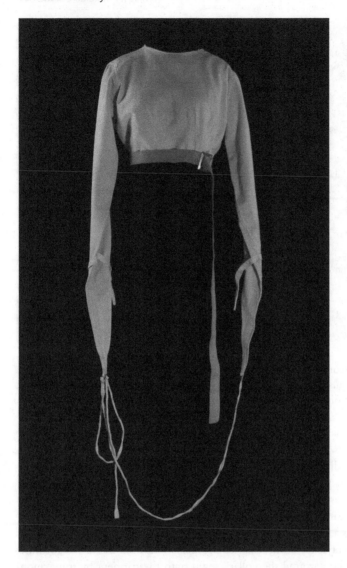

FIGURE 4.3 *strong* by Jane Fradgley. A women's straitjacket from Bethlem Museum of the Mind, *c.*1880–1920, in the 2012 exhibition, *held*. Jane Fradgley

psychiatric hospital this stitching served a double purpose, preventing a patient tearing or otherwise damaging her clothing. In the same collection a women's jacket – pictured in Figure 4.3 – features a short, darted bodice in the style of contemporary women's clothing, with an adjustable waist belt.[29] These features are easily missed when we approach such an item with the assumption that its purpose already tells us everything we need to know about it. As Karen Harvey recognises, historians are trained to focus on the content or meaning of a source, rather than its aesthetic qualities.[30] When exploring material culture, however, these aesthetic details can offer us new and unexpected information. Someone cared enough about the wearer of a straitjacket to 'make it a little more comfortable, a little softer and easier to wear'.[31] Restraints are not always the reminder of brutality that the collectors of psychiatry's material culture would have us believe.

Once we have examined the object itself for information, how can the historian situate the source within the wider context of psychiatric history? Often, the information gathered from material culture can help to enhance or challenge conventional narratives. The objects themselves might also prompt new questions. Why were these particular items kept by hospitals and institutions? What was their legal or therapeutic value? And what was their symbolic meaning to staff, patients, or visitors? Broadening the field of research beyond medical history is a helpful technique. The history of clothing and fashion design, as we have seen above, can help to illuminate the techniques of straitjacket manufacture. We can also read these objects alongside more traditional historical sources – published texts, medical journals, letters, and institutional records – to look for patterns or contradictions. Restraint was a prominent topic within psychiatry during the second half of the nineteenth century. While the creators of twentieth-century psychiatric museums retained these garments to shock and horrify, basing their claims to progress in contrast to a brutal past, the reality was much more complex. Indeed, while the straitjacket has come to be associated with nineteenth-century psychiatric hospitals in the popular imagination, most Victorian asylums claimed not to practice restraint at all. The non-restraint movement was begun by Robert Gardiner Hill, Superintendent of the Lincoln Asylum, and his mentor, Edward Parker Charlesworth, in 1838.[32] Hill claimed to have removed all forms of mechanical restraint – including chains, straps, belts, and straitjackets – from his institution.[33] By the early 1850s most asylums in England and Wales reported that they had followed suit.[34] 'I have the satisfaction of stating that the "Non-Restraint System" continues to be unreservedly adopted in this Hospital,' the new resident physician at Bethlem, W. Charles Hood, stated in his annual report for 1853, 'and, as far as my experience has gone, it has been attended with considerable success.'[35]

These reformers declared non-restraint to be the foundation of modern psychiatry: 'humane and enlightened principles' that had been 'recently discovered'.[36] This did not, of course, mean that every psychiatric patient was chained up before this time. Nor did it mean that patients suddenly had freedom afterwards, as emphasised by the prominent presence of institutional locks and keys in museum collections. This rhetoric does, however, suggest the origin of one of the symbolic associations the straitjacket retains today: that of brutality. In the later nineteenth century, asylum doctors in England frequently complained about the use of restraint in the community, citing improper treatment in the home as further evidence of the necessity – and benevolence – of medical institutions.[37] Patients admitted to hospital in chains or straitjackets were – according to official reports – immediately removed from such garments.[38] Even patients who requested that such measures were used were often denied them. Samuel S., admitted to Bethlem Hospital in 1889 with a diagnosis of melancholia, had bought himself a padlock and chain before admission, to prevent his incessant skin-picking. Two weeks after admission, Samuel 'continues to ask for the chain, finding himself unable to refrain from picking at the anus'. The request was denied.[39] The gothic horror of the straitjacket might also form the basis of a threat issued to those behaving improperly, by relatives or even servants. In 1898, Eliza M. wrote to Dr Hyslop during convalescence after her stay at Bethlem to complain about her housekeeper, Sallie. Sallie 'threatened me with a strait jacket which she read in "The Lancet" how to make', Mrs M. reported, an act of insubordination which sheds light on Victorian class relations and education, as well as popular views of psychiatry.[40] There is no evidence that *The Lancet* really did print some kind of template for straitjacket design; instead, this interaction illustrates the symbolic power the straitjacket held for patients and their carers by the late nineteenth century.

The non-restraint system, however, was not without controversy, and psychiatric collections can also shed light on the way restraint was viewed in the context of therapeutic practice and legal reform. Some doctors argued that dispensing with restraints might increase the risk of harm to patients, who would instead be manually restrained by ill-trained and badly paid attendants. Others suggested that alternative measures were being employed: increased use of seclusion, or sedatives to keep patients quiet. In 1844, a padded room was introduced at Hanwell, and these quickly became widespread.[41] Indeed, the very Bethlem report extolling the virtues of non-restraint admitted that, as a substitute, 'seclusion in the padded room is now resorted to'.[42]

Many psychiatric collections retain padded cells from this period – they can be found on display at Bethlem, Glenside, Wakefield, and the Science Museum among others. Most institutions would have had a number of these rooms, even one for each ward.[43] Those that remain are not necessarily representative, perhaps being merely the wall panels in best repair. Their scratched, discoloured surfaces and narrow observation slits are nonetheless evocative. Sometimes they reveal snapshots into the lives of patients who spent time within the walls. Padded panels may bear evidence of their protests or attempts to escape, indicating that the claimed benevolence of non-restraint was not necessarily experienced as such by psychiatric patients. The thick, heavy door of the padded cell in the Porirua Hospital Museum in New Zealand, for example, is marked on the inside 'where a bed end has been bashed against it'.[44]

Some patients wrote about their experiences of this treatment, describing the sensory nature of seclusion in a manner difficult to fully appreciate without reference to the heavy padded walls themselves. In 1897, for example, Graham W. wrote a letter to the superintendent at Bethlem from the padded cell. Locked up over seemingly mundane matters – as he reported it, an argument over cards and not being allowed any more jam at tea – Graham talked of the sounds and smells of the padded room. 'I constantly heard footsteps,' he reported, 'I called out, but no one would pay attention to me, though I begged for water.' All he could do, he said, was sit and smoke the remains of a torn cigarette in his pipe. 'Am I to sleep here again tonight?' he asked. 'If so it means another sleepless night. The stench of the India rubber etc. is unbearable.'[45]

In addition to his complaint about the padded room, Graham W. spoke in detail about the everyday objects he required for his health and comfort. 'I begged that I might at least be allowed to have my handkerchief and smelling salts, which I always carry with me,' he continued. He could not brush his teeth or hair 'for I would rather never brush it again than use the filthy brushes they provide here'. Yet he had brought with him to Bethlem 'shoes, nightshirt, a cake of vinolia soap, brushes & comb, also a writing case etc'. So far, he had been allowed only his nightshirt, 'for which I suppose I ought to return thanks to God, but just at present, I don't feel that way disposed'. It was not only instruments of coercion that gained additional meaning in the psychiatric institution, then. Everyday objects were imbued with new significance for patients and staff alike. For staff, ordinary items might become rewards or punishments, access to the everyday given following 'good' behaviour. For patients, they became an essential connection to the outside world, begged for from friends and relatives as well as carefully guarded. 'My dear Mother,' young Ernest G. wrote home in 1896, 'In spite of all my begging and praying I get no jam & I am out of tobacco & cigarettes. Do for God almighty's sake send me these things at once, I don't ask for them for amusement but because I really do want them.'[46]

Personal items in psychiatric collections thus often speak to removal from their original owners: the abandoned storage room at the Perray-Vaucluse hospital in the Paris region, or the hundreds of suitcases found in the attic of the former Willard Psychiatric Center in 1995, seemingly untouched since their owners were admitted many decades before.[47] In his mid twentieth-century study of institutional life, *Asylums* (first published in 1961), Erving Goffman noted the significance not only of everyday items but also the places where they might be kept: 'stashed' on the person in pockets or bags or in hidden 'fixed' stashes around the ward and grounds. Goffman interpreted this practice of stashing as generating a sense of self for patients. Although denied access to their own or collective items except on occasions decreed by staff, residents found their own methods of providing quick access to soap, playing cards, food, pens and paper, books, or clothes.[48] In modern ethnology, Fiona Parrott has written about the social significance of objects in secure psychiatric units, especially the way patients interpret them as a connection with their lives and relationships outside the institution.[49] Other sources thus become an essential way of framing psychiatric objects: when read alongside the items themselves, a focus on objects can reveal new ways of understanding institutional life and practices.[50]

What can psychiatric objects offer the historian?

While restraints and straitjackets were retained in institutional collections to support a progressive narrative of psychiatry, their presence or absence in psychiatric wards was more complicated. As we have seen above, a more detailed reading of such objects can complicate the story of psychiatry's progress to a humane and enlightened present by revealing the many slippages between rhetoric and practice.[51] Garments, sometimes made or embellished with care, do not show the unmitigated cruelty later claimed of them. Yet neither was the practice of non-restraint experienced as kind and benevolent by many institutional residents, who emphasised instead the everyday restrictions, constraints, and cruelties they experienced within the asylum walls. Institutional collections can thus help to reveal discrepancies between the claims of spokespeople and the practices and experiences inside the asylum. A homemade cudgel in the Charles Brothers collection in Australia, fashioned out of a piece of rubber hose by a member of staff, is 'clear evidence that the regulations were not always kept'.[52] As in England and Wales, Australian asylums had strict rules for ward staff. A lack of training and supervision, however, meant that these rules were often stretched. Many of the canvas garments in the Bethlem Museum of the Mind, meanwhile, date from the last decade of the nineteenth century, a period in which public asylums were growing rapidly in size but nonetheless still claiming to adhere to non-restraint. In 1888, Bethlem found itself at the centre of a controversy around this shift in practice when hospital governor and elderly psychiatrist John Charles Bucknill wrote to *The Times* newspaper to complain about the 'ill-treatment, as I think it, of the patients in Bethlem by the use of mechanical restraint'.[53] Since 1845 it had been mandatory for asylums to keep a register of the restraint used in the institution. While for decades this had largely referred to instances of seclusion, in the 1880s garments slowly began to return to the wards.

Over the following weeks, numerous asylum psychiatrists weighed in on either side. Some claimed that the canvas garments then in use – with such euphemistic titles as 'strong dresses', 'padded gloves', and 'side-arm dresses' – would not previously have been defined as restraint. Others used similar language to Bucknill, declaring restraint to be a degrading, cruel, and antiquated pastime, akin to witch-finding.[54] In his defence, the Superintendent of Bethlem, George Savage, reported that there 'are no straitwaistcoats, handcuffs, or what may be called true instruments of restraint in Bethlem'.[55] The bewildering array of garments referred to is hard to understand without examining the items found in the collection itself, such as the side-arm dress, in which the hands were enclosed in pockets, or featured sleeves sewn to the sides of the dress and closed at the ends. Collections can also help us to investigate the veracity of Savage's further statement that, at Bethlem, 'no patients are ever kept quiet by means of drugs'. Finally, on viewing the garments, we might also wonder if there was some truth in his claim that so-called 'strong dresses' increased the amount of 'personal freedom' given to some patients, who would otherwise be sedated or secluded in bedrooms or the padded cell. Indeed, such was the confusion over how restraint should be defined that, several years later, the Commissioners in Lunacy ruled that a dress in which the sleeves were sewn shut did not constitute restraint at all.[56] Investigating psychiatry's material culture thus prompts new questions and unexpected answers about the history of psychiatric practice.

Finally, exploring the material culture of psychiatry can help us to uncover the experiences of people in past societies who did not leave written records. Material culture has thus been a particular feature of scholarship in women's history. Sasha Handley's in-depth exploration of an early modern bed-sheet in the Museum of London collection draws attention to the woman who embroidered it – Anna Maria Radcliffe – after the execution of her husband in 1716.[57] Laura McAtackney's research on the Irish Civil War, meanwhile, uses prison graffiti and scrapbooks of female political prisoners to illuminate their stories, which are all but invisible in published form.[58] In asylums too, it is often easier to find out about the men – medical staff and patients – who populated them, especially those who were wealthy or well-educated. Women and working-class residents – including attendants – did not usually write down their stories or leave reports or publications. However, the tools they worked with in laundries and workshops remain. So too does their needlework, from the uniforms they mended to the decorative samplers they worked.[59] Some, perhaps for want of other means of self-expression, embellished their clothing.[60] While the items that were retained by collectors are usually the unique or unusual, reading them alongside everyday items – fabrics, clothing, and sewing materials – can generate micro-histories which help to shed light on the broader experiences of other women and working men in these institutions.[61]

Material culture: reflections on psychiatry past and present

Material culture has a fascinating capacity to reveal both past and present.[62] Psychiatric objects do not tell us merely about the time in which they were made or used. The addition of these items to collections and their changing display over time also reveals the meanings lost or gained during an object's 'biography'.[63] Take, for example, the shifting location of the famous statues of 'Melancholy' and 'Raving Madness' sculpted by Caius Gabriel Cibber for the Bethlem Royal Hospital in 1676. At first, these huge stone figures were displayed prominently above the gates of the institution in Moorfields – a visible symbol of its purpose and charity for patients, passers-by, and even tourists. When the hospital moved south in 1815 (to the building that now houses the Imperial War Museum), the statues moved too. Now, however, they were displayed inside the foyer, no longer advertising the hospital and its charity in the street.[64] By the second half of the nineteenth century the statues were assumed to be antiquated, even distressing, and covered by curtains. In the 1890s, the pair were formally consigned to Bethlem's past, with the removal to the Guildhall Museum cited above. Today, they inhabit the foyer of the Bethlem Museum of the Mind.

The way these and other psychiatric items are exhibited is often revealing of our modern assumptions about them, and their place in history. Upstairs in the Museum of the Mind, eighteenth-century manacles and early 1900s strong clothing are visible only in a mirror, distancing the viewer from them in the assumption that these are some of the most distressing objects in the collection. As we have seen in the history of restraint and the non-restraint movement, such items have long been read in this symbolic manner. When we encounter these objects today, our immediate and emotive reactions might tell us about our own preconceptions as a historian. What do we assume is right or wrong? What do we define as medical treatment and what do we view as coercion and control? Are these always two different things? And what do we mean by freedom itself? In asking these questions when we encounter an object or collection of objects, we begin to establish a more nuanced view of the past. Our modern views were not necessarily held by past actors. By exploring psychiatric objects in depth, we can attempt to move beyond the straightforward, progressive view of mental health history that the straitjacket has come to symbolise. Indeed, this may help to open up questions around psychiatry today. Restraint remains a concern in psychiatric hospitals – whether through the legal constraints on patients, the requirement to take certain forms of medication, or physical handling by members of staff.[65] Yet such is the power of psychiatry's past symbols that discussion of these issues can provoke kneejerk emotive responses. When the National Patient Safety Agency contacted a number of health care institutions to ask about their restraint policies in 2008, some replied that they had no such thing and 'would not tolerate restraint in their organisation in any circumstances'. One even referred to restraint as 'elder abuse'.[66]

In contrast, the tangible remnants of past psychiatric practice can open up discussion about mental health care and practice, past and present. Rather than using the existence of historic restraint devices as proof of psychiatry's humanitarian and benevolent future (as Victorian commentators did), we can find evidence to support a more nuanced or critical reading of these past assumptions. The way these items have been made or embellished indicates something of the complexity of discussions around restraint in the nineteenth century and beyond. By reading them alongside other sources – institutional reports and case books, legal statutes, newspapers, journal articles, and patient letters and diaries – we can begin to better understand when such garments were used, and when they were not. We can start to appreciate what the experience of restraint was like for patients, and how this compared or contrasted with other features of institutional life that placed constraints on the individual – a lack of access to everyday items or clothing, for example. We can explore the legal and therapeutic controversies surrounding restraint in various periods, and better understand what exactly the complex descriptions of restraint practices refer to. And, finally, we can understand the symbolic power that the straitjacket has gained over the past 200 years. While restraint in popular culture continues to imply dangerous madness, acknowledging the adaptations and adjustments to garments helps to humanise those who wore them. Read alongside the words of Graham W., Samuel S., Eliza M., and others, these garments show us a range of different experiences and a tiny window into the lives of the people who wore them.

While iconic, the straitjacket is by no means the only element of psychiatry's material culture that demands such analysis. Other items may seem straightforward but nonetheless benefit from a multi-layered approach to institutional life. Take the door key. At Glenside Museum, a display of vast numbers of keys across the years speaks to the importance of this item in daily life for those who could – and could not – access them. Yet some objects in the display again complicate the narrative of freedom and constraint. What of the master key, fashioned by a patient from wire, that supposedly opened every door in the hospital? Swiss psychiatrist Walter Morgenthaler collected 90 such fake keys in the early twentieth century.[67] Similarly, the heavy iron or garden rake can help to illuminate the experience of occupation – voluntary and enforced – in the institution. And, beyond this, what of the institutional environments themselves? What can the window, the door, the vaulted ceiling, or the dormitory tell us about the history of mental health care? A lot more, certainly, than at first glance we assume it can.

Notes

1 Tara Hamling and Catherine Richardson, 'Introduction', in David R.M. Gaimster, Tara Hamling, and Catherine Richardson (eds), *The Routledge Handbook of Material Culture in Early Modern Europe* (London: Routledge, 2017), pp. 1–23: p. 14.

2 Monika Ankele and Benoit Majerus, 'Material Cultures of Psychiatry', in Monika Ankele and Benoit Majerus (eds), *Material Cultures of Psychiatry* (Bielefeld: Transcript, 2020), pp. 10–29: p. 15.

3 Lisa W. Foderaro, 'Hospitals Seek an Alternative to Straitjacket', *The New York Times*, 1 Aug. 1994.

4 Royal College of Nursing, *'Let's Talk about Restraint': Rights, Risks and Responsibility* (London: Royal College of Nursing, 2008), p. 4.

5 For further examples, see Benoit Majerus, 'The Straitjacket, the Bed and the Pill: Material Culture and Madness', in Greg A. Eghigian (ed.), *The Routledge History of Madness and Mental Health* (Abingdon, Oxon: Taylor & Francis Group, 2017), pp. 263–76: p. 264.

6 Dolly MacKinnon and Catharine Coleborne, 'Seeing and Not Seeing Psychiatry', in Dolly MacKinnon and Catharine Coleborne (eds), *Exhibiting Madness in Museums: Remembering Psychiatry through Collections and Display* (New York and London: Routledge, 2011), pp. 3–13: p. 3.

7 Catharine Coleborne, 'Collecting Psychiatry's Past: Collectors and Their Collections of Psychiatric Objects in Western Histories', in MacKinnon and Coleborne, *Exhibiting Madness*, pp. 14–29: p. 15.

8 MacKinnon and Coleborne, 'Seeing and Not Seeing', p. 5.

9 Elizabeth Willis, 'Home but Away: Material Evidence of Lives in Victorian Asylum, 1850–1950', *Psychiatry, Psychology and Law*, 2, 2 (1995), pp. 111–6: p. 113.

10 Ankele and Majerus, 'Material Cultures', p. 17.

11 Monika Ankele, 'The Fabric of Seclusion: Textiles as Media of (Spatial) Interaction in Isolation Cells of Mental Hospitals', in Ankele and Majerus, *Material Cultures of Psychiatry*, pp. 140–58; Monika Ankele, 'Material Configurations of Nursing and Their Ethical Implications. The Prolonged Bath Treatment in Psychiatry', *European Journal for Nursing History and Ethics*, 2 (2020), pp. 101–23; Marianna Scarfone, 'Lives in Storage: Clothes and Other Personal Effects as a Way of Recovering Patients' Histories in a Psychiatric Hospital', in Ankele and Majerus, *Material Cultures of Psychiatry*, pp. 300–34: p. 304.

12 Hamling and Richardson, 'Introduction', p. 8.

13 Karen Harvey, 'Introduction: Historians, Material Culture and Materiality', in Karen

Harvey (ed.), *History and Material Culture: A Student's Guide to Approaching Alternative Sources* (Abingdon, Oxon: Routledge, 2018), pp. 1–26: p. 4.

14 Ankele and Majerus, 'Material Cultures', p. 17.

15 Willis, 'Home but Away', p. 113.

16 Some additional collections in Europe are listed in Ankele and Majerus, 'Material Cultures', p. 25, n. 1.

17 MacKinnon and Coleborne, *Exhibiting Madness*.

18 Rob Ellis, '"Without Decontextualisation": The Stanley Royd Museum and the Progressive History of Mental Health Care', *History of Psychiatry*, 26, 3 (2015), pp. 332–47: p. 333; Coleborne, 'Collecting Psychiatry's Past', p. 16.

19 For evidence of this context of nostalgia, see Coleborne, 'Collecting Psychiatry's Past', pp. 17–8; Sarah Chaney and Jennifer Walke, 'Mansions in the Orchard: Architecture, Asylum and Community in Twentieth-Century Mental Health Care', in Solveig Julich and Sven Widmalm (eds), *Communicating the History of Medicine: Perspectives on Audiences and Impact* (Manchester: Manchester University Press, 2020), pp. 138–61: pp. 147–9.

20 Bronwyn Labrum, '"Always Distinguishable from Outsiders": Materialising Cultures of Clothing from Psychiatric Institutions', in MacKinnon and Coleborne, *Exhibiting Madness*, pp. 65–83: p. 66. See also Ankele and Majerus, 'Material Cultures'.

21 Ellis, '"Without Decontextualisation"', p. 334. The Stanley Royd Museum Ellis refers to is the predecessor of today's Wakefield Mental Health Museum (also previously known as the Stephen G. Beaumont Museum).

22 MacKinnon and Coleborne, 'Seeing and Not Seeing', p. 5.

23 Daniel Hack Tuke, *Reform in the Treatment of the Insane: Early History of the Retreat, York: Its Objects and Influence, with a Report of the Celebrations of Its Centenary* (London: J. & A. Churchill, 1892), p. 6.

24 These are now held by the Science Museum, London. https://collection.sciencemuseumgroup.org.uk/objects/co134152, accessed 17 Jul. 2020.

25 The Royal Hospital of Bethlem, Edward Thomas Monro, and Alexander Morison, *The Physician's Report for the Year 1845: Ordered to Be Printed for the Use of Governors, March 9, 1846* (London: G.J. Palmer, 1846), p. 9.

26 MacKinnon and Coleborne, 'Seeing and Not Seeing', p. 6.

27 Willis, 'Home but Away', p. 115.

28 Beverley Lemire, 'Draping the Body and Dressing the Home: The Material Culture of Textiles and Clothes in the Atlantic World, c.1500–1800', in Harvey, *History and Material Culture*, pp. 89–105: p. 100.

29 Jane Fradgley, *strong* (2012).

30 Harvey, 'Introduction', p. 6.

31 Willis, 'Home but Away', p. 115.

32 Leslie Topp, 'Single Rooms, Seclusion and the Non-Restraint Movement in British Asylums, 1838–1844', *Social History of Medicine*, 31, 4 (2018), pp. 754–73: p. 756.

33 Robert Gardiner Hill, *A Concise History of the Entire Abolition of Mechanical Restraint in the Treatment of the Insane* (London: Longman, Brown, Green, and Longmans, 1857).

34 For more on this see Akihito Suzuki, 'The Politics and Ideology of Non-Restraint: The Case of the Hanwell Asylum', *Medical History*, 39, 1 (1995), pp. 1–17; Nancy Tomes, 'The Great Restraint Controversy: A Comparative Perspective on Anglo-American Psychiatry in the Nineteenth Century', in W.F. Bynum, Roy Porter, and Michael Shepherd (eds), *The Anatomy of Madness: Essays in the History of Psychiatry Vol. III* (London and New York: Tavistock Publications, 1985), pp. 190–225.

35 W. Charles Hood, Bethlem Royal Hospital, and Bridewell Royal Hospital, *General Report of the Royal Hospitals of Bridewell and Bethlem, and of the House of Occupations, for the Year Ending 31st December, 1853: Printed for Use of the Governors* (London: David Batten, 1854), p. 45.

36 Ibid., p. 41.

37 Akihito Suzuki, *Madness at Home: The Psychiatrist, the Patient, and the Family in England, 1820–1860* (Berkeley, CA: University of California Press, 2006).

38 Royal Hospital of Bethlem, Monro, and Morison, *Physician's Report*, p. 3; Anne Shepherd and David Wright, 'Madness, Suicide and the Victorian Asylum: Attempted Self-Murder in the Age of Non-Restraint', *Medical History*, 46, 2 (2002), pp. 175–96: p. 175.

39 Bethlem Royal Hospital, CB/136 Male Patient Casebook for 1889, Bethlem Museum of the Mind (hereafter referred to as BMotM), p. 13.

40 Bethlem Royal Hospital, CB/159 Female Patient Casebook for 1898, BMotM, p. 63.

41 Topp, 'Single Rooms', p. 772.

42 Hood, Bethlem Royal Hospital, and Bridewell Royal Hospital, *General Report*, p. 47.

43 Willis, 'Home but Away', p. 114.

44 Labrum, '"Always Distinguishable"', p. 73.

45 Bethlem Royal Hospital, CB/153 Male Patient Casebook for 1896, BMotM, p. 68.

46 Ibid., p. 21.

47 The Willard Suitcase Exhibit Online, http://www.suitcaseexhibit.org, accessed 15 Jul. 2020; Scarfone, 'Lives in Storage'.

48 Erving Goffman, *Asylums: Essays on the Social Situation of Mental Patients and Other Inmates* (Harmondsworth and New York: Penguin, 1975), pp. 222–3.

49 Fiona R. Parrott, '"Real Relationships": Sociable Interaction, Material Culture and Imprisonment in a Secure Psychiatric Unit', *Culture, Medicine, and Psychiatry*, 34, 4 (2010), pp. 555–70.

50 Hamling and Richardson, 'Introduction', p. 10.

51 For another example of this, see the discussion of prolonged bath treatments in Ankele, 'Prolonged Bath'.

52 Willis, 'Home but Away', p. 114.

53 John Charles Bucknill, 'Mechanical Restraint of the Insane: To the Editor of The Times', *The Times*, 22 Aug. 1888.

54 An Asylum Medical Officer, 'Letters to the Editor: The Mechanical Restraint of the Insane', *The Times*, 3 Sept. 1888.

55 George Savage, 'The Mechanical Restraint of the Insane', *The Lancet*, 132, 3398 (1888), pp. 738–9: p. 738.

56 R. Percy Smith, 'Mechanical Means of Bodily Restraint', *Journal of Mental Science*, 39, 166 (1893), pp. 469–70: p. 470.

57 Sasha Handley, 'Objects, Emotions and an Early Modern Bed-Sheet', *History Workshop Journal*, 85 (2018), pp. 169–94.

58 Laura McAtackney, 'Graffiti Revelations and the Changing Meanings of Kilmainham Gaol in (Post)Colonial Ireland', *International Journal of Historical Archaeology*, 20 (2016), pp. 492–505: pp. 500–3.

59 Such as Mary Heaton's samplers, held by the Wakefield Museum of Mental Health.

60 Gail A. Hornstein, *Agnes's Jacket: A Psychologist's Search for the Meanings of Madness* (New York: Rodale, 2009).

61 The same approach – especially to illuminate the relationship between gender and objects in the early modern era – is followed by many of the essays in Gaimster, Hamling, and Richardson's *Routledge Handbook of Material Culture in Early Modern Europe*. Sasha Handley's micro-history of an early modern bedsheet also takes this approach (Handley, 'Objects, Emotions').

62 Handley, 'Objects, Emotions', p. 188.

63 Hamling and Richardson, 'Introduction', p. 14.

64 For more on the statues see Jonathan Andrews, Asa Briggs, Roy Porter, Penelope Tucker, and Keir Waddington, *The History of Bethlem* (London: Routledge, 1997).

65 Mind, *Mental Health Crisis Care: Physical Restraint in Crisis. A Report on Physical Restraint in Hospital Settings in England* (Mind, 2013); J.A. Duxbury, 'The Eileen Skellern Lecture 2014: Physical Restraint: In Defence of the Indefensible?', *Journal of Psychiatric and Mental*

Health Nursing, 22, 2 (2015), pp. 92–101; Laura Allison and Joanna Moncrieff, '"Rapid Tranquillisation": An Historical Perspective on Its Emergence in the Context of the Development of Antipsychotic Medications – Laura Allison, Joanna Moncrieff, 2014', *History of Psychiatry*, 25, 1 (2014), pp. 57–69.
66 Royal College of Nursing, *'Let's Talk about Restraint'*, p. 11.
67 Martina Wernli, 'The Fake Three-Sided Key: Patient-Fabricated Duplicate Keys in Psychiatry around 1900', *European Journal for Nursing History and Ethics*, 1 (2019), pp. 67–86.

Select bibliography

Ankele, M. and Majerus, B. (eds), *Material Cultures of Psychiatry*, Bielefeld: Transcript, 2020.
Gaimster, D.R.M., Hamling, T., and Richardson, C. (eds), *The Routledge Handbook of Material Culture in Early Modern Europe*, London: Routledge, 2017.
Handley, S., 'Objects, Emotions and an Early Modern Bed-Sheet', *History Workshop Journal* 85, 2018, pp. 169–194.
Harvey, K. (ed.), *History and Material Culture: A Student's Guide to Approaching Alternative Sources*, Abingdon, Oxon: Routledge, 2018.
MacKinnon, D. and Coleborne, C. (eds), *Exhibiting Madness in Museums: Remembering Psychiatry through Collections and Display*, New York and London: Routledge, 2011.
Willis, E., 'Home but Away: Material Evidence of Lives in Victorian Asylum, 1850–1950', *Psychiatry, Psychology and Law* 2, 1995, pp. 111–116.

5

MEDICAL JOURNALS

Chris Millard

There is a type of historian's fantasy where, in dusty archives, they uncover a secret stash of uncatalogued, never-before-consulted documents that decisively settle a controversial historical question. Using medical journals as primary sources takes you about as far away from that fantasy as it is possible to be. These are among the most public, the most official, of sources. They have been digitised and made available online more than any other primary source in the history of psychiatry (although thanks to prohibitive paywalls, this does not necessarily make them any more accessible to members of the general public). They are often good places to start when looking for orientation in a new topic, such as the emergence of a new diagnosis, or the discovery of a new treatment. Many research articles come headed with abstracts (short summaries of the research) and many journals have indexes that mean finding, appraising, and sorting articles is a much faster process than having to trawl through them to find out whether they are worth closer reading. Thanks to text recognition software, many are keyword searchable too. Perhaps most usefully for historians, journals are almost always precisely dated (unlike much archival material) so establishing chronologies is relatively simple. In addition to the dates, a significant chunk of the content (research articles, letters) is also *attributable*, that is, it comes attached to a name or a set of names who have authored it.

For all their benefits, do not be lulled into a false sense of security. Medical journals are extremely complicated and rich sources, and they contain much more material than simply the research articles that make up their most obvious content. Remember that although *most* journals are *mostly* online, some are not; significant chunks of some journals are not digitised. Do not mistake the absence of online evidence for an absence of evidence. There are also gaps in what gets digitised – most obviously the advertisements that take up huge amounts of space in printed journals. This and other absences will be covered in more depth below. The formulaic nature of many journal articles (abstract, introduction, method, results,

DOI: 10.4324/9781003087694-6

discussion) can obscure as much as it reveals. But these difficulties are also op-portunities to reflect on what kinds of sources journals are, and how one might expect them to function as part of historical research into the history of psychiatry.

This chapter is focused upon the journal landscape in Britain, principally be-cause that is the expertise of the author, but also because it would be wildly impractical to attempt a much wider survey. The structure of journals of course varies from country to country, but English language journals in the nineteenth and twentieth centuries are relatively similar in the kinds of content they publish; the general points covered here hopefully have some use in other contexts. Medical journals now exist all over the world. They have had an important part to play in the creation and transmission of medical knowledge – which is not neutral or impartial, but heavily implicated in systems of colonialism, hygiene, racism, sexism, and classism. The chapter proceeds by looking at some of the major types of material found between the covers of medical journals: editorials, research ar-ticles, case reports, and letters. There is then an opportunity to cover some of the miscellaneous and less common kinds of text that crop up intermittently. Finally, absences are considered – things you might *not* find in medical journals (either online, or in physical copy) that are nevertheless relevant to the kinds of knowledge produced.

Types of journal

The term 'medical journal' is difficult to define, but in this chapter it means that a significant portion of the publication must contain peer-reviewed research articles relating to medicine.[1] In this sense the 'medical journals' considered here are 'scholarly' and 'academic'. That is, they contain many technical terms, and are written primarily for professionals in the field. Medical magazines also exist (*Medical World* and *Pulse* are two of the more famous ones in Britain), and these are still very useful for historians of psychiatry. However, these are more generally concerned with news and comment pieces. The medical journals most obviously useful for historians of psychiatry are those aimed at professional psychiatrists and psychologists, and two of the most influential are the *British Journal of Psychiatry* (often abbreviated as *BJPsych*) and *British Journal of Medical Psychology* (*BJMedPsychol*). However, in Britain in the nineteenth and twentieth centuries, psychiatry is considered as a (contested, ambiguous) part of general medicine. This means that general medical journals are also a rich seam to mine for historians of psychiatry. In Britain the two most famous general medical journals are the *British Medical Journal* (*BMJ*) and *The Lancet*. These journals often carry research articles or announcements about psychiatry or psychiatric treatments. To go into any detail about the vexed relationship between mental medicine and general medicine would very quickly swallow all of the space allowed for this chapter. However: the relationship between psychiatry and other branches of medicine is a valuable topic of research in its own right. It also means that any material that crops up in general medical journals about psychiatry will contain details (explicitly or not) about the ways in which the relationship between mental and general medicine is conceived.

The field of the journal tells you much about the intended audience of the content, and the expectations of those professionals. For example, surgery journals can turn up interesting articles on self-cutting or suicide attempts (both of which are normally analysed from a psychological standpoint). These are articles that focus upon the surgical repair of self-inflicted wounds, but still manage to convey interesting assumptions about the psychology behind the actions.[2] Similarly, journals of emergency medicine will have interesting insights into the treatment of cases of mental crisis, and the politics of the differences between psychiatry and other specialisms can be explored.[3] These 'outsider' perspectives on psychiatry are extremely useful for contextualising psychiatry and its relative professional prestige.

It is quite possible to write an academic article (or dissertation) entirely through the lens of one journal's output on a particular topic. For example, Chris Philo used the *Asylum Journal* to analyse nineteenth-century discussions around the best places to locate asylums.[4] The *Asylum Journal* is now the *British Journal of Psychiatry* – name changes can be confusing, especially for those unfamiliar with the field. This publication begins as *Asylum Journal* (1853–1855), then *Asylum Journal of Mental Science* (1855–1858), before a longer stint as simply *Journal of Mental Science* (1858–1963), and then *British Journal of Psychiatry* (1963–present). Attention to these changes is vital if you are not to miss valuable sources, and it is usually helpfully located in part of the bibliographic record for a journal in electronic library catalogues.

Most scholarship in the history of psychiatry that is based upon medical journal articles uses multiple journals. Liam Clarke is explicit in his 1993 paper, 'The opening of doors in British mental hospitals in the 1950s' that he 'relies on accounts largely taken from the *Lancet, Nursing Times* and *Nursing Mirror*'.[5] Frank van der Horst and René Van Der Veer have written about changing attitudes towards treating children in hospital (1940–1970). They write that:

> In order to be able to make our point, we went through all issues of the *British Medical Journal* and *The Lancet* from approximately 1940 to 1970, reasoning that if one wishes to convince medical doctors of the need for hospital reforms this is best accomplished by addressing them in the professional journals they read.[6]

They do use other sources, but the article is structured around the content of the two most influential general medical journals in Britain. It is also notable that even though they are looking at a primarily psychiatric issue (the influence of theories of child development on hospital practice), the journals are general medical ones. There are of course many other publications available should you want to explore some of the lesser-known medical literature. For example, the Victorian publications *Medical Times and Gazette*, *Medical Mirror*, and *Medical Press and Circular* have recently been used to great effect by Alison Moulds, who combines analysis of these with the more influential titles.[7]

Important unattributed pieces: editorials, leaders, annotations

Many journals have 'Leading Articles' or 'Editorials' that are not attributed to a particular person, but instead give the 'editorial line': supposed to be the view of the publication itself, rather than any single author. This is common practice with newspapers, most famously *The Times*. It is perhaps the most 'official' view one is likely to find about an issue; the fact that a particular issue has a 'leading article' written about it, is in itself evidence of its perceived importance. Of course, individual editors can have a strong and partisan stance obscured by the impersonal trappings of an editorial – another trap for the unsuspecting scholar.[8]

The various Acts of Parliament regulating psychiatric practice in the twentieth century are good examples of the kind of important topic that gets editorialised in the medical journals. Searching for 'Mental Health Act' and 'Mental Health Bill' in the 1950s in the various online journal archives returns huge numbers of results relevant to the Mental Health Act 1959 (in the UK, pieces of legislation are 'Bills' until they become law, and then they are 'Acts'). In the *BMJ* this includes commentary for General Practitioners (worried about the complexity of the Act's provisions),[9] and a number of instances of the important column 'Medical Notes in Parliament', charting the passage of the Bill through the two Houses of Parliament in the UK.[10] In *The Lancet,* there are other kinds of unattributed article, sometimes called 'Annotations' or 'Special Articles'. To pick one example at random for this topic, there is an interesting discussion in March 1960 of Nesta Roberts' pamphlet *Everybody's Business*, published by the National Association for Mental Health (later MIND) on how the new mental health law works in practice, because it 'relies largely on the expansion of community care for the mental patient'.[11] These articles can provide an initial orientation in a topic, or a pointer towards an important milestone, or influential publication. Staying in that same year, *Public Health* (The Journal of the Society of Medical Officers of Health) runs an editorial, 'Toward Mental Health', in August 1960 where the necessity of teamwork between public health doctors, psychiatrists, and general practitioners is discussed.[12] The competition and cooperation between different health professions in attending to the health needs of emotionally or psychiatrically vulnerable people is a vital strand of historical analysis, especially after the Second World War. As the asylum system is dismantled, the practice of mental health care becomes ever more diffuse, and psychological and psychiatric expertise is seen as valuable for people working in education, public health, paediatrics, general practice, the prison system, and more.[13] The different journals associated with all these professions (on top of the general medical ones) give vital insight to anyone attempting to piece these separate approaches together. The *British Journal of Psychiatric Social Work* (1947–1970) is a useful journal for this – full of evidence of psychiatry's influence on and position within social work. This journal also has indicative changes of title: it is the *Charity Organization Review* (1885–1921), *Charity Organization Quarterly* (1922–1939), and *British Journal of Psychiatric Social*

Work (1947–1970). It then merges with the journal *Social Work* (published separately from 1939 to 1970) and becomes *The British Journal of Social Work* (1971–present).

In any case, there is considerable ambiguity over what constitutes an editorial, or the 'line' of the publication, but there are many anonymous or unattributed pieces in these journals – reports, discussions, or special articles. This is especially so going back to the early twentieth century and before. Tracey Loughran's 2009 article, 'Shell-Shock and Psychological Medicine', makes a sophisticated argument about how far the First World War problem of 'shell-shock' transformed British psychiatry. A significant chunk of this article's bibliography is authored by 'Anon' contributors from *The Lancet* and *BMJ*: for example, a 1915 piece on 'War and Nervous Breakdown' or 'The Treatment of War Psych-Neuroses' from 1918.[14] These articles show some of the diagnostic confusion that characterises the whole shell-shock debate. Is it hysteria? Malingering? Is it physical shock or mental trauma? These go alongside the attributed articles, such as Charles Myers' first use of the term 'shell shock' in print (1915) or Grafton Elliott Smith's 'Shock and the Solider' (1916), both in *The Lancet*.[15] The journals carry these articles and they circulate amongst professionals, becoming part of a conversation in print. This conversation – disagreements, revisions, support of previous research – is a vitally important part of the history of psychiatry.

Research articles

The core of academic medical journals is the research articles. These are normally highly structured, in the way that physical science articles often are, with headings such as 'Methods', 'Results', 'Conclusion', and 'Discussion', each covering a different part of the analysis. Some of the most useful material for historians of psychiatry is contained in the introductory bits, and then the 'Methods' section, where you can see the researchers laying out what they actually *do*, in order to get the results they have. The discussion section puts the results in a context that is also vital to digest and understand for historians.

Revealing methods

Methods sections written by psychiatrists in the twentieth century are especially interesting if written by those who work outside of the asylum system. This is principally because a lot of the methodology is a given when conducting a study of people already admitted to a psychiatric hospital. The small but growing number of psychiatrists who were attached to general hospitals in the 1950s and 1960s have much to reveal about how psychiatry fitted in with general medicine (or failed to). During the late 1940s, psychiatrist Max Hamilton joined University College Hospital (UCH), where: 'At first, they didn't know what to do with me. After a while, I managed to establish a job in liaison psychiatry … word got around that somebody was available'.[16] This anecdote reveals much about the uncertain place of psychiatry within hospitals focused upon general medicine. It is a key part of the rather sprawling topic of the relationship between mental and general medicine (often referred to in association with the aspiration to achieve 'parity of esteem'). Medical journals can provide practical, specific insight here, because they contain not only the information they are trying to present to their readership (the results of a study, usually), but a whole host of material that is peripheral to their 'results' section.

For example, a number of articles are published in the mid 1960s about 'attempted suicide'. This contested and flexible term refers at this time to people who have harmed themselves in ways that look like they are attempting to end their lives, but who have survived the attempt and ended up in hospital. A cluster of research articles emerges from King's College Hospital (KCH), which is significant because it is a large general hospital, but it is across the road from psychiatric hospital and epicentre of British psychiatry in the twentieth century, the Maudsley Hospital. The proximity of the two hospitals is important because most psychiatric hospitals (formerly called mental asylums) were built far away from centres of population, and geographically isolated – but this one is not.[17] KCH has a number of technical relationships with the psychiatric institution across the road, but one of the more ephemeral is an 'Accident Service' in the mid to late 1960s, which prompts six research articles that touch upon attempted suicide, published between 1966 and 1969. Almost all mention the accident service, either in the opening section of the article, or in the methods section. For example, one of the early studies in 1966 states explicitly:

> In this study we have taken advantage of an accident service provided by King's College Hospital. Within a defined area of South-east London all patients using the emergency ambulance service are brought to the casualty department. Any patient who has made a suicidal attempt, however slight the medical danger, is admitted and referred for psychiatric opinion.[18]

This administrative arrangement, where the original proposal will be buried in obscure and inaccessible meeting minutes if preserved at all, is here preserved and digitised because it forms part of a research article published in a journal. It shows how any patients who use an ambulance will be referred for a psychiatric opinion if they seem to have harmed themselves – even if there is no physical danger. As psychiatrists in this period are increasingly interested in non-life-threatening self-harm, this arrangement is *extremely* useful both for the psychiatrists to be able to speak to increasing numbers of patients, and for historians of psychiatry who are looking for practical arrangements that allow psychiatrists to function effectively at general hospitals.

In methods sections it is also possible to see some work that might otherwise be hidden. A number of papers on 'self-cutting' are produced in the 1960s and 1970s, from psychiatric hospitals in North America. These articles are extremely invested in portraying self-cutting as a phenomenon of women rather than men. In one of the groups from an article published in 1967, it is mentioned that their sample was '21 females and one male'. Revealingly, '[t]he male, a 56-year-old dentist, was excluded from the study because we felt he was atypical'.[19] In another study, from Mount Sinai Hospital in New York City, it is remarked when discussing the methods that 11 male patients (out of a sample of only 35) were recorded as having a history of cutting, 'but the findings were so different from those of the women that they will be presented in a separate paper'.[20] I cannot find any evidence that this separate paper was ever published, but the traces of the work done to make the syndrome of self-cutting appear as a female affliction are still there in the journal articles for those who look.

These articles are useful in other ways. They provide evidence for the assumptions that psychiatrists are trying to investigate and establish. The authors from KCH investigate the significance of 'childhood parental loss' in the history of those who attempt suicide. They provide a definition ('loss or continuous absence of one or both natural parents for at least 12 months before the fifteenth birthday'[21]) which is revealing in its own way (the reference to 'natural parents', for example). But the key information is that this is considered a plausible contributing factor for those who end up in hospital having attempted to harm themselves. There are many other articles attempting to make similar connections from the 1950s to the 1970s, all in medical journals. This might help feed into a project on the post-1945 family, or how psychiatry reinforces normative familial relations by supposing (and establishing) a link between an attempt at self-harm and a disruption to a particular, conventional, family arrangement.

New diseases, syndromes, and treatments

Medical journals are extremely useful for charting the emergence of new insights, techniques, and therapies, as well as new diseases or syndromes. We have already seen this for 'shell-shock', but this is also true for the emergence of many other issues in the history of psychiatry. For example, the extremely controversial category of 'Borderline Personality Disorder' (BPD) can be traced through its emergence in print. BPD has been vehemently criticised by feminists for a number of decades, for pathologising women as emotionally manipulative, sexually promiscuous, and generally unstable.[22] Any historical criticism of this category *must* look at the emergence of the term 'borderline' in psychiatry in medical journals. Whether you pick Adolph Stern in the *Psychoanalytic Quarterly* (1938),[23] Robert Knight in the influential *Bulletin of the Menninger Clinic* (1953),[24] or Otto Kernberg in the *Journal of the American Psychoanalytic Association* (1967)[25] as the origin point for this category, all three have a claim to the formation of this particular psychiatric diagnosis. All these articles undertake definitional work, making it clear to the reader that this is a contested and new category. These three authors also use 'borderline' in different ways – opening up the possibility for a rich and nuanced analysis around the roots of the category, and when it might be reasonable to claim that the contemporary form of 'borderline personality disorder' finally emerges.[26]

All this work can be undertaken through close reading of medical journals – from a term that begins as 'borderline neurosis', and is attached to schizophrenia, to a term that signals the emergence of perhaps the most important of the 'personality disorders' (alongside 'psychopathy').[27]

A keyword search for the various commercial and generic names for one of the new psychiatric drugs of the 1950s (chlorpromazine, Thorazine [USA], Largactil [UK]) turns up a huge number of articles assessing the effects of these drugs.[28] There are also discussions of these and any number of other drugs used in psychiatry after 1945 – lithium, Selective Serotonin Reuptake inhibitors (SSRIs, including Prozac), barbiturates, and more.[29] Many journals are concerned with pharmacological treatment, rather than psychiatry specifically, but as with the general medical journals, the emergence of psychiatric concerns in fields that are not only concerned with psychiatry is an important point for discussion in itself.

The study of treatments in psychiatry through medical journals could include the emergence and development of Electro-Convulsive Therapy (ECT) or psychosurgery (lobotomy/leucotomy), as they appear in journals.[30] But this brings an important issue into focus. These treatments are today extremely controversial, and in the case of psychosurgery (now called Neurosurgery for Mental Disorder [NMD]) almost never practised any more.[31] However, if you look solely at the journal articles that first publicised them, and later articles that report on their efficacy, you will have an extremely partial picture of their effectiveness. This is due partly to different clinical standards for ethics and consent in the past (and the articles are themselves evidence of this). But it is also due to something called publication bias, which is an enormous issue to consider for anyone looking at medical journals.

Simply put, publication bias acknowledges that journals are much less likely to publish accounts of failed treatments. This does not mean that they never do so, or even that they rarely do so. In fact, publishing accounts of treatments that have had no effect, or damaging side effects, is a core part of scientific credibility. However, new treatments that impact positively upon diseases are far more likely to be written up by clinicians and far more likely to be published if they are a resounding success. Doctors rarely win prizes or acclaim for treatments that do not work, even if the demonstration of the lack of effect can be useful if a particular treatment has become popular rapidly. On the other hand, Egas Moniz, the pioneer of lobotomy, won a Nobel Prize (largely thanks to the lobbying of American psychiatrist and fervent psychosurgery advocate Walter Freeman).[32] This is perhaps the most important bit of contextual information to keep in mind when searching for evidence of a particular diagnosis, treatment, or institution. Journals are not neutral or transparent; journals are slanted towards successful outcomes, even if those successes are shaky or uncertain, or later thought to be hugely unethical and damaging.

Journal research articles are also formulaic, as mentioned above when talking about the various sections. This formula leads research articles to present discoveries as the only obvious logical outcome of the testing. However, decades of work in the history of science and medicine has shown how scientific work (which includes clinical drug trials, or assessments of other treatments, or the naming of a particular syndrome or illness) is highly contingent, uncertain, and ad hoc. Often, experiments are considerably less robust than they seem in the published literature. One of the most famous examples of this is Stanley Milgram's experiments on obedience to authority (in the field of psychology rather than psychiatry), where one researcher used Milgram's extensive preserved papers to cast doubt on the robustness of all of Milgram's findings.[33] Journal articles must be used with caution.

These articles are the outcome of a lot of labour, both in the performing and calibrating of experiments, the writing-up process, the peer review process, and any revisions required. The vast majority of this labour of work and revision is obscured by a simple, four- or five-page account with very few of the bumps in the road mentioned at all. At present, one journal – *Wellcome Open Research* – publishes and attributes all peer review reports, but it is an outlier, certainly in historical terms.[34] Journal articles might usefully be called teleological because they have a set end point established (the successful trial, or the decision on a set of diagnostic criteria honed over months), and the rest of the article is written backwards from that point. Thus, everything fits. Some of this work in the history of psychiatry might include writing, revising, and piloting a questionnaire, with critical changes made at every stage. These revisions make it 'more precise' (which might cynically be interpreted as 'the questions get the kinds of answers you are looking for'). This work in revision is extremely useful when thinking about developments in the history of psychiatry, but is often nowhere to be seen in the journal article that uses the questionnaire. As much as medical journals are po-lished, coherent, specific nuggets of information – one of the reasons they are so useful – this is also why they are so infuriatingly opaque. From this end of the publication process they make it difficult to ask or answer any other questions than the ones they ended up answering.

References

Almost all scholarly journal articles (whether in medical journals or not) have references. This acknowledges the other literature that is being built upon or contested. For historians these references can be incredibly useful for mapping out a particular field or sub-field concerned with a certain issue. In my work on self-harm, I located almost all the early works talking about a new form of 'delicate self-cutting' through the references of other articles.[35] Having found articles in this way, I was then able to scour their references in turn and locate further relevant sources. References in medical journals are intended as part of a conversation with other researchers, and historians can use them as evidence of the self-conscious connections that people are making between different medics and researchers. As always, these references do not give the whole picture. Especially during the nineteenth century, when psychiatry was considered more of a 'backwater', asylum superintendents might report their findings with no knowledge of or access to others working on similar problems. In these cases, a very partial picture will be portrayed in the references. If you, the historian, know that other workers were publishing similar things at a similar time, this absence becomes a kind of evidence of its own.

Letters pages

Letters pages are extremely useful. One of the most difficult issues for any published historical source is working out its *reception* – that is, what the people reading it thought of it. It is relatively straightforward to work out who the articles are *aimed* at, but much more difficult to see how articles are received by those who read them. Letters are very helpful here, as they contain commentary, correction, and reaction to previous issues of the journal. There is even a literature on the practice and significance of writing such letters.[36]

In 1951 Richard Asher is published in *The Lancet* naming a new syndrome after Baron Munchausen – a famous (fictionalised) teller of highly embellished tales.[37] Some patients, Asher claims, travel from hospital to hospital pretending to be acutely ill, having painful exploratory operations performed upon them, and leaving abruptly when they are unmasked as frauds. They then turn up a few days later in another hospital, often many miles away. In the issues that follow doctors write in with their own experiences of patients that 'hoodwink' them – or follow up on Asher's three example patients with more sightings, or providing alternate false names given.[38] There are also letters that speculate on the psychological reasons why people might do this – and it gets rather heated when some physicians argue that these patients need more care and sympathy than mocking.[39] People also write in with their own alternative names for these patients, or this condition: hospital hoboes, hospital addicts, thick chart syndrome, and more.[40] A new category of patient is created and debated across the letters pages of medical journals – not only in *The Lancet* in 1951 but in the *BMJ* in 1955.[41] These patients are seen as psychologically ill, but present at general hospitals (not asylums), and so once again they are a key contact point in the fraught relationship between psychiatric and general medicine. In another reading, these patients are routinely diagnosed across these letters as 'psychopaths', another important and troubling diagnosis in psychiatry that has antecedents in 'moral insanity' and which transforms into 'personality disorder'.[42]

There are numerous fantastic examples of the historical richness of letters to medical journals, but there is only space for one more example here. Tom Harrisson, anthropologist and founder of social research group Mass Observation writes to the *BMJ* in April 1941 to discuss what are called 'The Obscure Nervous Effects of Air Raids'. (All letters responding to him are printed in subsequent issues under the same heading, making it simple to track them down.) There are seven letters in all including responses and rejoinders, until the middle of June 1941.

Harrisson begins by setting out the contention that there has been 'a surprisingly low degree of nervous and shock response among the civilian population when subjected to heavy bombardment'. This supposed resilience is one part of what historian Angus Calder writes about in *The Myth of the Blitz*.[43] Harrisson is sceptical about this resilience, noting that as part of his work observing morale

> we have come across several cases of persons who, after a heavy bombard-
> ment, have left next morning, found a billet with friends or relatives or
> strangers, and then caved in. In some cases they have simply taken to bed
> and stayed in bed for weeks at a time. They have not shown marked
> trembling or hysteria, but an extreme desire to retreat into sleep and into
> being looked after, as if chronically ill.[44]

He further notes in his letter that these cases do not seem like normal presentations of nervous troubles, and that they are unlikely to be reported to doctors, and even less likely to reach psychiatrists. He thinks that there is potentially a psychological problem and it is not being picked up. A number of the responses to his letter push back against this assessment, and argue that this might not be a psychological problem, but a physical one. Hugh Crichton Miller argues that a rhinologist (nose specialist) would find that these cases had developed sinusitis as a result of the bomb blasts, or impact from the bombs.[45] Another clinician ventures that 'the pathology of both immediate and remote effects is essentially vascular',[46] and yet another that it is the force of the blast wave (rather than any other impact caused by being thrown around) in the nose or ear passages.[47] Harrisson responds that

> no one who has spent any time objectively studying behaviour in the
> 'blitztowns' ... could shut their eyes – however hard they try – to the very
> considerable effect that continuous raiding has on people's nervous system,
> irrespective altogether of the physical impacts.[48]

This back and forth, between emphasis on physical and mental damage, is characteristic of the debates around shell-shock in the First World War. Despite the widespread censorship of any information that might adversely affect morale, or show that there were problems with morale, the information in these letters gets through. This is partly because it is valuable information for the maintenance of morale, partly because it is expressed in highly technical (rather than alarmist) language, and also because care is taken to emphasise the general good state of morale ('The great majority of people behave with their normal calm and common sense, of course'[49]). Letters to the editor remain a huge trove of insight, response, and conversation that plugs into many important issues in the history of psychiatry.

Absences: advertisements, patient voices, and structural biases

Having substantially sung the praises of medical journals in this chapter, it is important to think very carefully about what is *not* there. Perhaps the most obvious absence for the history of psychiatry is the advertising that tends to be removed when binding the volumes for storage in libraries, and the lack of scanning adverts when digitising. Much of the post-1945 history of psychiatry is bound up with pharmaceutical drugs, and in the UK, advertising of medication to consumers remains prohibited.[50] Thus the advertisements are exclusively aimed at clinicians, and it is therefore logical to place them in medical journals. Some studies have been attempted, but when browsing online issues of medical journals, it is vital to remember that one of their chief revenue streams is obscured, and a key part of what clinicians might have read at the time of publication is not there.[51] It is still possible to study the history of advertising and medication, of course, even if it is difficult to access bound journals with the advertisements included. Some are kept at the British Library Reading Room at Boston Spa, but getting in touch with archivists first and asking questions is to be recommended here. Another option is to access the digitised and publicly available full run of *Chemist and Druggist*, the leading trade journal for pharmacists in the UK. This covers more than simply psychiatric treatments, and is a very useful resource.[52]

Another aspect of medical journals that is absolutely central to the history of psychiatry is the absence of patient/service user/survivor voices (for more on this issue, see Steffan Blayney's chapter in this volume). It has been argued that 'one of the most important and striking changes in the history of post-war British mental health care has been the rise of the service user perspective'.[53] There have also been multiple attempts to analyse and historicise service user experience in the history of psychiatry.[54] Given medical journals are written by (and for) clinicians, one would rightly expect little from service users to surface. However, there are some examples (including medical journal articles) in published *bibliographies* of service user experiences, including two by Sommer and Osmond as far back as 1960 in the *Journal of Mental Science*.[55] For example 'Mrs. F.H.' wrote 'Recovery from a Long Neurosis' which was published in *Psychiatry* in 1952, and Jonathan Lang wrote 'The other side of hallucinations' which made it into the *American Journal of Psychiatry* in 1938.[56] These first-person accounts of mental illness are often presented with explicit justifications as to why they have been included in medical journals. For example, Lang's article is prefaced with the assertion that 'The report of the psychotic patient provides the basic data concerning halluci-natory phenomena' and that because the writer 'still retained a certain amount of intelligence, and who has some knowledge of general psychiatric literature, the writer feels that an account of the phenomena which he has experienced might be of some value.'[57] The accounts themselves are hugely rich and useful – and the justifications are yet another layer of important information about the perceived value of patient testimony across time. Patient testimony in mental health might be usefully traced as far back as John Thomas Perceval's account published in 1830, and even before.[58]

Angela Woods has written about how, in 1979, the journal *Schizophrenia Bulletin* 'started to include among its experts people with a subjective experience of schizophrenia, publishing short pieces'.[59] The inclusion of these kinds of accounts should not be taken at face value – as some kind of raw 'patient experience' to be harvested by scholars and clinicians alike. As Lucy Costa et al. have argued in general about 'service user experience':

> We seek to question the use and propagation of personal narratives, and elucidate how our stories are increasingly being used as a way to harness support, funding, or press coverage for the systems that we recognize as being part of the problem.[60]

The telling of stories is not a neutral act, and certainly the publication of particular accounts in medical journals is a political act with an intended outcome. There is always a politics to the disclosure of 'experience'.[61] The same is true of those accounts published as stand-alone books, but the parameters around format, justification, and publication are all different.[62]

Finally, when thinking about absences more generally, there are omissions on more general lines of race, class, and gender here. The medical profession cannot exist outside of the societies in which it is embedded, and these societies are strafed by inequalities and prejudices. Medical journals represent a particular set of interests, and are the outcome of a set of gendered, raced and classed barriers to the medical profession. In Britain, especially in the nineteenth and twentieth centuries, the medical profession (and thus its scholarly journals) has been overwhelmingly white, male, and upper middle class.[63] When using medical journals to interrogate the history of psychiatry, these inequalities must be born in mind. There is much work on race and psychiatry, much of it issuing from the USA, which can contextualise and expose this absence in journals.[64]

Miscellaneous

There are many other kinds of article or series in medical journals; some are ephemeral, others longstanding. There is a column in *The Lancet* called 'In England Now' which formed a set of rather whimsical observations and commentaries connected to medicine in England.[65] In the *BMJ* there has been a longstanding set of reminiscences by clinicians called 'In My Own Time' which reflects upon past practice.[66] There are 'reports of societies' where some of the cutting-edge controversies in medicine and psychiatry are debated – for example a report on Child Guidance from Liverpool, published in the *BMJ* in the early 1930s, shows how 'advances in psychology' are aiding the understanding of mental stress, misbehaviour, and how this might intersect with the physical health of children.[67] There are also obituaries, which along with Munk's Roll and the output of various other professional societies, provide vital biographical details for psychiatrists and other clinical workers.[68] There are short case reports that might detail a puzzling or interesting case, with either a plea for more work in a particular area, or a direct appeal for diagnostic help.[69] There is plenty more between the covers of medical journals, and sometimes browsing the bound copies is the only way to really get one's head around all the valuable material.

Conclusions

Medical journals are public, official, and aimed at professionals. They are one of the first ports of call for any historian of psychiatry. They have mostly been digitised and are keyword searchable. There is no excuse not to use them extensively for background and context, even when the main thrust of the project is different (for example, oral history interviews or activist pamphlets). There is no escaping the medical journal in the history of psychiatry – but this is all the more reason to subject it to sustained critique. It should always be held in mind that there is much that is hidden from view: from the teleological structure of most research articles, to the vast hidden conflicts and revisions of the peer review process. There are many absences – some practical (advertisements) and some structural (race, class, and gender disparities). Medical journals are a complicated and rich source base, as a central or contextual part of any project in the history of psychiatry, especially in the twentieth century and beyond.

Notes

1 'Peer review' loosely means assessment by other competent professionals, which has existed for scientific publications for centuries; mandatory and systematic peer review for scientific journals only emerged in the 1970s. See Melinda Baldwin, 'Scientific Autonomy, Public Accountability, and the Rise of "Peer Review" in the Cold War United States', *Isis*, 109, 3 (2018), pp. 538–58.
2 R.M. Goldwyn, J.L. Cahill, and H. Grunebaum, 'Self-Inflicted Injury to the Wrist', *Plastic and Reconstructive Surgery*, 39 (1967), pp. 583–9.
3 For example: Katarina Bilén, Carin Ottosson, Maaret Castrén et al., 'Deliberate Self-Harm Patients in the Emergency Department: Factors Associated with Repeated Self-Harm among 1524 Patients', *Emergency Medicine Journal*, 28 (2011), pp. 1019–25.
4 Chris Philo, '"Fit localities for an Asylum": The Historical Geography of the Nineteenth-Century "Mad-Business" in England as Viewed through the Pages of the *Asylum Journal*', *Journal of Historical Geography*, 13, 4 (1987), pp. 398–415.
5 Liam Clarke, 'The Opening of Doors in British Mental Hospitals in the 1950s', *History of Psychiatry*, 4, 16 (1993), pp. 527–51.
6 Frank Van der Horst and René Van Der Veer, 'Changing Attitudes towards the Care of Children in Hospital: A New Assessment of the Influence of the Work of Bowlby and Robertson in the UK, 1940–1970', *Attachment & Human Development*, 11, 2 (2009), pp. 119–42: p. 120.
7 Alison Moulds, 'The 'Medical-Women Question' and the Multivocality of the Victorian Medical Press, 1869–1900', *Media History*, 25, 1 (2019), pp. 6–22.
8 See for example Michael Brown's work on *The Lancet* and its editor Thomas Wakley: Michael Brown, '"Bats, Rats and Barristers": *The Lancet*, Libel and the Radical Stylistics of Early Nineteenth-Century English Medicine', *Social History*, 39, 2, (2014), pp. 182–209.
9 Anon., 'The Mental Health Act 1959: A Practitioner's Guide', *British Medical Journal* [*BMJ*], 2, 5164 (1959), pp. 1478–9.
10 For example Anon., 'Medical Notes in Parliament', *BMJ*, 2, 5145 (1959), pp. 196–7.
11 Anon., 'Annotations: In and By the Community', *The Lancet*, 1, 7126 (1960), p. 689.
12 Anon., 'Toward Mental Health', *Public Health*, 74, 11 (1960), pp. 401–2.
13 Greg Eghigian, 'Deinstitutionalizing the History of Contemporary Psychiatry', *History of Psychiatry*, 22, 2 (2011), pp. 201–14.

14 Anon., 'The War and Nervous Breakdown', *The Lancet*, 1, 4769 (1915), pp. 189–90; Anon., 'The Treatment of War Psycho-neuroses', *BMJ*, 2, 3023 (1918), p. 634, cited in Tracey Loughran, 'Shell-Shock and Psychological Medicine', *Social History of Medicine*, 22, 1 (2009), pp. 79–95.

15 Charles Samuel Myers, 'A Contribution to the Study of Shell-Shock', *The Lancet*, 1, 4772 (1915), pp. 316–20; Grafton Elliott Smith, 'Shock and the Soldier', *The Lancet* 1, 4833 (1916), pp. 813–7, 853–7.

16 Richard Mayou, 'The History of General Hospital Psychiatry', *British Journal of Psychiatry*, 155 (1989), pp. 764–76: p. 774.

17 For more on the Maudsley and its place within British psychiatry, see Edgar Jones, Shahina Rahman, and Robin Woolven, 'The Maudsley Hospital: Design and Strategic Direction, 1923–1939', *Medical History*, 51, 3 (2007), pp. 357–78; Rhodri Hayward, 'Germany and the Making of "English" Psychiatry: The Maudsley Hospital 1908–1939', in Volker Roelcke, Paul Weindling, and Louise Westwood (eds), *International Relations in Psychiatry: Britain, Germany, and the United States to World War II* (New York: University of Rochester Press, 2010), pp. 67–90.

18 S. Greer, J.C. Gunn, and K.M. Koller, 'Aetiological Factors in Attempted Suicide', *BMJ*, 2, 5526 (1966), pp. 1352–5: p. 1352.

19 H. Graff and R. Mallin, 'The Syndrome of the Wrist Cutter', *American Journal of Psychiatry*, 124 (1967), pp. 36–42: p. 36.

20 R. Rosenthal, C. Rinzler, R. Wallsch, and E. Klausner, 'Wrist-Cutting Syndrome: The Meaning of a Gesture', *American Journal of Psychiatry*, 128 (1972), pp. 1363–8: p. 1363.

21 Greer, Gunn, and Koller, 'Aetiological Factors in Attempted Suicide', p. 1353.

22 For example Lisa Appignanesi, *Mad, Bad and Sad: A History of Women and the Mind Doctors* (New York and London: W.W. Norton & Co., 2008).

23 Adolph Stern, 'Psychoanalytic Investigation of and Therapy in the Border Line Group of Neuroses', *Psychoanalytic Quarterly*, 7 (1938), pp. 467–89.

24 Robert P. Knight, 'Borderline States in Psychoanalytic Psychiatry and Psychology', *Bulletin of the Menninger Clinic*, 17 (1953), pp. 1–12.

25 Otto Kernberg, 'Borderline Personality Organization', *Journal of The American Psychoanalytical Association*, 15 (1967), pp. 641–85.

26 Some of this lineage is taken from Elizabeth Lunbeck, 'Borderline Histories: Psychoanalysis Inside and Out', *Science in Context*, 19, 1 (2006), pp. 151–73, which relies heavily on medical journal articles. The most significant part of this chronology is taken from a grant application on this topic by Åsa Jansson, included with the author's permission.

27 See David W. Jones, *Disordered Personalities and Crime: An Analysis of the History of Moral Insanity* (London: Routledge, 2015); Susanna Shapland, 'Defining the Elephant: A History of Psychopathy, 1891–1959.' Doctoral thesis, Birkbeck, University of London, 2019.

28 For example Else B. Kris and Donald M. Carmichael, 'Follow-Up Study on Patients Treated with Thorazine', *American Journal of Psychiatry*, 112 (1956), p. 1022

29 For example Dennis S. Charney, J.H. Krystal, P.L. Delgado, and G.R. Heninger, 'Serotonin-Specific Drugs for Anxiety and Depressive Disorders', *Annual Review of Medicine*, 41 (1990), pp. 437–46.

30 One of the earliest reports of the effectiveness of what became ECT was L. Bini, 'Experimental Researches on Epileptic Attacks Induced by the Electric Current', *American Journal of Psychiatry*, 94 (1938), pp. 172–4; one of the earliest reports on psychosurgery was A.E. Moniz 'Essai d'un traitement chirurgical de certaines psychoses [A trial of surgical treatment for certain psychoses]', *Bulletin de l'Académie de Médecine (Paris)*, 115 (1936), pp. 385–92.

31 https://www.mind.org.uk/information-support/drugs-and-treatments/neurosurgery-for-mental-disorder-nmd/about-nmd/, accessed 23 Mar. 2021.

32 For a recent account of this see Anne Harrington, *Mind Fixers: Psychiatry's Troubled Search for the Biology of Mental Illness* (New York: W.W. Norton & Co., 2019), pp. 32–73.

33 Gina Perry, *Behind the Shock Machine: The Untold Story of the Notorious Milgram Psychology Experiments* (London: Scribe UK, 2013).

34 See https://wellcomeopenresearch.org/, accessed 23 Mar. 2021.

35 Chris Millard, 'Making the Cut: The Production of "Self-Harm" in Post-1945 Anglo-Saxon Psychiatry', *History of the Human Sciences*, 26, 2 (2013), pp. 126–50.

36 Peter P. Morgan, 'How to Write a Letter that the Editor Will Want to Publish', *Canadian Medical Association Journal*, 132 (1985), p. 1344; N. Papanas et al., 'Letters to the Editor: Definitely Not Children of a Lesser God', *International Angiology*, 28, 5 (2009), pp. 418–20; N.W. Goodman, 'How to Write a Critical Letter and Respond to One', *Hospital Medicine*, 62, 7 (2001), pp. 426–7; E. Tierney, C. O'Rourke, and J.E. Fenton, 'What Is the Role of "The Letter to the Editor"?', *European Archives of Oto-Rhino-Laryngology*, 272, 9 (2015), pp. 2089–93.

37 Richard Asher, 'Münchhausen syndrome', *The Lancet*, 1, 6650 (1951), pp. 339–41.

38 Between the publication of Asher's article on 10 February 1951 and a letter from a Swedish physician on 12 May 1951, there are 21 letters published in *The Lancet*.

39 D. Bardon, 'Munchausen's Syndrome', *The Lancet*, 2, 7706 (1957), p. 1170.

40 For example E. Clarke and S.C. Melnick, 'The Munchausen Syndrome or the Problem of Hospital Hoboes', *American Journal of Medicine*, 25, 1 (1958), pp. 6–12; J.C. Barker, 'Hospital and Operation Addiction', *British Journal of Clinical Practice*, 20, 2 (1966), pp. 63–8.

41 Between 29 October 1955 and 26 November 1955 in the *BMJ*, there are 13 letters on this topic.

42 Jones, *Disordered Personalities and Crime*.

43 Angus Calder, *The Myth of the Blitz* (London: Jonathan Cape, 1991).

44 Tom Harrisson, 'Obscure Nervous Effects of Air Raids', *BMJ*, 1, 4188 (1941), pp. 573–4: p. 573.

45 H. Crichton-Miller, 'Obscure Nervous Effects of Air Raids', *BMJ*, 1, 4190 (1941), p. 647.

46 F.A. Pickworth, 'Obscure Nervous Effects of Air Raids', *BMJ*, 1, 4194 (1941), p. 790.

47 D. Whitteridge, 'Obscure Nervous Effects of Air Raids', *BMJ*, 1, 4194 (1941), pp. 790–1: p. 791.

48 Tom Harrisson, 'Obscure Nervous Effects of Air Raids', *BMJ*, 1, 4195 (1941), p. 832.

49 Ibid.

50 Two general histories of psychiatry that are centrally concerned with drugs and psychiatric medication – in very different registers – are Harrington, *Mind Fixers*, and Edward Shorter, *A History of Psychiatry: From the Era of the Asylum to the Age of Prozac* (New York and Chichester: Wiley, 1997).

51 For example C. Hanganu-Bresch, '"Treat Her with Prozac": Four Decades of Direct-to-Physician Antidepressant Advertising', in Robert C. MacDougall (ed.), *Drugs & Media: New Perspectives on Communication, Consumption and Consciousness* (New York: Continuum, 2012), pp. 166–92; Mat Savelli and Melissa Ricci, 'Disappearing Acts: Anguish, Isolation, and the Re-Imagining of the Mentally Ill in Global Psychopharmaceutical Advertising (1953–2005)', *Canadian Bulletin of Medical History*, 35, 2 (2018), pp. 247–77.

52 See https://wellcomelibrary.org/item/b19974760#?c=0&m=0&s=0&cv=0&z=-1.3203%2C-0.0921%2C3.6406%2C1.8421, accessed 21 Mar. 2021.

53 John Turner, Rhodri Hayward, Katherine Angel, Bill Fulford, John Hall, Chris Millard, and Mathew Thomson, 'The History of Mental Health Services in Modern England: Practitioner Memories and the Direction of Future Research', *Medical History*, 59, 4 (2015), pp. 599–624: p. 612.

54 Tehseen Noorani, 'Service User Involvement, Authority and the "Expert-by-Experience" in Mental Health', *Journal of Political Power*, 6, 1 (2013), pp. 49–68; Diana

Rose, 'Service User/Survivor-Led Research in Mental Health: Epistemological Possibilities', *Disability & Society*, 32, 6 (2017), pp. 773–89.

55 Robert Sommer and Humphry Osmond, 'Autobiographies of Former Mental Patients', *Journal of Mental Science*, 106, 443 (1960), pp. 648–62; Robert Sommer and Humphry Osmond, 'Autobiographies of Former Mental Patients: Addendum', *Journal of Mental Science*, 107, 451 (1961), pp. 1030–2.

56 Anon. [Mrs F.H.], 'Recovery from a Long Neurosis', *Psychiatry*, 15, 2 (1952), pp. 161–77; Jonathan Lang, 'The Other Side of Hallucinations', *American Journal of Psychiatry*, 94 (1938), pp. 1089–97.

57 Anon. [Aaron Rosanoff?], 'Introduction' to Lang, 'Other Side of Hallucinations'.

58 John Thomas Perceval, *Perceval's Narrative: A Patient's Account of His Psychosis, 1830–1832*, ed. Gregory Bateson (Oxford: Oxford University Press, 1961).

59 Angela Woods, 'Rethinking "Patient Testimony" in the Medical Humanities: The Case of *Schizophrenia Bulletin*'s First Person Accounts', *Journal of Literature and Science*, 6, 1 (2012), pp. 38–54: p. 38.

60 Lucy Costa, Jijian Voronka, Danielle Landry, Jenna Reid, Becky Mcfarlane, David Reville, and Kathryn Church, '"Recovering Our Stories": A Small Act of Resistance', *Studies in Social Justice*, 6, 1 (2012), pp. 85–101: p. 98.

61 See Scott's classic account: Joan W. Scott, 'The Evidence of Experience', *Critical Inquiry*, 17, 4 (1991), pp. 773–97.

62 For example Barbara O'Brien, *Operators and Things. The Inner Life of a Schizophrenic* (London: Elek Books, 1960); Clifford W. Beers, *A Mind that Found Itself. An Autobiography* (New York: Longmans, Green & Co., 1907).

63 https://www.ethnicity-facts-figures.service.gov.uk/workforce-and-business/workforce-diversity/nhs-workforce/latest, accessed 23 Mar. 2021.

64 For work in Britain see for example, Suman Fernando, *Cultural Diversity, Mental Health and Psychiatry: The Struggle Against Racism* (Hove: Brunner-Routledge, 2003); H. Bhui, 'Race, Racism And Risk Assessment: Linking Theory To Practice With Black Mentally Disordered Offenders', *Probation Journal*, 46, 3 (1999), pp. 171–81; R. Cochrane, 'Race, Prejudice and Ethnic Identity', in D. Bhugra and R. Cochrane (eds), *Psychiatry in Multicultural Britain* (London: Royal College of Psychiatrists, 2001), pp. 80–1; Jayasree Kalathil and Alison Faulkner, 'Racialisation and Knowledge Production: A Critique of the Report "Understanding Psychosis and Schizophrenia"', *Mental Health Today* (2015), pp. 22–3. For the USA the literature is huge, but two good starting points are Jonathan M. Metzl, *The Protest Psychosis: How Schizophrenia Became a Black Disease*, (Boston: Beacon Press, 2010) and Martin Summers, *Madness in the City of Magnificent Intentions: A History of Race and Mental Illness in the Nation's Capital* (Oxford: Oxford University Press, 2019). There is also a good (US-focused) section in the bibliography of Harrington's *Mind Fixers*.

65 A collection of these 'In England now' columns was published in 1989: G.A.C. Binnie, R.L. Sadler, W.O. Thomson, D.M.D. White, and D.W. Sharp (eds), *In England Now: Fifty Years of Peripatetic Correspondence in the Lancet* (London: The Lancet/Hodder & Stoughton, 1989).

66 W.H. Trethowan, 'In My Own Time: Suicide and Attempted Suicide', *BMJ*, 2, 6185 (1979), pp. 319–20.

67 'Reports of Societies – Child Guidance', *BMJ*, 2, 3805 (1933), p. 1074–5. This feeds into histories of child guidance e.g. John Stewart, *Child Guidance in Britain, 1918–1955: The Dangerous Age of Childhood* (London: Routledge, 2015), as well as studies of ideas of child bonding, attachment and psychology, e.g. Marga Vicedo *The Nature and Nurture of Love: From Imprinting to Attachment in Cold War America* (Chicago: University of Chicago Press, 2013).

68 Munk's Roll is the informal name for the series of obituaries of members of the Royal College of Physicians, which used to be called 'Lives of the Fellows' and is now called

'Inspiring Physicians': https://history.rcplondon.ac.uk/inspiring-physicians, accessed 23 Mar. 2021.
69 One such appeal from John Lorber, a paediatrician at Sheffield's children's hospital, turns out to be a case of Munchausen Syndrome by Proxy: John Lorber, 'Unexplained Episodes of Coma in a Two-Year-Old', *The Lancet*, 2, 8087 (1978), pp. 472–3; John Lorber, J.P. Reckless, and J.B. Watson, 'Nonaccidental Poisoning: The Elusive Diagnosis', *Archives of Disease in Childhood*, 55, 8 (1980), pp. 643–7.

Select bibliography

Eghigian, G., 'Deinstitutionalizing the History of Contemporary Psychiatry', *History of Psychiatry* 22, 2011, pp. 201–214.

Fernando, S., *Cultural Diversity, Mental Health and Psychiatry: The Struggle against Racism*, Hove: Brunner-Routledge, 2003.

Harrington, A., *Mind Fixers: Psychiatry's Troubled Search for the Biology of Mental Illness*, New York: W.W. Norton & Co., 2019.

Lunbeck, E., 'Borderline Histories: Psychoanalysis Inside and Out', *Science in Context* 19, 2006, pp. 151–173.

Millard, C., 'Making the Cut: The Production of "Self-Harm" in Post-1945 Anglo-Saxon Psychiatry', *History of the Human Sciences* 26, 2013, pp. 126–150.

Moulds, A. 'The 'Medical-Women Question' and the Multivocality of the Victorian Medical Press, 1869–1900', *Media History* 25, 2019, pp. 6–22.

Rose, D., 'Service User/Survivor-Led Research in Mental Health: Epistemological Possibilities', *Disability & Society* 32, 2017, pp. 773–789.

Scott, J.W. 'The Evidence of Experience', *Critical inquiry* 17, 1991, pp. 773–797.

Van der Horst, F. and Van Der Veer, R., 'Changing Attitudes towards the Care of Children in Hospital: A New Assessment of the Influence of the Work of Bowlby and Robertson in the UK, 1940–1970', *Attachment & Human Development* 11, 2009, pp. 119–142.

Woods, A. 'Rethinking "Patient Testimony" in the Medical Humanities: The Case of *Schizophrenia Bulletin*'s First Person Accounts', *Journal of Literature and Science* 6, 2012, pp. 38–54.

6

EXPERIMENTS IN LIFE: LITERATURE'S CONTRIBUTION TO THE HISTORY OF PSYCHIATRY

Melissa Dickson

In his 1907 reading of Wilhelm Jensen's novel *Gradiva*, Sigmund Freud declared creative writers to be 'valuable allies' to the discipline of psychiatry, whose 'knowledge of the mind' was 'far in advance of us everyday people, for they draw upon sources which we have not yet opened up for science'.[1] Freud's insistence here, that literature discloses and gives artistic expression to the workings of the subconscious, emphasised a close alliance between literature and psychoanalysis in their shared interest in the human mind. Given that the fields of literature and psychiatry are both deeply invested in the nature of individual subjectivity, agency, and mental states, as well as the shaping force of unconscious operations on the construction of identity, it is perhaps not surprising that each provides a different form of evidence, from different sources, of psychological operations. However, the notion that literature has the capacity not only to reflect and imaginatively to illustrate psychiatric cases, but also to anticipate and actively inform the science of the mind, renders it a valuable source in the history of psychiatry and, more specifically, a critical source in the formation and formulation of psychiatric theories and categories.

This chapter focuses on the close exchange of ideas and terminologies across literary and psychiatric discourses of nineteenth-century Britain, demonstrating how such productive exchanges with literature have informed the emergence and the evolution of psychiatry as a discipline. During this period, as the human mind increasingly became an object of empirical and scientific, rather than philosophical, investigation, the new science of the mind shared the challenges of the nineteenth-century novelist in rendering consciousness in language.[2] Confronted with the question of how to know, represent, and understand another mind, mental scientists found inspiration in and borrowed from the formal structures and narrative properties of literary works, whilst novelists drew upon the latest developments in psychiatry in their imaginative constructions of other selves, and the

DOI: 10.4324/9781003087694-7

forces that drive them. This confluence makes much literature of the period a valuable, at times even indispensable, source for our understanding of the history of psychiatric science. Taking up George Eliot's *Daniel Deronda* (1876) as my main case study, I explore this exchange of influence in relation to the Victorian practice of Realism, before turning to Robert Louis Stevenson's *Dr Jekyll and Mr Hyde* (1886), and the more metaphoric frameworks of investigation of the unconscious that are to be found in the fantastic and the Gothic modes. In each case, I will argue, the persistently fluctuating boundaries between scientific theories and cultural representations of the mind mean that literary works themselves played an essential role in the development of the emergent psychiatry, and so can make apparent to us different perspectives on the discipline that remain latent in 'purely' scientific discourse.

Realist constructions of the self

Victorian Realism, in its dedication to faithful representations of life, explores a range of consciousnesses and natures in true-to-life situations in the recognition that, as George Levine has noted, 'there are ways of thinking, feeling, desiring and suffering that we haven't experienced, and have trouble understanding'.[3] The nineteenth-century novel sought to provide these experiences vicariously, meticulously attending to the details of daily life while allowing readers imaginatively to access the thoughts, feelings, and desires that occupied other minds and other lives. This project gave rise, for example, to the so-called condition-of-England novels of Elizabeth Gaskell, Charles Dickens, Benjamin Disraeli, and Charles Kingsley, who worked to detail the unique stresses and strains of individual lives caught up in the mass urbanisation and industrialisation of the era, and thus comment upon larger social and political trends. Some novels of the period, like Dickens' *Great Expectations* (1860–61) and Charlotte Brontë's *Jane Eyre* (1847), adopted the model of first-person autobiography to explore the social, familial, and environmental factors that mediate and contribute to the individual's formation of a sense of self. Others, like Anne Brontë's *The Tenant of Wildfell Hall* (1848), addressed more specific social ills, in this case the limited legal rights and sustained emotional and psychological sufferings of an abused wife.

While recognising the impossibility of truly presenting an unmediated reality in language, Victorian Realism nonetheless aspires to transcend the limits of the individual's egocentric perspective, and thereby establish a more fulsome understanding of others. Such a project requires a degree of what Levine – himself drawing on the field of psychoanalysis – terms 'imaginative self-transference', in first recognising the existence of an 'other' consciousness and then attempting to understand their experience and perspective.[4] It thus shared with the new mental sciences a dedication to penetrating those internal forces which constitute individual subjectivity and influence behaviour. In this sense, as the French critic Hippolyte Taine declared in his 1871 *History of English Literature*, the novelist 'is a psychologist, who naturally and involuntarily sets psychology at work', and the emergent field of psychiatry provided fruitful conceptions for the novelist's imaginative explorations of selfhood in this moment.[5] Contemporary definitions of monomania, and self-management, for instance, actively informed Charlotte Brontë's explorations of female identity and sexuality, while Charles Dickens' ongoing fascination with current theories of memory, trauma, and the nature of dreaming played out in the many instances of haunting, repetition, and the return of the repressed in his writing.[6] As their works 'thrust the reader into an intimacy with possibilities well beyond the limits of the self who reads', their provocative and realistic representations of the workings of the human mind provided complex case studies for psychiatric investigation.[7]

For George Eliot, the Realist novel was, quite explicitly, a form of psychological and philosophical experiment, one that was actively engaged with the workings of individual lives and individual minds. In January 1876, a few weeks before the commencement of the serial publication of her final novel *Daniel Deronda*, Eliot wrote to a bereaved friend on what she understood to be her role as a novelist:

> But my writing is simply a set of experiments in life—an endeavour to see what our thought and emotion may be capable of—what stores of motive, actual or hinted as possible, give promise of a better after which we may strive—what gains from past revelations and discipline we must strive to keep hold of as something more sure than shifting theory. I become more and more timid—with less daring to adopt any formula which does not get itself clothed for me in some human figure and individual experience, and perhaps that is a sign that if I help others to see at all it must be through that medium of art.[8]

Writing fiction is cast here as an investigative process, which poses hypotheses relating to human nature, and then tests them through intimate observation of the individual experiences of human figures, as they operate within their particular social, economic, and political environments. For Eliot, this work of attempting to 'see', and thus to know and understand, has a clear ethical function: to find models of human behaviour that might become guiding principles for life. However, it also requires both empirical and imaginative engagement with those forces, thoughts, and emotions which comprise the human psyche, and in focusing so intently on the inner lives, 'actual or hinted', of her characters, her novels offer rich fields of play for the latest developments in Victorian psychology and neurology.

Gwendolen Harleth, the heroine of *Daniel Deronda*, is a key figure in that experimental field. Gwendolen exhibits the kind of pre-Freudian, '"deep" complicated self', and the 'implicit dialogue between different layers, currents or sections of the mind' that Jenny Bourne Taylor has shown was developing in the nineteenth century as writers and scientists sought to explore the complex relations between consciousness and unconsciousness.[9] With her 'very common egoistic ambition' and her 'favourite key of life – doing as she liked', Gwendolen aspires to self-determination and the domination both of those around her and her own inner forces and impulses.[10] While her masterful ego struggles to maintain her self-image, she nonetheless finds herself subject to periodic 'fits of spiritual dread', which fill her with shame and seem 'like a brief remembered madness, an unexplained exception from her normal life'.[11] What Gwendolen fears, as Jill Matus observes, is that intrusive, 'dark, shadowy self beyond the control of her will', and her moments of intense dread constitute fleeting intimations of that self.[12] When, for example, she is in despair at having lost all her money, and pawns a necklace only to discover that Daniel has redeemed and returned it to her, the 'movement of mind which led her to keep the necklace' is 'not much clearer to her than why she should sometimes have been frightened to find herself in the fields alone'.[13] She is similarly confused by her own feelings of terror when, while she is performing a charade with her sister and cousins, the movable panel at Offendene suddenly gapes open to reveal a fleeing figure pursued by the apparition of a pale, grotesque 'dead face'.[14] Although she seeks to evade, or repress, those impulses which cannot be accommodated within her self-image, the workings of Gwendolen's 'wonderfully mixed consciousness' trouble the boundaries between consciousness and unconsciousness, and between social, somatic, and psychic selves. After her marriage to the psychological tyrant Mallinger Grandcourt, dread of her husband manifests as a 'nightmare of fear', suggestive of the fragile, porous boundaries between the psychic layers of the mind.[15] Tormented by persistent images of Grandcourt's death, Gwendolen fears that her hatred will erupt into violence, while frequently imagining her husband's white hands strangling her. Through such chronicling of the 'play of various, nay, contrary tendencies' within her heroine, Eliot draws upon and offers insight into contemporary psychological theories of unconscious and neural processes.[16]

Eliot provides us with a particularly clear example of the reciprocal influences at work between literary art and the science of the period. Just as the narrator of *Daniel Deronda* insists that 'there is a great deal of unmapped country within us which would have to be taken into account in an explanation of our gusts and storms', Eliot's partner, the philosopher and amateur physiologist George Henry Lewes, upheld the view in his *Physiology of Common Life* (1859) that 'nothing is more certain than that we have many sensations which are not perceived at all, of which we are said to be wholly "unconscious"'.[17] In seeking to navigate those sensations, Lewes adopted a holistic and organicist approach to consciousness as one element of the broader spectrum of human sentience. 'Consciousness', he wrote, is 'the sum total of all our sensibilities'; it 'is not an agent but a symptom' of the larger mental processes and activities of the mind.[18] Consciousness does not function in opposition to, but exists on a spectrum with, unconsciousness: 'Unconsciousness struggles with, blends with, and replaces Consciousness in the organism, and is a positive state of the sentient organism, not to be confounded with a mere negation of Sentience; above all, not to be relegated to merely mechanical processes.'[19]

Lewes's conceptualisation of the self as capable of recording impressions and sensations of which it is both conscious and unconscious, and acting on repressed impulses and memories as well as known desires, corresponds to Eliot's imaginative scrutiny of that 'insignificant thread in human history' that comprises the 'consciousness of a girl, busy with her small inferences of the way in which she could make her life pleasant'.[20] *Daniel Deronda* thus offers an intimate portrait of the inner turmoil and deep interconnections of the individual mind and body, in dialogue with contemporary sciences of the mind. The literary text is never self-contained and does not take shape in isolation; rather, it emerges from, and is embedded within, larger social and cultural fields, such as the scientific disciplines that inform Eliot's work. Unlike the scientific and medical literature in which Eliot was so well versed, however, Eliot dramatises these theories, using them to develop, explore, and complicate her depictions of human beings in action. The illusion of consciousness Eliot seeks to create draws upon then cutting-edge models of the workings of the mind, allowing us to view in practical terms the consequences of these models, as they would have been understood by practitioners of the time, medical or otherwise.

In a cultural moment when, as Richard Menke observes in the context of nineteenth-century experiments in vivisection, 'physiologists could catalog heartbeats but not thoughts' and 'administer electric shocks but not emotional ones', Eliot 'appropriates the framework of Victorian physiology to go where science itself could not, to develop her own novelistic techniques for the close analysis of imaginary minds and bodies'.[21] From the novel's opening line, 'Was she beautiful or not beautiful? And what was the secret of form or expression which gave the dynamic quality to her glance?' – an unspoken line of thought emerging from the mind of Daniel as he watches Gwendolen gamble – the novel maps, in minute detail, the changing thoughts and feelings of its characters from one moment to the next.[22] As readers, we observe the hidden impulses that lie behind the individual's overt behaviour, symptomised, for example, by Gwendolen's 'spiritual dread' and 'world nausea'; Mirah Lapidoth's suicidal impulses when, in despair, she finds 'my thoughts were stronger than I was', or Daniel's own extreme sensitivity, which allows him to drift into 'forgetting everything else in a half-speculative, half-involuntary identification of himself with the objects he was looking at'.[23] By scrutinising and cataloguing these inner workings and desires, Eliot explores new, medicalised assumptions about pathologies of the mind and body and the broader dynamics of social, cultural, and economic exchange. In constructing images of minds, rather than analysing real ones, and placing them within representations of society (as opposed to society itself), Eliot's art lays bare the ways in which the science of her contemporaries was envisaged as connecting to lived experience. Her texts thus offer us insight into the implicit aims and social agendas of the wider projects of medical science.

Critics of *Daniel Deronda* have delineated many convincing links between Eliot's fictional creations and nineteenth-century psychiatric fields of inquiry. David Trotter, for example, has identified Gwendolen's inexplicable terror of solitude in wide open places, which 'impressed her with an undefined feeling of immeasurable existence aloof from her', as a form of agoraphobia, a condition associated with the pressures and pathologies of modern life that had only recently been defined by the German professor Carl Friedrich Otto Westphal in 1871.[24] Jane Wood, in interrogating *Daniel Deronda*'s relationship to George Henry Lewes's investigations of the connections between body and mind, argues that 'Gwendolen's discontinuity and alarming compulsion to determine all outside objects towards the self' is a formation of the contemporary 'rhetoric of hysterical neurosis'.[25] Margaret Loewen Reimer argues that Gwendolen's seemingly disproportionate hysterical outbursts and paralysing dread, culminating in the suggestively phrased 'insistent penetration of suppressed experience' on her wedding night, are the result of sexual abuse at the hands of her stepfather, Captain Davilow, which the novel points to but never explicitly reveals.[26] By approaching Eliot's fiction as a useful source in the broader landscape of nineteenth-century investigations into the workings of mind and body, such studies demonstrate how fiction can absorb and reflect, but also challenge and critically re-interpret scientific and psychiatric constructs. If we understand Eliot's characters in the context of the models that informed their development, the means by which they are developed in turn furthers our understanding of how those models were conceived.

It is important to recognise, too, that literature does not simply mirror science, or current hypotheses regarding the workings of the conscious and unconscious mind; it can also play a constitutive role in the formulation of psychiatric theories and categories. It was not unusual for medical texts of the period to draw upon literary works for their psychological case studies.[27] We see such an interaction at work in the Scottish psychiatrist T.S. Clouston's 1880 essay, 'Puberty and Adolescence Medico-Psychological Considered'. Seeking to define the various stages of psychological development from childhood to adolescence and then adulthood, Clouston turns here not to any known medical case, but to the imaginary figure of Gwendolen Harleth. Eliot, Clouston writes,

> is by far the most acute and subtile [*sic*] psychologist of her time, and certainly the character I have mentioned is most worthy of study by all physicians who look on mind as being in their field of study or sphere of action.[28]

Choosing a series of quotations from the novel to illustrate Gwendolen's 'subjective egoism tending towards objective dualism', her selfishness, and her 'organic craving to be admired', Clouston contends that Gwendolen is the epitome of the female adolescent.[29] This fictional creature, although she is in fact in her early twenties, provides the psychiatrist with a complex study of the constantly fluctuating thoughts and feelings of a young woman, from one moment to the next. Such references to fiction and fictional characters, as well as reviews of the latest literary works, are surprisingly common in the medical press of the time, and constitute valuable sources of information on the ways in which literary texts were received in discussions that dovetailed with constructions of the modern self. Searching major medical and psychiatric periodicals of the period, such as the *British Medical Journal*, the *Lancet*, the *Journal of Mental Science* (forerunner of the *British Journal of Psychiatry*), and *Mind*, for the names of authors, publications, and even individual characters, will regularly turn up analyses of fictional works and concepts by medical professionals, from the perspective of their own disciplines and training. Literature provided an accessible and familiar site at which the complexities surrounding the dynamic mind and body in general, and in the case of Gwendolen Harleth the female psyche in particular, might be articulated and negotiated.

The framework for Eliot's psychiatric investigations is, of course, an imaginative one, but it is very much in keeping with the methodologies of mid nineteenth-century scientific materialists such as George Henry Lewes, John Tyndall, and William Clifford, who sought to access a world of pulses, particles, and vibrations which lay beyond the reach of any available microscope, stethoscope, or telescope. 'It is plain', wrote the physicist Tyndall, 'that beyond the present outposts of microscopic inquiry lies an immense field for the exercise of the imagination', and he tasked the imagination with moving between presence and absence, materiality and the immaterial, the visible and the invisible in order to 'grapple with the ultimate structural energies of nature'.[30] 'The truth is', Lewes affirmed in *Problems of Life and Mind* (1874), 'that science mounts on the wings of imagination into regions of the Invisible and Impalpable, peopling those regions with Fictions more remote from fact than the phantasies of the Arabian Nights are from the daily occurrences in Oxford Street'.[31] Eliot, with her brand of Victorian Realism, recognised the necessity of employing the imagination when confronted with the prospect of a realm beyond the human senses, and she dedicated her narratives to tracing those metaphoric heartbeats, vibrations, and palpitations that signify psychological struggles within so much of her oeuvre. Beyond the bounds of the Realist novel, however, literary explorations of the invisible and impalpable recesses of the human psyche in this period took other, more fantastic forms.

Metaphors of mind

When the curious young Alice chases a white rabbit into its vast warren under a hedge, she finds that 'the rabbit-hole went straight on like a tunnel for some way, and then dipped suddenly down, so that Alice had not a moment to think about stopping herself before she found herself falling down a very deep well'.[32] Ultimately, of course, this intricate labyrinth of tunnels opens out into Wonderland, a dream realm where time, logic, and the properties of material objects follow different rules.[33] As the Cheshire Cat announces, 'we're all mad here', and the story is, in many ways, an insight into contemporary attitudes to psychiatric disorder.[34] However, beyond the fictional representations of insanity we find throughout this deceptively simple story, we might consider the spatial and temporal structures of Wonderland symbolically, as representative of contemporary theories of the mind's operations.

It is the moment of Alice's initial tumble, a physical movement from surface to depth, from the known to the unknown, which draws the reader's attention to the stratification of her mind and the drama of psychological discovery upon which she is embarking. *Alice's Adventures in Wonderland* (1865), which, significantly, was originally called *Alice's Adventures Underground*, deliberately uses a potent archaeological metaphor in suggesting Alice's movement from consciousness to unconsciousness – her falling asleep – as a literal fall through the layers of the earth. Robert Douglas-Fairhurst also notes that the cupboards, bookshelves, maps, pictures, and marmalade she encounters on her way down indicate that, as she falls, 'she is also reviewing her past in a series of muddled snapshots: her maps and pictures come from the schoolroom; the marmalade comes from the breakfast table'.[35] The underground cavern, or rabbit-hole, represents the threshold between waking and sleeping, for just as the material relics of the past are buried within the layers of the earth, so, it seems, the contents of the psyche are preserved within its depths.

Alice's fall down the rabbit-hole draws on a familiar model of the period in conceptualising the psychological movement between the layers of the mind as a form of archaeological excavation. Her descent into Wonderland mirrors the archaeologist's movement between the surface and depths of the earth, whereby the material traces of earlier times are physically (re)located to the present. Widely understood as being concerned with 'uncovering and revealing structures and artefacts that have been hidden for centuries', the discipline of archaeology, as Julian Thomas has demonstrated, emerged and took shape during a period of fundamental shifts in the character of knowledge, which drew attention to the hidden structures underpinning reality, and led to the development of structural thought in the nineteenth and twentieth centuries.[36] Moreover, archaeology 'provided a metaphor through which that thought could articulate itself'.[37] In so doing, it also provided an extremely potent series of metaphors, frequently deployed in fictions like Carroll's, for evoking notions of the repressed, the subconscious, the stratification of the mind, and the operations of buried memories, each of which is 'often spatialised in terms of the relationship between depth and surface'.[38]

Freud himself made extensive use of this metaphoric template in his descriptions of the unconscious, and the impulses and drives that lie beneath the surface of the individual's mind. Freud's own fascination with archaeology has been well documented.[39] As Donald Kuspit has observed, the distinctions that Freud made throughout his career between 'surface and depth, manifest and latent, adult and infantile, civilised and uncivilised, historic and prehistoric', in his descriptions of the mind as a series of psychic layers built up within the individual from childhood, explicitly drew upon the language of archaeology.[40] Archaeology, like his own practice of psychoanalysis, was figured by Freud as a potential mode of recovering and reconstructing the individual's childhood, the distant past, the mysterious, and the mythic. Archaeology is, in this sense, a wonderful 'adventure underground' with the capacity to unearth past, or repressed, knowledge and experiences.

Much of Freud's work both drew on and was inspired by works of fiction, and he openly acknowledged the impact of Gothic literature on the ideas and metaphors deployed in his field. Certainly, literary explorations of the darker recesses of the human psyche in the nineteenth century are most readily apparent in the Gothic mode, in which fictional expeditions into haunted houses, castles, dungeons, cloisters, caves, and crypts become physical manifestations of psychological operations. Descent into such spaces quickly becomes the stuff of nightmares. In Ann Radcliffe's *The Mysteries of Udolpho* (1794), for example, young Emily D'Aubert finds herself locked within the chamber of a ruined castle housing a bloody cadaver and various instruments of torture, her obvious physical entrapment serving as an indicator of her mental realisation that she has been caught up in powerful forces beyond her control. The homicidal narrators of Edgar Allan Poe's 'The Tell-Tale Heart' (1843) and 'The Black Cat' (1843) actively seek to repress their own manic fury and sense of guilt by burying the bodies of their victims in underground spaces – spaces clearly suggestive of the unconscious mind – only to find themselves haunted and ultimately destroyed by what they have done. Poe's 'The Fall of the House of Usher' (1839), 'The Premature Burial' (1844), and 'Some Words with a Mummy' (1845), as well as Edith Nesbit's later story 'The Five Senses' (1909), also trouble the boundary between consciousness and unconsciousness through their accounts of individuals who are buried alive. Gothic accounts of live burial in this period harnessed and amplified the growing popular fear of waking from a trance or other state of unconsciousness to find oneself prematurely interred with the dead. Literary descriptions of the abject terror and powerlessness of such a state, as Andrew Mangham has demonstrated, provided the Italian psychiatrist Enrico Morselli with the vocabulary and diagnostic tools he needed to identify and define taphephobia – the fear of being buried alive – in 1891. Such was the influence of this literature on scientific discussions of the mind that '[t]he awakening of the condition, as a medical diagnosis', Mangham shows, 'could never have occurred without the complex, phenomenological understandings of fear and obsession that emerged from the Gothic'.[41] While we must exercise caution in drawing connections between different fields of practice purely on the basis of analogous activities and investigations, such moments of explicit interaction – when psychiatrists turn to literature or writers take up psychiatric concepts and categories – demonstrate that literary works have formed part of an ongoing negotiation between psychiatric theories and cultural representations of the mind and its operations. That process of negotiation is now continued by many historians of Victorian psychology, such as Anne Stiles in *Popular Fiction and Brain Science in the Late Nineteenth Century* (2012), Roger Smith in *Free Will and the Human Sciences in Britain, 1870–1910* (2013), and Alison Winter in *Mesmerized: Powers of Mind in Victorian Britain* (1998), who each attend to the social and cultural constructions and contexts of psychological phenomena.[42]

The Gothic, as Robert Miles has noted, 'worries over a problem stirring within the foundations of the self', and it has thus remained 'embroiled within a larger, theoretically complex project: the history of the "subject"'.[43] In the latter decades of the nineteenth century, Gothic writing remained deeply enmeshed in the history of psychiatric research, as traditional motifs of ruined castles and subterranean passageways gave way to new, updated configurations of the self and the mind. Late Victorian Gothic was, in Roger Luckhurst's words, 'fascinated by forms of psychic splitting, trance states, and telepathic intimacies', as well as serving as 'the primary locus for discussion of degeneration'.[44] Robert Louis Stevenson's *Dr Jekyll and Mr Hyde* (1886) is perhaps the most famous literary exploration of the individual's capacity for psychic splitting.[45] Welcomed by *The Times* as either 'a flash of intuitive psychological research, dashed off in a burst of inspiration' or 'the product of the most elaborate forethought, fitting together all the parts of an intricate and inscrutable puzzle', the novella constituted a very active, creative intervention in late Victorian debates about multiple personalities, subliminal consciousness, and the dual hemispheres of the brain.[46] Here, the seemingly respectable London-based medic Dr Henry Jekyll, as the autobiographical narrative concluding the tale relates, becomes increasingly aware that he is not a coherent, unified self. There is a kind of radical doubleness, or 'profound duplicity' within his consciousness, which he senses is at 'perennial war' with itself.[47] The precise nature of that part of himself which ultimately adopts the persona of Mr Hyde is unclear, although the name Hyde is a clear pun on the word 'hide', and reflects the notion that this is a concealed, inner self that Jekyll, with a 'morbid sense of shame', seeks to repress.[48] What is clear, however, is that each part of his dual nature comprises an authentic, if contradictory, aspect of the self and, as he says, 'I was no more myself when I laid aside restraint and plunged in shame than when I laboured, in the eye of day, at the furtherance of knowledge or the relief of sorrow and suffering'.[49] This sense of a deeply unstable, internally contradictory self reflects developments in psychiatric thought of the 1880s and 1890s, which posited that the mind, rather than being divided only between layers of consciousness, might in fact contain multiple selves, or personalities.[50]

Registering the cultural anxieties induced by this new understanding of an inherently divided self, Stevenson's novella explores the dystopian possibilities of the separation of these components of individual identity. The concoction of powders, tinctures, and salts that allows the degenerate aspects of Dr Jeykll to be split off from his consciousness in the form of Mr Hyde is, in many ways, a fictional variant of the plethora of new medical remedies that were increasingly glutting the Victorian pharmaceutical marketplace in the latter decades of the century. Certainly, popular tonics and stimulants, which emphasised the value of strengthening the nervous system and restoring firmness and vigour to overwrought bodies, were frequently patented and publicly embraced throughout this period. However, Jekyll's chemical concoction is also a speculative premise for the purposes of illustrating current theories of the mind's operations. It responds to psychological cases like that of Louis Vivet, who was found to have eight separate personalities, each of which seemingly had a separate memory, or the young hysteric known as Félida, who the *Cornhill Magazine* had reported in 1875 experienced a 'peculiar secondary state of mind' which alternated with her usual state of being, while questioning whether 'the promptings of evil and the voice of conscience resisting these promptings present themselves as the operation of two brains, one less instructed and worse trained than the other'.[51]

Stevenson's novella asks, in such a context, what is the precise nature of these two brains, how do they inform and influence one another in comprising the individual mind, and what might be the possibilities and effects of disaggregating the multiple selves within one consciousness? Indeed, the work's full title, *The Strange Case of Dr Jekyll and Mr Hyde*, invites us to read it as a form of thought experiment, or psychological case study. Certainly, the psychical researcher Frederic William Henry Myers (1843–1901) read the work as such, and he afterwards wrote to Stevenson to offer him a series of detailed notes and corrections which he believed might assist him in achieving greater psychological accuracy in exploring this premise.[52] Writers' correspondence, as we saw in George Eliot's reflections on the art of fiction above, may also offer insights into the connections between literary projects and the wider social, cultural, scientific, and medical networks in which they operate.[53] The subsequent correspondence between Myers and Stevenson constitutes a mutual exploration of psychic spaces and psychic splittings from their varying perspectives and, as part of this ongoing dialogue between literature and psychiatry, Stevenson's final letter on the subject was included in Myers' later work, *Human Personality and Its Survival of Bodily Death* (1903). Myers was not alone in finding *Dr Jekyll and Mr Hyde* a productive provocation: the influential evolutionary psychologist James Sully recorded in his 1918 memoirs that his interactions with Stevenson and his work had influenced his own theories of the unconscious.

These instances of mutually-affirming interaction between nineteenth-century literary and psychiatric discourses proffer intricate case studies of the cross-disciplinary negotiations which worked to structure perceptions and understandings of the individual self and the mind in the long nineteenth century. Nineteenth-century theories and treatments of mental processes and pathologies were not only deeply embedded in social and cultural operations; literary explorations and modifications actively constructed and were deployed within psychiatric discourse. Such negotiations are not unique to the nineteenth century, or the decades before Freud. Throughout the twentieth century, the diagnosis and understanding of conditions such as gaslighting, a term drawn from Patrick Hamilton's 1938 play *Gaslight* and used in psychiatric literature since the 1960s, continue to draw on both psychiatric and broader cultural fields.[54] We might think, too, of the Superman Complex, a term first used by psychiatrist Fredric Wertham in his 1954 testimony before a Senate Subcommittee on juvenile delinquency. Literature, as it moves between the self and its environment, between the operations and pathologies of the mind and the broader dynamics of social, cultural, and economic exchange, performs a crucial intermediary role in establishing and exposing new, medicalised assumptions about the workings of the mind and individual identity.

Using literature to explore the history of psychiatry, then, requires not only an examination of mental states and conditions as they are represented *within* literature, but also the patient investigation of those broader operational fields *outside* the text, with which it is in conversation. What psychiatric studies or cases, for example, was the author reading at the time they were writing? What ideas and concepts of the period have been drawn upon, experimented with, or challenged in a fictional framework? How was the work received and engaged with within the medical sphere and by scientific periodicals? To answer such questions, we look to the author's own notes, diaries, and correspondence during the period leading up to the publication of their novel, in order to gain insight into the research and reading they were undertaking alongside their creative outputs. We might also search contemporary newspapers and the medical and scientific press for current debates on the ideas and concepts that have provided the subject matter for fictional exploration and experimentation. Tracking psychiatric concepts and categories – such as trauma, repression, or multiple personality disorder – as they are represented, re-framed, and debated in wider culture, demonstrates not only how different societies construct and formulate notions of selfhood and mental health, or illness, more broadly, but also how cultural and literary contexts become deeply embedded within institutionalised understandings of physiological and psychological identity.

Notes

1 Sigmund Freud, 'Delusions and Dreams in Jensen's *Gradiva*', *The Standard Edition of the Complete Psychological Works of Sigmund Freud*, trans. and ed. James Strachey, 24 vols (London: Hogarth, 1959), vol. 9, pp. 7–93 p. 8.
2 The terms 'psychology' and 'psychiatry' were not in common use until the twentieth century. The terms 'mental science' or 'science of the mind' were typically used to describe these emergent fields, and so I employ them throughout this chapter.
3 George Levine, *Realism, Ethics, and Secularism: Essays on Victorian Literature and Science* (Cambridge: Cambridge University Press, 2008), p. 4.
4 Levine, p. 250.
5 Hippolyte Taine, *History of English Literature*, 5 vols (Edinburgh: Edmonston and Douglas, 1871), vol. 2, p. 390.
6 Sally Shuttleworth, *Charlotte Brontë and Victorian Psychology* (Cambridge: Cambridge University Press, 1996); Catherine Bernard, 'Dickens and Victorian Dream Theory', in James Paradis and Thomas Postlewait (eds), *Victorian Science and Victorian Values: Literary Perspectives* (New Brunswick, NJ: Rutgers University Press, 1986), pp. 197–216; Athena Vrettos, 'Defining Habits: Dickens and the Psychology of Repetition', *Victorian Studies*, 42, 3 (1999/2000), pp. 399–426.
7 Levine, p. viii.
8 George Eliot, 'GE to Dr. Joseph Frank Payne, London, 25 January 1876', in Gordon S. Haight (ed.), *The George Eliot Letters, Vol. 6: 1874–1877* (New Haven, CT: Yale University Press, 1954), pp. 214–5.
9 Jenny Bourne Taylor, 'Obscure Recesses: Locating the Victorian Unconscious', in J.B. Bullen (ed.), *Writing and Victorianism* (London: Longman, 1997), pp. 137–79: p. 141.

10 George Eliot, *Daniel Deronda,* ed. Graham Handley, intro. K.M. Newton (Oxford: Oxford University Press, 2014), p. 43, 112.

11 Eliot, *Daniel Deronda,* p. 52, 51.

12 Jill Matus, *Shock, Memory and the Unconscious in Victorian Fiction* (Cambridge: Cambridge University Press, 2009), p. 149.

13 Eliot, *Daniel Deronda,* p. 232.

14 Ibid., p. 49.

15 Ibid., p. 585, 378.

16 Ibid., p. 33.

17 Ibid., p. 233. George Henry Lewes, *The Physiology of Common Life,* 2 vols (Leipzig: Bernhard Tauchnitz, 1860), vol. 2, p. 49, 44.

18 G.H. Lewes, *Problems of Life and Mind, Third Series* (London: Trübner and Co, 1879), p. 365.

19 G.H. Lewes, *Problems of Life and Mind, Second Series* (Boston: James R. Osgood, 1877), p. 405.

20 Eliot, *Daniel Deronda,* p. 101. For a detailed study of Eliot's and Lewes's conceptualisation of consciousness and the mind, as well as the broader psychological field Eliot is drawing on, see Sally Shuttleworth, *George Eliot and Nineteenth-Century Science: The Make-Believe of a Beginning* (Cambridge: Cambridge University Press, 1984).

21 Richard Menke, 'Fiction as Vivisection: G.H. Lewes and George Eliot', *ELH,* 67, 2 (2000), pp. 617–53: p. 636.

22 Eliot, *Daniel Deronda,* p. 3.

23 Ibid., p. 52, 237, 185, 158.

24 Ibid., p. 52. David Trotter, 'The Invention of Agoraphobia', *Victorian Literature and Culture,* 32, 2 (2004), pp. 463–74.

25 Jane Wood, *Passion and Pathology in Victorian Fiction* (Oxford: Oxford University Press, 2001), p. 158.

26 Eliot, *Daniel Deronda,* p. 298. Margaret Loewen Reimer, 'The Spoiled Child: What Happened to Gwendolen Harleth?', *Cambridge Quarterly,* 36, 1 (2007), pp. 33–50. Shelley's *The Cenci* (1820), a tale of a victim of incest who finally murders her sexually abusive father, is, as Reimer notes, explicitly referenced in *Daniel Deronda.*

27 Shakespearean characters such as King Lear, Hamlet, and Ophelia were particularly popular choices for psychiatric analysis, while Dickens provided a more up to date literary reference for doctors. Sally Shuttleworth has demonstrated that the key text in emerging debates of educational overpressure in Britain was not a medical but a literary one, as the compelling fictional account of the forced education and premature death of little Paul Dombey in Dickens's *Dombey and Son* (1848) 'passed rapidly into psychiatric literature as a defining case study' of the period. See Sally Shuttleworth, *The Mind of the Child: Child Development in Literature, Science, and Medicine, 1840–1900* (Oxford: Oxford University Press, 2010), p. 107.

28 T.S. Clouston, 'Puberty and Adolescence Medico-Psychological Considered', *Edinburgh Medical Journal,* 26 (1880), pp. 5–17: p. 14.

29 Ibid.

30 John Tyndall, *The Scientific Use of the Imagination* (London: Longmans, Green, and Co., 1870), p. 31.

31 G.H. Lewes, *Problems of Life and Mind, First Series, The Foundations of a Creed* (London: Trübner and Co., 1874), p. 289. On the importance of the imagination to the scientific ideals of Lewes, Eliot, and their community, see George Levine, *Realism, Ethics and Secularism: Essays on Victorian Literature and Science* (Cambridge: Cambridge University Press, 2008), pp. 25–50.

32 Lewis Carroll, *Alice's Adventures in Wonderland, and Through the Looking Glass,* ed. Peter Hunt (Oxford: Oxford University Press, 2009), p. 10.

33 On Wonderland's relationship to the mathematical and scientific cultures of the period, see Gillian Beer, *Alice in Space: The Sideways Victorian World of Lewis Carroll* (Chicago,

IL: University of Chicago Press, 2016). On Carroll's sustained engagement with Victorian psychiatry, see Franziska Kohlt, "'The Stupidest Tea-Party in All My Life": Lewis Carroll and Victorian Psychiatric Practice', *Journal of Victorian Culture*, 21, 2 (2016), pp. 147–67.

34 Carroll, *Alice's Adventures*, p. 58.

35 Robert Douglas-Fairhurst, 'Working Through Memory and Forgetting in Victorian Literature', *Australasian Journal of Victorian Studies*, 21, 1 (2016), pp. 1–13: p. 2.

36 Julian Thomas, *Archaeology and Modernity* (London: Routledge, 2004), p. 149.

37 Ibid., p. 70.

38 Ibid., p. 149.

39 On Freud's long-standing interest in archaeology, see, for example, Paul Ricoeur, *Freud and Philosophy: An Essay on Interpretation*, trans. Denis Savage (New Haven, CT: Yale University Press, 1970), Sarah Kofman, *The Childhood of Art: An Interpretation of Freud's Aesthetics*, trans. Winifred Woodhull (New York: Columbia University Press, 1988), and Donald Spence, *The Freudian Metaphor: Towards Paradigm Change in Psychoanalysis* (New York: Norton, 1987).

40 Donald Kuspit, 'A Mighty Metaphor: The Analogy of Archaeology and Psychoanalysis', in Lynn Gamwell and Richard Wells (eds), *Sigmund Freud and his Art: His Personal Collection of Antiquities* (New York: N. Abrams in conjunction with London: Freud Museum, 1989), pp. 133–51: p. 135.

41 Andrew Mangham, 'Buried Alive: The Awakening of Taphephobia', *Journal of Literature and Science*, 3, 1 (2010), pp. 10–22: p. 20.

42 For an excellent review article on interdisciplinary approaches to the Victorian sciences of the mind, which includes many other examples of studies which take this kind of approach to the history of psychiatry, see Suzy Anger, 'The Victorian Mental Sciences', *Victorian Literature and Culture*, 46, 1 (2018), pp. 275–87.

43 Robert Miles, *Gothic Writing 1750–1820: A Genealogy* (London: Routledge, 1993), pp. 1–2.

44 Robert Luckhurst, *The Invention of Telepathy, 1870–1901* (Oxford: Oxford University Press, 1993), p. 185.

45 Examples of other literary explorations of multiple personalities in this period include Dostoyevsky's *The Double* (1846), James Hogg's *Private Memoirs and Confessions of a Justified Sinner* (1824), Henry Harland's *Two Women or One?* (1890), and Rudyard Kipling's short story 'Wireless' (1902).

46 'Strange Case of Dr Jekyll and Mr Hyde', *The Times*, 25 Jan. 1886.

47 Robert Louis Stevenson, *Dr Jekyll and Mr Hyde and Other Stories*, ed. Jenni Calder (London: Penguin, 1979), p. 81.

48 Ibid.

49 Ibid., p. 82.

50 For more on medical conceptions of double consciousness in the Victorian era, see Anne Harrington, *Medicine, Mind and the Double Brain: A Study in Nineteenth-Century Thought* (Princeton, NJ: Princeton University Press, 1987) and Ian Hacking, *Rewriting the Soul: Multiple Personality and the Sciences of Memory* (Princeton, NJ: Princeton University Press, 1995).

51 R.A. Proctor, 'Have We Two Brains?', *Cornhill Magazine*, 31, 182 (1875), pp. 149–66: p. 157. For a detailed analysis of this article as a source for *Dr Jekyll and Mr Hyde*, see Anne Stiles, 'Robert Louis Stevenson's "Jekyll and Hyde" and the Double Brain', *Studies in English Literature, 1500–1900*, 46, 4 (2006), pp. 879–900.

52 Roger Luckhurst provides a detailed summary of these notes in *The Invention of Telepathy*, pp. 190–6.

53 Writers' correspondence is now frequently to be found in edited editions of their collected letters. The website *Archives Hub* is also an invaluable resource for identifying relevant archives and collections relating to individual figures: https://archiveshub.jisc.ac.uk/.

54 The term's initial appearance in print in this context was in the American-Canadian writer Anthony Francis Clarke Wallace's 1961 book *Culture and Personality*, in which Wallace noted that 'it is also popularly believed to be possible to "gaslight" a perfectly healthy person into psychosis by interpreting his own behavior to him as symptomatic of serious mental illness'. See Anthony Wallace, *Culture and Personality* (New York: Random House, 1961), p. 183.

Select bibliography

Anger, S., 'The Victorian Mental Sciences', *Victorian Literature and Culture* 46, 2018, pp. 275–287.

Bourne Taylor, J., 'Obscure Recesses: Locating the Victorian Unconscious', in J.B. Bullen (ed.), *Writing and Victorianism*, London: Longman, 1997, pp. 137–179.

Harrington, A., *Medicine, Mind and the Double Brain: A Study in Nineteenth-Century Thought*, Princeton, NJ: Princeton University Press, 1987.

Levine, G., *Realism, Ethics, and Secularism: Essays on Victorian Literature and Science*, Cambridge: Cambridge University Press, 2008.

Mangham, A., 'Buried Alive: The Awakening of Taphephobia', *Journal of Literature and Science* 3, 2010, pp. 10–22.

Matus, J., *Shock, Memory and the Unconscious in Victorian Fiction*, Cambridge: Cambridge University Press, 2009.

Menke, R., 'Fiction as Vivisection: G.H. Lewes and George Eliot', *ELH* 67, 2000, pp. 617–653.

Miles, R., *Gothic Writing 1750–1820: A Genealogy*, London: Routledge, 1993.

Stiles, A., *Popular Fiction and Brain Science in the Late Nineteenth Century*, Cambridge: Cambridge University Press, 2012.

Wood, J., *Passion and Pathology in Victorian Fiction*, Oxford: Oxford University Press, 2001.

7

SOURCES AND METHODS IN THE HISTORIES OF COLONIAL PSYCHIATRY

Sloan Mahone

Introduction

In 1997, historian Shula Marks gave her Presidential Address to the Society for the Social History of Medicine to ask: 'what is "colonial" about "colonial medicine"?' In doing so, she attributed this steady rise in interest to a number of concurrent 'impulses' within history including the development of social history as an academic field; the influence of Foucault and social constructionist theory; developments in medical anthropology, and understandings of health and disease as social metaphor, particularly in light of modern pandemics such as AIDS.[1] We might adapt Marks' question for 'colonial psychiatry' which has also seen significant growth over the last several decades to become a robust field for historians. Some of our concerns echo those of Marks who has herself written about the political economy of health under apartheid, mental health nursing, and South Africa's uneven and racialised psychiatric history. This chapter engages with the great breadth and diversity of sources and approaches in the history of psychiatry under colonialism. Although my own area of specialisation is Africa, I will endeavour to incorporate examples from across the globe. The themes in this chapter will cover ways of approaching this broad subject with an aim to show the diversity of sources and methods historians have employed to tell increasingly personal, rather than institutional, stories. I will close the chapter with a brief case study from my own work on psychiatry in late colonial East Africa.

A well-developed historiography

From where we now stand, there is a rich sub-field in history for the study of the practice of western psychiatry in colonial settings. Growing up alongside this, however, are related interests in local resistances to colonial practices and

DOI: 10.4324/9781003087694-8

institutions, local systems of mental healing that worked in opposition to, or entangled with, western ideas and technologies, and patient-centred histories, where possible, that may provide a glimpse into the social dynamics of the everyday with local concerns and internal politics and cosmologies. While you will find that most primary sources have been produced from the perspective of the 'coloniser' not the 'colonised', there is a growing body of scholarship that attempts to tease out more balanced stories. The study of medical auxiliaries, for example, has been instructive within the history of colonial medicine overall, and is no less important for the history of psychiatry where both language skills and competence in understanding local concerns and beliefs were crucial for doctors and administrators. In most of these cases the influence of intermediaries, such as translators, drivers, and medical orderlies went uncredited. Scholars such as Lynette Schumaker, writing about the history of anthropology, as well as a more recently edited volume on colonial public health work, have pulled these important stories out of the shadows and the most up-to-date historical work would be remiss in relying on colonial voices and interpretations alone.[2]

The political and cultural disconnect that existed between colonial institutions and the patients they kept (sometimes with patient consent, but often not) sits at the heart of the seminal work by Megan Vaughan which put into motion decades of new research on what psychiatric and psychological ideas can tell us about the anxieties and fragilities of the colonial state and its justifications for rule. Vaughan's 1983 article 'Idioms of Madness', taken from the writings of doctors at the Zomba Lunatic Asylum in Nyasaland (now Malawi) exposes the ways in which psychiatric diagnoses can be fraught with deeply held prejudices about race, ethnicity, religion, or gender. Vaughan reflects on colonial interpretations of African 'madness' and what she terms the 'double othering' that occurs in colonial settings where pathology was attributed both to 'being African' and to 'being mad'.[3] Colonial administrators' fears that the imposition of the modern world, or 'civilisation', would destabilise African personalities (and thus whole populations) had real world implications for colonised peoples whose aspirations for self-governance were deemed to be psychologically deviant.[4] One notorious example of the oppressive uses of psychological theory can be seen in an influential government-commissioned document, *The Psychology of Mau Mau* (1954) authored by Dr J.C. Carothers, the psychiatrist formerly in charge of Mathari Mental Hospital in Nairobi, Kenya. This policy document provided the British government with a scientific rationale for characterising the Kenyan war for independence as a movement led by fanatics who controlled a psychologically unstable population.[5] The influence of the 'East African School' of psychiatry has been the subject of a number of studies fuelled in part by the voluminous material produced by a succession of doctors posted to hospitals in Kenya.[6]

The deep politicisation of psychiatry amongst oppressed people has been well documented within important anti-colonial writings as well. Frantz Fanon, a revolutionary thinker as well as a practicing clinical psychiatrist, starkly criticised psychiatry in Algeria, characterising it as a failure at best, and a sinister, degrading, and oppressive force at its worst. Fanon likened the abuses he witnessed in North Africa to the racism inherent in the medical knowledge produced by psychiatrists like Carothers. His famous philosophical works about colonial oppression, such as *The Wretched of the Earth* (1961), are notable for the inclusion of chapters on the influence of medicine and psychiatry.[7] We might compare a contemporary of Fanon, the western-trained Nigerian psychiatrist, Thomas Adeoye Lambo (commonly referred to as T.A. Lambo) who worked within the colonial system and internationally to develop innovative forms of psychiatric treatment in Nigeria. Lambo published widely and was a leader of international congresses on psychiatry that sought to modernise the profession across Africa.[8] Recognising the need for mental health services to work in tandem with Nigerian ideas about healing, Lambo founded the Aro Village hospital as a model for outpatient care that was considered a potential blueprint for mental health across Africa. In a very welcome addition to the historiography, historian Matthew Heaton has published a study of T.A. Lambo's important career and legacy, as well as the broader network of psychiatrists he engaged with, in a 2013 monograph, *Black Skin, White Coats* which might serve as a model for a deeply contextualised history that reaches beyond 'doctor' or 'hospital'.[9] Newer work, like that from Yolana Pringle, takes a similar approach, introducing what she calls the 'Africanisation' of psychiatry with the influence of Ugandan psychiatrist Stephen Bosa in the forefront.[10]

The historiography of colonial psychiatry is equally strong for the Indian subcontinent, with important work by Waltraud Ernst and James H. Mills high-lighting British colonial structures and policies, but also Indian agency.[11] Christiane Hartnack has centred her work around the development of psycho-analysis in colonial India, a subject also covered for diverse colonialisms in the edited volume, *Unconscious Dominions: Psychoanalysis, Colonial Trauma, and Global Sovereignties* (2011).[12] Comparative case studies can be instructive as they highlight over-arching themes that may be helpful in your own work, alongside country-specific contexts that highlight the importance of the politics of place.[13] Monographs that provide in-depth studies of single colonial contexts or hospitals include Leonard Smith's study of the Caribbean, Lynette Jackson on Ingutsheni Hospital in colonial Zimbabwe, and Richard Keller's work on French North Africa.[14]

Working in the archives

It is no surprise that many studies, such as those mentioned above, focus on the documents and published materials produced by hospitals whose records and re-lated correspondences may be deposited in national archives in both the metropole and former colonial territories themselves. Additional material may be gleaned from the extensive reporting systems of colonial government medical departments' annual reports, sanitation and public health reports, or the far more interesting, if you can find them, 'handing over reports' which are decidedly 'unofficial' in tone, but relay what the departing administrator thought his successor should know about the region. Such unofficial reports and letters often eschew statistics and 'factual' analysis for observation and opinion about what local officials *believed* to be happening in their district. If London is your starting point, you can access the records of the former Colonial Office at The National Archives at Kew, which will provide you with a broad range of reports and correspondence for your country of interest.[15] If you are able to visit archives in former colonial cities you may find similar records but you may have the most luck by doing keyword searches for relevant hospital names, district medical officers, or individuals who were prominent locally. Broad search terms such as 'mental health', 'insanity', or 'ministry of health' might also give results. Keep in mind that some local archives and databases may not operate in ways that you expect. I have had luck by intentionally misspelling common words or place names ('Mathare Hospital' instead of 'Mathari', for instance) as not all databases are intuitive. Communicating clear questions to archivists and librarians by email or in person is a good starting point. They are the experts and can often suggest document series that you may be unaware of or which may be hard to find in catalogues.

Many documents and published materials show that colonial administrators often felt confident about their own observations and interpretations of local populations, and records are replete with opinions about the 'psychology' of the people they governed. Physicians and non-physicians alike frequently used psychological language to describe local troublemakers, but they might also attempt to engage with the colony's few psychiatrists to give a more definitive ruling on individuals or whole regions.[16] Non-medical staff often used language that 'medicalised' social or political problems. Anxieties about the ability of prophets or diviners to influence anti-government sentiment, or to foment real revolt, was an overriding concern for officials who sought orders to confine the most intractable, and psychologically unpredictable, rebels. Robert Edgar and Hilary Sapire's account of the Xhosa prophetess Nontheta Nkwekwe (1875–1935) depicts the critical role of prophets in helping communities navigate internal societal tensions as well as necessary engagements with the occupying state.[17] But prophecies were frequently seen as subversive and were labelled as 'mad' or dangerous, or both. In such cases, the prophet might be arrested, but their confinement might entail a lengthy stay in the colony's mental hospital rather than the prison. Indeed, the histories of colonial asylums and colonial prisons, or of other institutions for the marginalised, such as leprosaria, were often intertwined particularly in the early period, Robben Island being one prominent example.[18]

While the colonial asylum may be the most useful starting point for your research (there may be only one significant psychiatric hospital in the colony or region of your study), a broader goal would be to engage with the social and political contexts that surround the hospitals and the practice of psychiatry. Annual reports (in any field) tend to be regimented and dry, but they are useful for understanding scale, financial resources (and perhaps the material conditions for patients), lists of diagnoses and deaths, treatments and pharmaceutical use, disciplinary cases, and other technical matters. There are also general comments or qualitative sections of reports that describe the key concerns or trends observed by doctors. Annual medical reports are useful as a starting place, but no historical study should rely on them as the core primary source: they provide the nuts and bolts of institutions, but are not, on their own, a basis for an in-depth social or political history.

Diagnosing the insane

Hospital reports and medical statistics will generally include lists of diagnoses and causes of death. Reports may give some general useful impressions about the types of cases that took up doctors' time, but these categories will vary widely in terms of reliability. It may be safe to assume that doctors understood what they were seeing when listing advanced syphilis (or General Paralysis of the Insane) as contributing to deaths, but what should the historian do with categories such as 'mania' or schizophrenia? Retrospective diagnoses pose difficulties within the history of medicine in general, but psychiatric diagnoses, with complications of language, cultural familiarity, the imposition of racial pseudo-science, and contentious politics can alter the diagnostic picture significantly. Historical examples abound for retrospective diagnoses within the history of psychiatry, psychology, and neurology. Epilepsy has frequently been associated with historical figures, including religious figures such as St Teresa of Avila, St Paul (in particular, his revelations on the road to Damascus), and Joan of Arc. These are generally speculative pieces, sometimes written by physicians, that suggest that what contemporaries may have witnessed may be related to epileptic auras or convulsive seizures.[19] Anorexia is another condition that has captured the imagination of medical historians who have attempted to contextualise the religious fasting of young girls in relation to modern understandings of a psycho-medical condition.[20] Historians of medicine have begun to challenge (or give context for) the practice of retrospective diagnosis in pieces most recently by neurologists A.J. Larner (2019) and Osamu Muromoto (2014), and historians Katherine Foxhall (2014) and Adrian Wilson (2000).[21] It might be most useful to gain a full understanding of the ways certain psychiatric diagnoses and terminologies have evolved over time. The meticulous work of German Berrios, tracing the descriptive psychopathology of modern psychiatry, is especially useful.[22]

Finding the patient voice

Despite their limitations, hospital reports and their diagnostic categories can offer up some interesting points to consider. For instance, did the hospital record frequent cases of psychiatric problems related to diseases like malaria? Do reports contain information about diagnostic tests (such as blood tests) or do they rely on assumptions about race, innate traits, or theories that address 'capacity' or 'backwardness'? You may find that some medical reports, correspondence, publications, and memoirs might depict genuine attempts by colonial psychiatrists to understand local approaches to diagnosing mental ill health as well as associated healing practices. In some cases, letters (including official correspondence between doctors, or between doctors and colonial administrators), will include notes about the interactions between doctors and patients. These will certainly not be verbatim, and can be severely lacking in detail or nuance, but they may help to paint a picture about individual lives before a person came to be a 'patient'. Were individuals brought to the hospital by their families or by the police? Did they indicate why or how they came to be ill? Did they believe themselves to be ill or bewitched or wrongly imprisoned? Did they pinpoint a moment when they felt their lives changed (my wife died and then I became mad)? In some cases, doctors' notes about what a patient said about their own condition can bring us a bit closer to the 'patient voice' and may provide some insight into their life circumstances. While they cannot be considered exact quotes (and may well have been translated from a local language), such passages may be incorporated into your narrative as a means of bringing the patient's sense of agency into perspective. In many cases a patient's sense of self and their own illness (my uncle bewitched me and then I became ill) may sit in opposition to a doctor's diagnosis (patient is delusional or schizophrenic).

While we are generally constrained by the sources we have, we can endeavour to historicise an era or region by cross-referencing official documents from institutions with materials that were not written for broad consumption. Catharine Coleborne's innovative study *Madness in the Family* (2010) provides an interesting methodological case study in using the intimate content of letters between the families of patients and asylum doctors in colonial Australasia.[23] The ephemeral nature of private letters presents the historian with a snapshot of personal circumstances, desperate concerns, and private emotions. The picture that emerges, at least for the 215 families that Coleborne looks at, is one of poverty, isolation, and extreme emotional vulnerability – not only of patients but of those concerned with their care. The intimacy in the thoughts, pleas, and doctors' responses complicate any attempts to see clearly demarcated lines between 'powerful' and 'powerless'. The patient voice may not be pristine in most of these cases, but such sources can give us a degree of context for the emotional lives of patients and their closest carers.

Alternatives to western psychiatry

Colonial doctors brought their knowledge, methods, and perceptions (some more rigid than others) to their encounters with local patients, but they also interacted on a daily basis with local medical systems and beliefs. Responses to local or 'traditional' healing methods could vary widely, but they were not always as dismissive as might be assumed. When engaging with the medical history of a colonial territory, a first step might be to identify anthropological writing from the period and era – in some cases, anthropologists and doctors were contemporaries occupying the same spaces. Early twentieth-century anthropology for Africa might offer some context for beliefs about ill health, mental illness, approaches to healing, and forms of sorcery or witchcraft that could have an impact on wellbeing. Some officers in the Colonial Service wrote book-length impressions of their experiences and observations. An example of one prolific author would be C.W. Hobley, who penned *Bantu Beliefs and Magic with Particular Reference to the Kikuyu and Kamba Tribes of Kenya Colony* in 1922. British anthropologist and psychiatrist Margaret J. Field wrote about approaches to healing in Ghana (formally the Gold Coast colony) based on her fieldwork from the 1930s to the 1960s. Her remarkable monograph, *Search for Security* (1960), is a detailed account of healing shrines and is replete with individual and community case studies of mental illness and healing. While some of the views expressed by early twentieth-century anthropologists, or the 'armchair' ethnologists of the Colonial Service, might appear ethnocentric by today's standards, they may still include useful descriptions of events, customs, and beliefs for a particular point in time.[24] It is also instructive to read contemporary professional reactions from book reviews, often published in anthropological, medical, or psychiatric journals. These were often written by prominent figures in their respective fields and might give an indication as to whether the views expressed in these studies were widely praised or controversial.

Historians have also given a *longue durée* perspective on the nuances of belief and practice throughout the colonial period. Julie Parle has approached this through early twentieth-century accounts of an 'epidemic' of spirit possession in South Africa, highlighting the ways psychological distress may be articulated in some communities even as they shift, adapt, and emerge with new purpose.[25] This case study also draws from locally produced scholarship such as anthropologist Harriet Ngubane's *Body and Mind in Zulu Medicine* (1977), allowing Parle to put a series of events into a broader context of thought and practice. Reading beyond the strict confines of medical history for your region of interest is critical for understanding the context for the emergence of colonial hospitals and the intellectual output for colonial psychiatry.

Working with archives and databases

Locating as many relevant archives as possible will be an early step in your research. In truth, you may continue to identify new collections and sources throughout the research and writing process, and you may find that you need to revisit archives as you go along. Logically, you might begin with the large national or university archives which will usually have online finding guides and searchable databases. Places to start in the UK might include: The National Archives in Kew, London, The Wellcome Library, London, and the Bodleian Libraries at the University of Oxford. Libraries at the University of Cambridge, the School of Oriental and African Studies (SOAS, University of London) and the London School of Hygiene and Tropical Medicine (LSHTM) may also be relevant. The Museum of the Mind (of the former Bethlem Hospital) in southeast London holds materials related to the history of psychiatry (although with fewer colonial sources), and the Imperial War Museum in London might provide contextual sources for colonial empires.

Online databases are also sources for an extensive range of materials. While some colonial doctors aspired to publish in leading medical journals from the metropole, such as *The Lancet* or the *Journal of Mental Science* (now the *British Journal of Psychiatry*), many others published in regional medical journals, such as the *East African Medical Journal*, or the *Indian Medical Gazette*. Increasingly, these types of sources are digitised, even dating back to their inaugural issues from the nineteenth century. The PubMed database allows for title and keyword searches of medical publications. It also includes a list of digitised journals that is extremely useful.[26] The *Indian Medical Gazette* is available online (1866–1955) through the PubMed Central database. The *South African Medical Journal* dates back to 1884 and is available through a number of online portals. The *Eugenics Review* (1909–1968) was concerned with matters of race difference and published material sent in from colonial territories and is also available from PubMed. Perusing complete issues of these journals will allow you to access additional useful material such as minutes from medical meetings, announcements about the profession, obituaries, letters to the editor, as well as the names of the editors who were likely influential within the profession. If key journals are not available in digital form, it is worth doing a search in major university libraries, medical association libraries, or the Wellcome Library. The University of Oxford's Bodleian Library has a near complete run of the *East African Medical Journal* (from 1932), as well as copies of its earlier version, the *Kenya and East African Medical Journal* (1927–1932). Chris Millard's chapter on journals in this volume will provide more depth here, but do keep in mind the importance of these sources published during the colonial era, as they are key for identifying the most prominent (or sometimes notorious) medical voices concerned with the psychology of colonial subjects.

Periodising medical knowledge (and access to that knowledge) is important when placing medical policies and doctors' decision-making into context. While the key medical textbooks published before or during the years of a physician's service may offer some context, it is also helpful to try to understand what other sorts of materials were accessed or favoured by the doctors you are writing about. This would include any texts that are referenced in their own bibliographies, correspondence, or memoirs. These references are often not very comprehensive, nor are they always up to date, but they may reveal much about a particular line of thinking, point of view, or influence. Colonial physicians often read anthropology, psychology, or educational studies about their region – some of which was infused with theoretical positions about local populations. Eugenics could easily come to the fore as physicians and non-physicians alike personally assessed their subjects – in some cases, such colonially produced materials were outdated even for their time. Colonial physicians such as H.L. Gordon and J.C. Carothers, for instance, reignited outmoded theories of race science to fit what they believed to be true for Kenya if not for the whole of Africa.[27]

An additional useful source for the later colonial period and the early period of independence are conference reports or *Proceedings* from international psychiatry congresses. International meetings of psychiatrists and related disciplines such as anthropology or sociology convened to discuss the future of psychiatry for the African continent, as well as enduring questions about the universality of mental illness or problems specific to the continent. The published conference reports can read like a 'who's who' for research at the time. Proceedings like the *First Pan-African Psychiatric Conference* (edited by T.A. Lambo) held in Abeokuta, Nigeria in 1961 are generally not available online but should be accessible in university libraries. Nigerian psychiatrist S.T.C. Ilechukwu published (in 1991) a review essay that includes a summary and bibliography of many of the early African psychiatric conferences and reviews.[28]

Fieldwork

While archival research may feel quite straightforward, it is important to note that the very nature of doing research *from* a former colonial power *about* a former colonial territory requires some sensitivity to local politics and historical legacies. If you are able to conduct fieldwork overseas, do read beyond your very focused historiography so that you have a good sense of the current political and social dynamics. Visiting the place you are writing about, even if archival holdings there are sparse, can add depth to your work. Official documents and archives are likely to be sited in the UK or Europe, often with additional support from well-stocked university libraries and specialist archives holding private papers, missionary collections, and full print runs of relevant publications. If you are starting your research from *within* a former colonial city, you will likely still wish to access the voluminous material available from colonial office records, medical and university libraries, and museums. Fieldwork and archival research trips can throw many unexpected problems and obstacles in your path, not the least of which is expense and the fact that they can be time consuming. The key to successful research trips is advance planning to the extent possible and flexibility once you are there.

When planning fieldwork you will naturally begin with an application for ethical clearance from your home institution (if relevant), but you will also need to take advice on any legal requirements for the country of your study. Foreign institutions may require research permits, sponsorship of a local institution or academic contact, or an application and fee for their national archives. In some cases, you may be required to send a copy of your dissertation or published work. Keep in mind that the archives may vary greatly in terms of access policy, quality of organisation and preservation of materials, hours and personnel, and resources and amenities. It is critically important to gather as much information as possible about what an archive requires before you visit. This will also be true for your home country. You may also be in a position to visit the site of a former colonial hospital, some of which may still be in operation. You may not be able to make suitable contacts in advance of your trip, but you may be able to show up with your contact details and a brief abstract of your proposed work and make an appointment to speak with a medical director, public engagement officer, or physician. Do keep in mind that working hospitals have an important job to do and their time may be limited, but it has been my experience that courteous visitors are very welcome. Speaking to local psychiatrists can add much more nuanced insights to materials you have collected or the secondary literature you have absorbed. While rare, there are occasions when you may come upon un-catalogued material that has been stored for years in a back room. It is important to assess the appropriateness of accessing some materials, especially material that identifies individual patients and their medical status. Finally, as some scholarship may only be published locally, perusing local bookshops is often very interesting and fruitful.

You may also be able to correspond online with some overseas contacts. This can be an effective way to add local perspectives, just be sure to have a concise description of your research project and clear questions in mind so that you use your (and their) time efficiently. Apart from the hospitals themselves, local university libraries, museums, and research institutes (and their associated researchers) are also a useful resource and it may be here that you gather the best advice about additional primary sources or interview contacts. With a research permit or letter of introduction from your home institution, you should be able to access these resources.

Case study: photography and psychiatry, the Margetts collection

Colonial histories, the history of anthropology, and the history of medicine under colonialism are often visual histories. There are a wealth of studies that focus on key collections, and others that more broadly contextualise how colonial subjects were depicted on film or in photographs. This discussion of photography in the history of psychiatry is developed more fully by Beatriz Pichel in this volume, but I will highlight some considerations for working with photographs in colonial (medical) contexts by introducing a primary source from my own research on photography and psychiatry. Much of my work over the last decade has engaged with the Canadian psychiatrist, Edward Margetts, the doctor in charge of Mathari Mental Hospital in Nairobi in the mid 1950s. Margetts published widely from his time in Kenya as well as later postings at the World Health Organisation in Geneva and the University of British Columbia in Vancouver. As an enthusiastic amateur photographer, he left behind photographs, negatives, and film clips which on their own are visually interesting, but when studied alongside his extensive note-taking, correspondence, published works, and personal diaries, the photographs provide a deeply contextualised glimpse of 1950s Kenya.

While Margetts did photograph patients at Mathari Hospital and other in-stitutions across Africa, he also took his camera on his frequent journeys across Kenya and other colonial settings as he investigated a wide range of medical and non-medical subjects. He photographed individuals of note, often writing impressions of them in his diaries. In some cases, he described his encounters in letters to district medical officers or editors of medical journals and his photographs often appeared in his published articles and chapters. This provides a unique opportunity to understand the photographer's perspectives on the photographs, showing his intent, interpretation, and belief that the photograph is an accurate reflection of a diagnosis. When working with photographs, pay particular attention to any captions as a means of gauging what the photographer felt was important. If you do have original photographs (these are sometimes found in archive files), it is instructive to see how they differ (by editing, cropping, or captioning) in their raw and published forms.

Edward Margetts also made an effort to document a wide range of healing practices he encountered. In some cases, he published accounts of healing rituals with photographs that he captioned for various international psychiatry conferences. Helpfully, the doctor also photographed the exhibits as they were mounted and he kept the accompanying caption cards in his personal records, giving a sense of the movement and uses of these photographs as artefacts in their own right. As with the use of captions in published works, the exhibit cards highlight what the photographer wanted to impart to his colleagues. Captions can themselves be revealing glimpses into the attitudes and theoretical perspectives of the time.

The doctor's documentation of a healing session in Kenya in 1958 (Figure 7.1) appears with the caption title 'The Magic Circle – Protective Fence' in a photographic exhibit displayed at international psychiatric conferences he attended. The photograph also appears published in a review article for the *Canadian Psychiatric Association Journal* with the caption 'Healer at work'.[29] Margetts describes in some detail the healing ritual and the differentiation of 'white' and 'black' (or good and evil) forms of magic. A similar photograph from the same visit also appears in an article about Margetts published in the Canadian newspaper supplement, *Weekend Magazine*. With the doctor (and not the medicine) now the subject, the article is entitled 'A Canadian Psychiatrist Meets the Witch Doctors' with an accompanying caption 'In the Kenya countryside, Dr Edward Margetts saw the dark forces of superstition and sorcery at work'.[30] The interview style of the article and the many quotes it incorporates allows us to contextualise the photograph, albeit with a one-sided narration and the ethnocentric view of a western medical professional. Lastly, the doctor's own diaries of his travels describe how he came to the moments he photographed. In the diary entry he wrote after witnessing the Kamba healing ritual, Margetts reported: 'We watched Kinyuma treat a pt [patient] who believed himself to have been bewitched by *dawa* being placed in his path ... The 'U' is a type of magic 'O', "so witchcraft will not come in from outside"'.[31] Within this entry, the doctor remarks upon the difficulty of observing and taking notes while also taking photographs. He gives the names of the healer as well as place names. The entry also includes a careful drawing of the

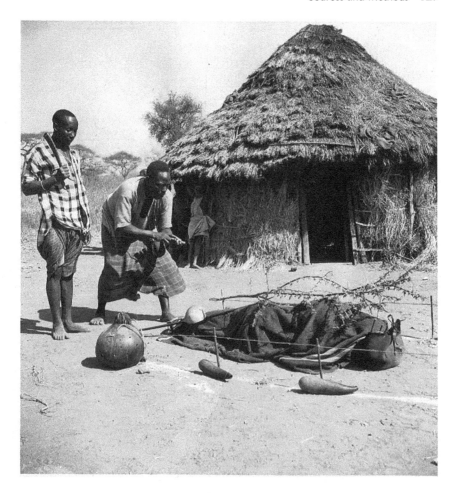

FIGURE 7.1 Photograph published by Edward Margetts of a healing session in Kenya, 1958. Author's own collection

U-shaped set-up and various items used by the healer as depicted in his photograph (Figure 7.2).

This brief case study brings forward a multitude of methodological questions and approaches. First and foremost, we see what may be learned by cross-referencing our sources and understanding how the photograph itself was 'put to work'. When using photographs, as Pichel emphasises in this volume, it is important to move beyond the most obvious visual representation to ask questions about production, movement, manipulation, and competing interpretations. Was the photograph staged by the photographer or was it impromptu? Patients, or 'actors' pretending to be patients were often asked to 'act out' a diagnosis for the purposes of a photograph. What does this say about the authenticity of the photograph or even of the medical diagnosis it aims to represent? Does the

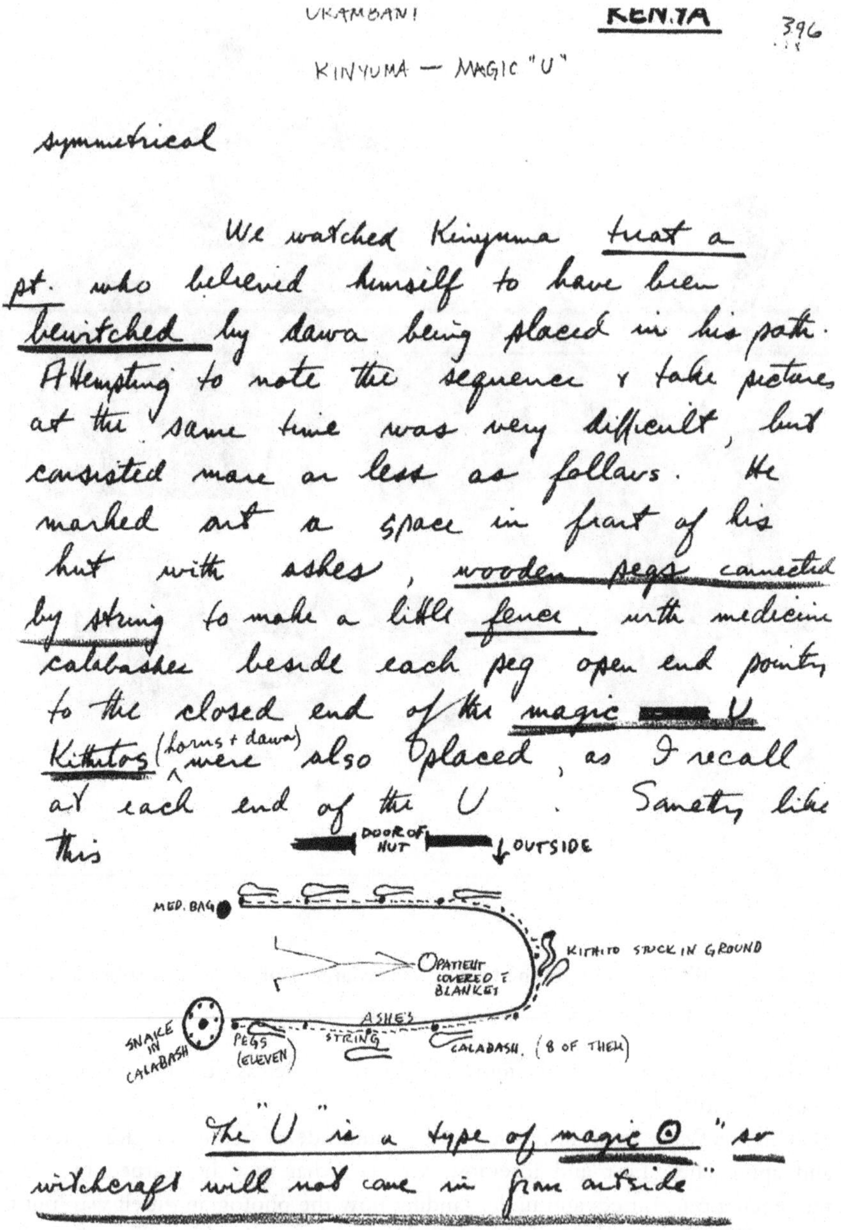

UKAMBANI   **KENYA**   396

KINYUMA — MAGIC "U"

symmetrical

We watched Kinyuma treat a pt. who believed himself to have been bewitched by dawa being placed in his path. Attempting to note the sequence & take pictures at the same time was very difficult, but consisted more or less as follows. He marked out a space in front of his hut with ashes, wooden pegs connected by string to make a little fence, with medicine calabashes beside each peg open end pointing to the closed end of the magic U. Kithitos (horns + dawa) were also placed, as I recall at each end of the U. Something like this

DOOR OF HUT / OUTSIDE
MED. BAG
PATIENT COVERED & BLANKET
KITHITO STUCK IN GROUND
SNAKE IN CALABASH
PEGS (ELEVEN)
ASHES
STRING
CALABASH. (8 OF THEM)

The "U" is a type of magic ⊙ "so witchcraft will not come in from outside"

FIGURE 7.2 Extract from the diaries of Edward Margetts, recounting the 'magic U' healing session from his photographic series; Kenya, 1958. Author's own collection

photograph appear to depict stereotypes (of race, gender, disability)? Where was the photograph displayed and what was the nature of its intended audience(s)? In the case of the photograph shown here, the photographic artefact can be shown to have multiple 'lives' and multiple audiences. The photographer comments upon the creation of the photograph and describes what it represents. He is also integral to how and where the photograph is recreated and for what purpose. The history of psychiatry has a long association with visuality (including paintings). Photography, from its inception, has been an important element in the depiction of psychiatric diagnoses and in conversations about the nature of mental illness.

Conclusion

While the history of psychiatry has always needed to address the impact of the 'medical gaze' (in language, practice, and visual materials) and the unequal power dynamics that often existed between patient and physician, there are additional sensitivities to be aware of when studying this dynamic under colonial rule. Katie-Kilroy-Marac's recent monograph, *An Impossible Inheritance* (2019), on the Fann Psychiatric Clinic in the former French colony of Senegal, includes excellent reflections on methodology and perspective when conducting historical and ethnographic work. Key concepts such as 'culture' are revisited for their modern relevance (or lack thereof) as she incorporates postcolonial perspectives and memory into her study.[32] Reflections on the imperial roots of much research, knowledge production, and history writing can also be seen in Linda Tuhiwai Smith's *Decolonizing Methodologies* (second edition, 2012) which refers specifically to the Maori, but offers a strong philosophical and social justice approach that is relevant to all research.[33] Similarly, Antoinette Burton's edited collection, *Archive Stories* (2005) comprises thematic case studies in how to approach archives sensitively, including colonial archives, official narratives versus counter narratives, family archives, queer archives, and the archives of cyberspace.[34] While not specifically 'colonial' in many cases, these interrogations of method are extremely useful when dealing with histories that involve contested narratives and sensitive topics. There are no hard and fast rules here, but it is important to heed diverse perspectives from the post-colony, which may themselves differ depending on gender, race, religion, or generation. A fascinating 'colonial' history may be someone else's contested or painful history. The history of colonial psychiatry and medicine can be replete with concepts and labels, diagnoses, and treatments. However, the most profound insights can come from digging deeper into the sources to find personhood at the centre of the colonial history.

Notes

1 Shula Marks, 'What is Colonial about Colonial Medicine? And What Has Happened to Imperialism and Health?', *Social History of Medicine*, 10, 2 (1997), pp. 205–6.
2 See Lynette Schumaker, *Africanizing Anthropology: Fieldwork, Networks, and the Making of Cultural Knowledge in Central Africa* (Durham, NC: Duke University Press, 2001); Ryan Johnson and Amna Khalid (eds), *Public Health in the British Empire: Intermediaries, Subordinates, and the Practice of Public Health* (London: Routledge, 2012).

3 Megan Vaughan, 'Idioms of Madness: Zomba Lunatic Asylum, Nyasaland, in the Colonial Period', *Journal of Southern African Studies*, 9, 2 (1983), pp. 218–38. See also Megan Vaughan, *Curing Their Ills: Colonial Power and African Illness* (Stanford, CA: Stanford University Press, 1991).

4 Sloan Mahone, 'The Psychology of Rebellion: Colonial Medical Responses to Dissent in British East Africa', *Journal of African History*, 47, 2 (2006), pp. 241–58.

5 J.C. Carothers, *The Psychology of Mau Mau* (Nairobi: Government Printer, 1954).

6 See Jock McCulloch, *Colonial Psychiatry and 'the African Mind'* (Cambridge: Cambridge University Press, 1995); Chloe Campbell, *Race and Empire: Eugenics in Colonial Kenya* (Manchester: Manchester University Press, 2012). At least two doctoral dissertations, including my own, have focused on Mathari Hospital in Nairobi: Gail C. Beuschel, 'Shutting Africans Away: Lunacy, Race and Social Order in Colonial Kenya, 1910–1963.' Doctoral thesis, SOAS, University of London, 2001; available online at https://ethos.bl.uk/OrderDetails.do?uin=uk.bl.ethos.392750, accessed 29 Mar. 2021; Sloan Mahone, 'The Psychology of the Tropics: Conceptions of Tropical Danger and Lunacy in British East Africa.' DPhil thesis, University of Oxford, 2004.

7 Frantz Fanon, *The Wretched of the Earth*, trans. Constance Farrington (New York: Grove Press, 1981 [1961]), p. 302. See the full Fanon canon for his writings on psychiatry and medicine under colonialism.

8 T.A. Lambo (ed.), *First Pan-African Psychiatric Conference, Abeokuta, Nigeria* (Ibadan: Government Printer, 1961).

9 Matthew M. Heaton, *Black Skin, White Coats: Nigerian Psychiatrists, Decolonization, and the Globalization of Psychiatry* (Athens, OH: Ohio University Press, 2013). Heaton's work follows on from an earlier study by Jonathan Sadowsky, *Imperial Bedlam: Institutions of Madness in Colonial Southwest Nigeria* (Berkeley, CA: University of California, 1999).

10 Yolana Pringle, *Psychiatry and Decolonisation in Uganda* (London: Palgrave Macmillan, 2019).

11 Wartraud Ernst, *Mad Tales from the Raj: Colonial Psychiatry in South Asia, 1800–58* (London, New York, New Delhi: Anthem Press, 2010); James Mills, *Madness, Cannabis and Colonialism: The 'Native-Only' Lunatic Asylums of British India, 1857–1900* (Basingstoke: Palgrave Macmillan, 2000).

12 Christiane Hartnack, *Psychoanalysis in Colonial India* (New Delhi: Oxford University Press, 2001); Warwick Anderson, Deborah Jenson, and Richard C. Keller, *Unconscious Dominions: Psychoanalysis, Colonial Trauma, and Global Sovereignties* (Durham, NC: Duke University Press, 2011).

13 See Dinesh Bhugra and Roland Littlewood, *Colonialism and Psychiatry* (Oxford: Oxford University Press, 2001); Sloan Mahone, and Megan Vaughan, *Psychiatry and Empire* (Basingstoke: Palgrave Macmillan, 2007).

14 Leonard Smith, *Insanity, Race and Colonialism: Managing Mental Disorder in the Post-Emancipation British Caribbean, 1838–1914* (Basingstoke: Palgrave MacMillan, 2014); Lynette Jackson, *Surfacing Up: Psychiatry and Social Order in Colonial Zimbabwe, 1908–1968* (Ithaca, NY: Cornell University Press, 2018); Richard C. Keller, *Colonial Madness: Psychiatry in French North Africa* (Chicago, IL: University of Chicago Press, 2007).

15 Search for: Records of the Colonial Office, Commonwealth and Foreign and Commonwealth Offices, Empire Marketing Board, and related bodies. These records are demarcated in the archives as CO series.

16 Mahone, 'Psychology of Rebellion'.

17 Robert R. Edgar and Hilary Sapire, *African Apocalypse: The Story of Nontetha Nkwenkwe, a Twentieth-Century South African Prophet* (Athens, OH: Ohio University Press, 2000).

18 Harriet Deacon, 'Madness, Race and Moral Treatment: Robben Island Lunatic Asylum, Cape Colony, 1846–1890', *History of Psychiatry* 7, 26 (1996), pp. 287–97.

19 Examples abound, but see for instance Edward L. Murphy, 'The Saints of Epilepsy', *Medical History*, 3, 4, (1959), pp. 303–11; Marcella Biro Barton, 'Saint Teresa of Avila: Did She Have Epilepsy?', *The Catholic Historical Review*, 68, 4 (1982), pp. 581–98; D. Landsborough, 'St Paul and Temporal Lobe Epilepsy', *Journal of Neurology, Neurosurgery, and Psychiatry*, 50, 6 (1987), pp. 659–64; Elizabeth Foote-Smith and Lydia Bayne, 'Joan of Arc', *Epilepsia*, 32, 6 (1991), pp. 810–15.

20 Randolph M. Bell, *Holy Anorexia* (Chicago, IL; University of Chicago Press, 1985); Joan Jacobs Brumberg, *Fasting Girls: The History of Anorexia Nervosa*, revised and updated edn (New York: Vintage Books, 2000).

21 There is an extensive literature on the retrospective diagnosis of medical and psychiatric conditions. See, for example: A.J. Larner, 'Retrospective diagnosis: Pitfalls and purposes', *Journal of Medical Biography*, 27, 3 (2019), pp. 127–8; Osamu Muramoto, 'Retrospective Diagnosis of a Famous Historical Figure: Ontological, Epistemic, and Ethical Considerations', *Philosophy, Ethics, and Humanities in Medicine*, 9, 10 (2014); Katherine Foxhall, 'Making Modern Migraine Medieval: Men of Science, Hildegard of Bingen and the Life of a Retrospective Diagnosis', *Medical History*, 58, 3 (2014), pp. 354–74; Adrian Wilson, 'On the History of Disease-Concepts: The Case of Pleurisy', *History of Science*, 38, 3 (2000), pp. 271–319.

22 German E. Berrios, *The History of Mental Symptoms: Descriptive Psychopathology Since the Nineteenth Century* (Cambridge: Cambridge University Press, 1996); German E. Berrios and Roy Porter (eds), *A History of Clinical Psychiatry: The Origin and History of Psychiatric Disorders* (London: Athlone, 1995).

23 Catharine Coleborne, *Madness in the Family: Insanity and Institutions in the Australasian Colonial World, 1860–1914* (Basingstoke: Palgrave Macmillan, 2010).

24 Margaret Joyce Field, *Search for Security. An Ethno-Psychiatric Study of Rural Ghana* (London: Faber & Faber, 1960).

25 Julie Parle, 'Witchcraft or Madness? The Amandiki of Zululand, 1894–1914', *Journal of Southern African Studies*, 29, 1 (2003), pp. 105–32.

26 PubMed Central is accessed through the National Library of Medicine in the United States, at: https://www.ncbi.nlm.nih.gov/pmc/. The PMC digitised journal list may be found here: https://www.ncbi.nlm.nih.gov/pmc/journals/

27 H.L. Gordon, a neurologist and avowed eugenicist, sat at the helm of Mathari Mental Hospital in Nairobi in the 1930s before the arrival of J.C. Carothers. Gordon was an enthusiastic author and published in the *East African Medical Journal*, *Eugenics Review*, and other British journals. For a history of eugenics in Kenya, see Chloe Campbell, *Race and Empire: Eugenics in Colonial Kenya* (Manchester: Manchester University Press, 2012). See also Sloan Mahone, 'East African Psychiatry and the Practical Problems of Empire', in Mahone and Vaughan, *Psychiatry and Empire*, pp. 41–66.

28 S.T.C. Ilechukwu, 'Psychiatry in Africa: Special Problems and Unique Features', *Transcultural Psychiatric Research Review*, 28, 3 (1991), pp. 169–218.

29 Edward L. Margetts, 'African Ethnopsychiatry in the Field', *Canadian Psychiatric Association Journal*, 13, 6 (1968), pp. 521–38.

30 M. Whitelaw, 'A Canadian Psychiatrist Meets the Witch Doctors', *WEEKEND Magazine*, 10, 12 (1960), pp. 30–3.

31 Diaries of Edward Margetts, III, 1958–1959. In the possession of the author.

32 Katie Kilroy-Marac, *An Impossible Inheritance: Postcolonial Psychiatry and the Work of Memory in a West African Clinic* (Oakland, CA: University of California Press, 2019).

33 Linda Tuhiwai Smith, *Decolonizing Methodologies: Research and Indigenous Peoples*, 2nd edn (London: Zed Books, 2012).

34 Antoinette Burton (ed.), *Archive Stories: Facts, Fictions, and the Writing of History* (Durham, NC: Duke University Press, 2005).

Select bibliography

Coleborne, C., *Madness in the Family: Insanity and Institutions in the Australasian Colonial World, 1860–1914*, Basingstoke: Palgrave Macmillan, 2010.

Edgar, R. and Sapire, H., *African Apocalypse: The Story of Nontetha Nkwenkwe, a Twentieth-Century South African Prophet*, Athens, OH: Ohio University Press, 2000.

Ernst, W., *Mad Tales from the Raj: Colonial Psychiatry in South Asia, 1800–58*, London: Anthem Press, 2010.

Heaton, M., *Black Skin, White Coats: Nigerian Psychiatrists, Decolonization, and the Globalization of Psychiatry*, Athens, OH: Ohio University Press, 2013.

Jackson, L., *Surfacing Up: Psychiatry and Social Order in Colonial Zimbabwe, 1908–1968*, Ithaca, NY: Cornell University Press, 2005.

Keller, R., *Colonial Madness: Psychiatry in French North Africa*, Chicago, IL: Chicago University Press, 2007.

Kilroy-Marac, K., *An Impossible Inheritance: Postcolonial Psychiatry and the Work of Memory in a West African Clinic*, Oakland, CA: University of California Press, 2019.

Mahone, S., 'The Psychology of Rebellion: Colonial Medical Responses to Dissent in British East Africa', *Journal of African History* 47, 2006, pp. 241–258.

Mahone, S. and Vaughan, M. (eds), *Psychiatry and Empire*, Basingstoke: Palgrave Macmillan, 2007.

McCulloch, J., *Colonial Psychiatry and 'the African Mind'*, Cambridge: Cambridge University Press, 1995.

Mills, J., *Madness, Cannabis and Colonialism: The 'Native Only' Lunatic Asylums of British India, 1857–1900*, New York: St. Martin's Press, 2000.

Patton, A., *Physicians, Colonial Racism and Diaspora in West Africa*, Gainesville, FL: University of Florida, 1996.

Sadowsky, J., *Imperial Bedlam: Institutions of Madness in Colonial Southwest Nigeria*, Berkeley, CA: University of California, 1999.

Vaughan, M., *Curing Their Ills: Colonial Power and African Illness*, Stanford, CA: Stanford University Press, 1991.

8

LEGAL SOURCES IN THE HISTORY OF PSYCHIATRY

Janet Weston

Psychiatry and law

Psychiatry since 1800 has been intimately connected with the law. The building, filling, and later, emptying of asylums was governed by legislation, and those dissatisfied with the way in which psychiatry was practised have often targeted mental health law reform through campaigns and legal challenges of their own. But the relationship between law and psychiatry runs deeper still. Legal systems are not only concerned with psychiatry as a profession to be regulated: the judiciary has increasingly drawn upon psychiatric expertise since 1800 to help resolve quandaries of its own. 'Wherever there are legal relations between people', as lawyer and historian Peter Bartlett has put it, 'there is a legal issue as to how those relations are affected by the insanity of one of the parties'.[1] Whether that relation is an attempted murder, a marriage, or a business deal, legal questions about responsibility, culpability, autonomy, and insanity have generated responses from medical experts. For some scholars, legal demands and decisions have not simply engaged with psychiatry; they have 'constructed and reconstructed' it, shaping its every aspect.[2]

Despite these connections between law and psychiatry, legal sources themselves are relatively rarely used by historians. One goal of this chapter is to address some of the potential barriers to their fuller exploitation, building on Peter Bartlett's valuable introduction to legal sources for histories of madness in the nineteenth century, published in the *Social History of Medicine* journal in 2001.[3] Assuming that one major barrier is still a lack of familiarity amongst historians, who are rarely trained in law, this chapter begins with a discussion of three specific kinds of legal source that merit attention: case law, court records, and legislation. In describing and giving examples of these sources and the ways in which they have been used in recent decades, this chapter considers what kinds of information they can provide and what strategies might be useful for interpreting them. Some of these

DOI: 10.4324/9781003087694-9

points are then illustrated with a case study from the archives of the Court of Protection of England and Wales. The chapter concludes with a brief reflection on some further questions that legal sources pose for historians of psychiatry.

What is a legal source?

Understanding different types of legal source requires some familiarity with legal systems, which can vary hugely from place to place as well as over time. The distinction between 'common law' and 'civil law' systems is particularly important, not least because one of the primary sources of law itself in common law systems, alongside statutes passed by government, is the judgements handed down in past cases. These judgements are known as 'case law'. The central role played by case law is why many common law systems refer to rules or principles set down in previous legal proceedings, rather than any rules to be found in legislation. One example is the test in England and Wales for determining whether an individual has capacity to make a valid will. This test was set down as part of the court's decision in the 1870 case of Banks v Goodfellow, in which the validity of the late John Banks's will was confirmed despite his history of delusions and confinement in an asylum.[4] In contrast, 'civil law' systems rely upon a systematic written code which sets down the legal principles and procedures that must be followed. The Napoleonic Code, introduced in France in 1804, is one such example. Each case within a civil law jurisdiction is then decided on its own merits in accordance with the code, paying no attention to other, similar cases that may have been heard before.

European colonisers tended to take their laws and legal systems with them, disrupting or displacing existing legal systems entirely. Indeed, it is possible that legal systems and methods, rather than asylums and psychiatry, played a primary role in responding to and shaping ideas of madness in colonised regions of the world.[5] Since 1800, the legal systems of many nations have changed dramatically as a result of colonialism. Civil law systems can be found today across most of continental Europe and South America, parts of Northern Africa, and much of East Asia. Common law systems based upon that of England and Wales are present in Australia, New Zealand, most of the United States, and much of Canada, with elements of English common law also found in countries including India, Pakistan, Nigeria, and Israel. This chapter will focus on common law systems, and particularly that of England and Wales. Some of what follows can be applied much more broadly, particularly to other common law jurisdictions, but inevitably different legal systems will bring their own challenges and opportunities in terms of documentation and interpretation.

Case law is unfamiliar territory for historians and very rarely mentioned in histories of psychiatry, despite being a cornerstone of common law legal systems and a potentially rich source. The source itself will generally take the form of a reported judgement. This is the published record of the decision in a specific case, usually including a statement of the relevant facts as well as the judicial conclusions reached. Figure 8.1 gives an example of the first page of a mid twentieth century

P.   PROBATE DIVISION.   89

that would have been a different matter. In such a case, as we said in
Barnard v. *Barnard*,[4] the best way of seeing whether the offer is genuine
is to accept it and see whether he will take her in, but the wife did not
suggest here that the offer was not genuine in that sense. There is no
doubt that the husband wanted her back. She only said that she was
justified in not going back because of his previous cruelty. That ought
to be alleged and proved, and it was not even alleged. Her only proper
course would have been to charge cruelty.

It is open to her, no doubt, to bring another petition now charging
cruelty, but I certainly would not wish to encourage it. I agree that
the appeal should be allowed.

SINGLETON L.J. I agree that the appeal should be allowed.

> *Appeal allowed.*
> *Decree nisi set aside and petition dismissed.*

Solicitors: *Sharpe, Pritchard & Co. for T. D. Windsor Williams,
Neath, Glam.*

   [4] (Unreported): November 18, 1952 (Final List of Appeals, No. 17).

IN THE ESTATE OF PARK, DECD.   PARK *v.* PARK.

[1951 P. No. 1348.]

*Husband and Wife — Marriage — Capacity to enter into marriage
contract — Requisites — Previous probate action — Party sued as
" widow " — Jury's finding that deceased mentally incapable of
executing will made on marriage day—Estoppel—Jury's finding not
binding on court considering mental capacity to marry.*

A mere comprehension of the words of the promises exchanged
at a ceremony of marriage is not sufficient to establish capacity of
the parties to consent to the marriage at the time. The minds
of the parties must also be capable of understanding the nature of
the contract into which they are entering free from the influence
of morbid delusions on the subject; and the essence of the contract
is an engagement between a man and a woman to live together and
to love each other to the exclusion of all others. Submission on
the part of the woman may no longer be an essential part of the
contract; but so far as the husband is concerned there is still the
duty to maintain and to protect.

The defendant in this probate action sought to establish that the
deceased was at the time of his marriage to the plaintiff incapable
of appreciating the nature of the marriage contract, and the duties
and responsibilities which it created, and that accordingly there
was no consent to the marriage; and he asked the court to declare
the marriage null and void and to pronounce in solemn form for
a will executed before the ceremony. The plaintiff, the widow of

FIGURE 8.1   First page of the reported judgement from May–June 1953, in the case of
Park v Park [1954] P. 89. Incorporated Council for Law Reporting of England and
Wales, reproduced with kind permission.

reported judgement. Law reporting has its own complex history,[6] but probably the most important point to bear in mind is that judgements are only reported when they are of particular *legal* interest, or heard in the most senior courts. This is a minority of all cases heard by the courts. Given their important status as case law within common law systems, reported judgements are carefully preserved in law libraries, for which legal librarians will be able to provide navigational advice, and also in digital repositories of varying quality and accessibility.[7]

As case law is particularly unfamiliar to historians, it is worth giving an example in some detail. The mid twentieth century case of *Park v Park* is still occasionally cited today in disputes over mental capacity. The Park family dispute began shortly after the death of London businessman Mr Park in June 1949. Aged 78, having lost his wife of 50 years in 1948 and then suffered a stroke, Mr Park had remarried and made a will in favour of his new wife just two weeks before his death. His sons brought claims that neither the marriage nor the will could be valid, as their father had not been of sound mind. A fortune of over £120,000 was at stake, and Mrs Park, unsurprisingly, disputed these claims. The claim regarding the validity of the will was heard in the High Court in 1950 and was reported in *The Times*, which was (and is) considered a 'newspaper of record', meaning that, in a legal context, its accounts of court proceedings will be relied upon by jurists where no other report exists. *The Times* is often a valuable legal source, especially for the nineteenth century when law reporting was less systematic than it later became. The importance of newspapers as a form of legal source is discussed further below. The second claim in *Park v Park* dealt with the validity of the marriage. At first instance, in May/June 1953, the marriage was found to be valid. This decision was appealed, and in October 1953 the Court of Appeal considered the case and dismissed the appeal. Both of these judgements were published in 1954.[8]

In legal terms, the judgement from the Court of Appeal in October 1953 is perhaps the most interesting. It was the final word on the matter, and it considered the legal tests for capacity to marry in detail. For historians of psychiatry, though, the judgement from the proceedings in May and June may be more useful. It gives the circumstances surrounding the case in greater depth and describes the evidence from many witnesses. Notably, this judgement gives much more time and space to the evidence of lay witnesses rather than doctors. For this judgement, the most significant contribution from Dr Urwick, Mr Park's regular medical attendant, was that his patient's mental condition would vary a great deal from day to day, and even hour to hour. Dr Urwick was not a specialist: Mr Park did see another doctor following his stroke, but only on a few occasions and the contribution of this medical witness is summarised quickly and then not mentioned again. In contrast, the evidence of Lady Greer, a close friend of Mr Park's for many decades, and Mr Starkey, the long-established caretaker of the block of flats where Mr Park lived, was explored in much more detail and described as particularly valuable. Its significance was rooted in these witnesses' long familiarity with Mr Park and their regular everyday encounters with him. The account of Mr Starkey's evidence concerning his interactions with the late Mr Park, 'the deceased', is highly evocative not only of the trial and the evidence itself but also of the way in which judgements are typically written, and it is worth quoting a section of this in full:

> Starkey was not, in my view, a man with great gifts of verbal expression, but he described by gesture rather than words the demeanour of the deceased and the conversations which took place after his stroke. Starkey said the deceased looked right through him and up and down and then stood still and vacant. Starkey demonstrated in the box by a piece of natural but convincing acting the vacant look and the rigid position of the body which he observed in the deceased. Starkey added, in homely but striking language, that if his own father had acted like the deceased he would have got someone to see about his head. In spite of his limitations, I thought Starkey was a shrewd observer of the deceased's condition.[9]

As this passage indicates, reported judgements do not pretend to reproduce evidence verbatim or to give a complete and impartial account of legal proceedings from start to finish. They are carefully constructed by their writer – likely to have been an enterprising lawyer in the nineteenth century, and thereafter, the judge – to persuade the reader of the final verdict. This imagined reader was a future jurist, not the witnesses or even the feuding parties themselves – although judgements or sections of judgements may be written with different audiences in mind, including the media and, recently, those directly affected by the case.[10]

This exercise in persuasion can be quite detailed, discussing everyday life and medical care, who was called to give evidence, whose evidence was given the greatest weight, and the kinds of behaviours or events that were influential in determining mental state. There are opinions and insights from a range of commentators, including but not limited to expert medical witnesses, brought together to illuminate and support the judge's eventual decision. In Mr Park's case, the judge concluded that Mr Park was capable of entering into a marriage notwithstanding his evident mental infirmity. What was important was that consent to a marriage did not require a high 'intellectual standard', and Mr Park had repeatedly (and apparently convincingly) talked to many witnesses about his profound loneliness after his wife's death, and his wish to remarry. The judgement is of course not a full account of Mr Park's life and state of mind, only that aspect which troubled his sons enough to go to court. Nevertheless, as Claudia Verhoeven has pointed out with reference to court records in general, 'the key concepts used to make sense of the unprecedented will reveal that culture's presuppositions about what constitutes ordinary and/or acceptable behavior'.[11] Put very simply, Mr Park's wish for companionship made sense.

Since the vast majority of cases are not reported, insight into more everyday legal events will usually require the records generated by courts themselves. But court records present a number of difficulties. As James Moran has suggested, court archives may have been more vulnerable to destruction than asylum archives, and even where records survive, those of interest to historians of psychiatry are usually embedded within much larger archives of legal proceedings which can make them extremely difficult to trace.[12] Discussion of mental illness might appear almost anywhere: marriage and inheritance disputes, as we have seen; criminal proceedings of any type; divorce proceedings; contested insurance claims; disagreements over contracts, deeds, or trusts, and more. In addition, for historians of the twentieth century there are often access restrictions. In Scotland, for example, the records of civil cases in the Sheriff courts are only available to researchers after 100 years.[13] Lastly, even where court records can be identified within national or local archives and access is granted, they may not contain a great deal of interest. There is some variation in terms of content, which is often shaped by whether a particular court is 'adversarial' or 'inquisitorial'. 'Adversarial' courts are closely associated with common law systems, and here, two opposing parties will gather their own evidence, identify and question their own witnesses, and generally fight their own corner, with the court acting as an impartial referee. Evidence was (and is) often given orally, and court archives might contain little more than a note of the name, date, and outcome of a case. In contrast, within inquisitorial systems, it is the court itself that investigates and gathers evidence, identifies witnesses, and requests information – including expert evidence – to inform its deliberations. This often produces a much fuller paper trail.[14]

Digitisation projects offering more accessible and searchable archives may provide some solutions to the problems posed by court records, as does a little creative thinking. For criminal proceedings, the archives of state bodies engaged in bringing criminal prosecutions, such as the police or the Director of Public Prosecutions (DPP) in England and Wales, sometimes include copies or originals of the evidence gathered, including the reports of psychiatric experts and legal commentary on these and other materials.[15] Institutional and personal archives may also contain records of expert psychiatric evidence, and where these can be identified they will likely offer a rich resource.[16] For particularly high-profile cases, full transcripts were sometimes published for mass consumption, albeit with editorial interventions that may not be immediately obvious.[17] The Proceedings of the Old Bailey were regularly published and contain quite detailed accounts of criminal cases heard there from the seventeenth to early twentieth centuries.[18] By the nineteenth century, though, newspaper coverage of the courts at national and local level was increasingly extensive, and plenty of excellent work on forensic psychiatry relies upon newspaper reporting of court cases, rather than court records.[19] The Times generally covers high profile or legally interesting cases, while local papers will provide insight into more prosaic legal proceedings in their area, albeit often with a focus on criminal cases.

There is one additional note of caution to sound, regarding both case law and court records. In legal proceedings of any type, the stakes are high and there are usually sharply competing views, carefully assembled in line with specific rules (of evidence, procedure, and law itself). One result of this, as Carolyn Steedman puts it, is that the 'narratives they purport to be are often not true, in the everyday and historical sense of "true"'.[20] These sources may contain knowing lies; there may also be omissions, distortions, and adjustments of the facts to meet the rules, to achieve specific goals, and even simply to accommodate the template documents of legal institutions. This does not mean that these sources are useless, only that they require the same critical thinking and attention to purpose and context as any other. One possible reading strategy for court records, taking this into account, is offered in the case study at the end of this chapter.

Finally, legislation itself is an important legal source, and not only legislation that mentions 'lunacy' or 'mental health'. Poor laws and those concerning health systems in general, for example, may be extremely relevant to historians of psychiatry.[21] As well as the words of the statutes themselves, historians might look at the circumstances that prompted them, the political debates that surrounded their passage into law, and the policies, rules, and codes of conduct that flowed from them. For the twentieth century, there are also international laws to consider as well as 'soft law' instruments, meaning declarations and commitments to which nations become signatories: the United Nations Declaration on the Rights of Mentally Retarded Persons 1971 is one such example. Like any source, laws and legal instruments have their limitations. A new piece of legislation might be unpopular, unclear, or in other ways unusable, meaning that what looks like a dramatic change has little or no practical impact. In the Republic of Ireland, for example, the Health (Mental Services) Act of 1981 set out to reform the processes and safeguards surrounding involuntary admission to psychiatric hospitals, but was never implemented.[22] Equally (and not unusually), new laws might reflect changes that have already taken place, whether in terms of public mood or common law, policy, and practice. The English Infanticide Acts of the early twentieth century, for example, appeared to create a new kind of offence and offender for which mental abnormality was a necessary precondition, but arguably did little more than formalise ideas and practices that had become firmly established decades earlier.[23] Sometimes, new laws are not new at all – perhaps especially in common law jurisdictions, where a great many legal principles exist separately from specific pieces of legislation, and a new or amended Act might state nothing more than the legal status quo.[24] For most historical enquiries, careful attention to laws in context will be invaluable.

Using legal sources

How have these kinds of sources been used by those interested in the history of psychiatry? Since the 1960s, legal sources have been used to explore three overlapping topics: the relationship between psychiatry and law, how mental illness has been perceived and understood, and policy responses to mental illness. As approaches to the sources have changed, so, too, have the conclusions reached. The relationship between psychiatry and law was initially characterised as hostile – or at the very least, one of irreconcilable difference. Nigel Walker's *Crime and Insanity in England* (1968) drew on a variety of legal proceedings in which insanity was argued, and paid close attention to evidence from psychiatrists and its reception.

This and Roger Smith's comprehensive *Trial by Medicine* (1981) identified a great deal of tension between expert medical witnesses and jurists within court proceedings, attributed to the fundamentally conflicting views of human nature upon which each profession drew. Law depended upon the principle that individuals were in possession of rational free will; medicine increasingly supposed that other forces were at work in determining human behaviour. As a result of this, these historians concluded, legal practitioners 'considered medical theory pretentious and showed little sympathy with medical men who tried to explain the grounds on which they based their opinions'.[25] Scholarship concerning forensic psychiatry in other jurisdictions also took up the theme of adversarial relations between the disciplines.[26]

Since the 1990s, historians of psychiatry have revisited Victorian court proceedings with greater sensitivity to the context in which they were produced, and have perceived a much less combative relationship between law and psychiatry. This was, after all, an adversarial legal system that required, by definition, the production and public performance of disagreement. Using Old Bailey court records and thinking about the kinds of cases in which psychiatric evidence was introduced and what effect it seemed to have upon sentencing, Joel Eigen argued that the two disciplines more often collaborated than competed. Psychiatric ideas were not resented, but rather, were eagerly adopted by defence lawyers and by (some) courts keen to find a reason to reduce the severity of punishments, especially for minor crimes.[27] Historians have also begun to look beyond the nineteenth-century insanity defence and towards the role of forensic psychiatry in the twentieth century, particularly in relation to sexual offenders. Using not only expert evidence in criminal proceedings and new legislation, but also the wider criminological literature and debate, this work tends to see a good deal of ambivalence about the role of psychiatry within criminal law, from psychiatrists and the judiciary alike. It also emphasises strategic uses of psychiatric knowledge, with ambiguous concepts such as the 'sexual psychopath' deployed to deliver both indeterminate detention and non-custodial punishments alike.[28]

This relates to the second topic for which legal sources have been used: understanding how mental illness has been perceived. Early case studies tended to focus on the evidence of experts, but later work has paid attention to the wider range of opinion that might be voiced within legal sources. Eigen's scrutiny of court records suggested that lay ideas of madness remained influential throughout the first half of the nineteenth century, and indeed, that these ideas strongly influenced psychiatry. Delving more deeply into descriptions and determinations of mental illness within legal sources, Peter Bartlett found that delusions became central to what it meant to be insane in law – not least because it was a relatively flexible idea that could bend to meet both medical and legal frameworks. James Moran's use of 'lunacy trials' in New Jersey also highlights frequent reference to delusions amongst witnesses, along with accounts of violent behaviour. But, as he observes, this could reflect a pragmatic use of lunacy law by families and communities to deal with violence amongst their members, rather than a belief that violence necessarily indicated lunacy. In this light, how might lay and legal models of madness influence one another, over time?[29]

Legal scholars adopting socio-historical approaches have offered a different perspective again. From close readings and careful contextualisation of reported judgements and court proceedings, they have analysed and explained changing legal models of mental infirmity, which were to some extent influenced by psychiatry but also deeply responsive to wider social change. Work on civil competence not only highlights the varied and conflicting views of self and sanity that litigants and judges presented, but also the political salience of these kinds of disputes, as Susanna Blumenthal has shown. Along with Arlie Loughnan's study of mental capacity in the criminal context, this close attention to a broad range of legal events provides an illuminating perspective on the uses and limitations of medical ideas in legal contexts, identifying both continuity and change within legal models of the rational or responsible individual.[30]

The third topic, policy responses to psychiatry and mental illness, makes intensive use of legislation and the debates that surround it, rather than case law or court records. New laws are often read as signs of a desire (if not always fully realised) to change policy and practice. Early histories, such as those by Kathleen Jones, charted new mental health laws and their implementation in order to describe the evolution of mental health policy over two centuries. This was not quite a tale of progress, since it picked up on the theme of medico-legal incompatibility and described each law in terms of a pendulum swinging between 'law' and 'medicine'; in Jones's view progress only occurred when the pendulum swung towards medicine.[31] Readings of legislation as another medico-legal battlefield have lingered on, but increasingly, historians using mental health legislation have considered these laws as indicators of changing ideas of citizenship and the role of the state.[32] Here, legislation is just one aspect of a much broader picture of political, professional, and popular concerns.

These three recurring topics – the relationship between psychiatry and law, perceptions of mental illness, and policy responses – can all be identified within the archives of the Court of Protection of England and Wales, to which we now turn. Using a file from this archive as a case study, the next section suggests a close reading that responds to the context and factual flexibility of legal records, and draws out these themes as they shaped the mid-twentieth century case of Miss Jean Carr.

A case study: Jean Carr and the Court of Protection

One of the least well-trodden paths in the use of legal sources is determinations of civil competency, 'marginal in the history of modern law and madness to the point of being almost ignored'.[33] Can someone with dementia make a will? Can someone with anorexia refuse treatment? Should someone with a severe mental illness (or learning disability) be prevented from selling their home, or giving their money to friends instead of paying their bills? Some of the difficulties in locating legal sources where these questions are addressed have been discussed above, but it remains a potentially rich field with scope for illuminating the management of mental illness, medico-legal relationships, and wider cultural beliefs. In England and Wales, the Court of Protection (and its precursor institutions) has overseen determinations of civil competency - usually known as mental capacity, in this context - in relation to financial decision-making for centuries. Its archives are patchy, but for the mid-twentieth century a good sample of case files has been retained. It is from this archive that my case study is drawn.[34]

Miss Jean Carr (1913–1992) was an artist and art lover from the south of England. She was independently wealthy; her father's family had made their fortune in biscuit manufacturing, and as both her father and an uncle had died during Jean's childhood and left her legacies in their wills, she inherited a sub-stantial fortune on her twenty-first birthday. As this birthday approached, Jean's mother applied to the Court of Protection (or Management and Administration Department, as it was then known) to have Jean declared incapable of managing her property and affairs by reason of infirmity caused by disease. Mrs Carr asked to be appointed as Jean's 'receiver', meaning that she would have day-to-day control over Jean's money.

The law governing this process is indicated by the heading of the form that Mrs Carr had to complete: '53 Vic C 5 and Amending Acts'. This refers to the fifth Act passed during the session beginning in the 53rd year of Queen Victoria's reign: the Lunacy Act of 1890. This Act is mainly known for its impact upon admission to and governance of asylums, but the legal proceedings within this archive indicate the potential importance of the Act in other circumstances too. Mrs Carr's ap-plication had nothing at all to do with asylum care. Jean's file states that she came under the auspices of the Court in accordance with section 116 (d) of the 1890 Act, meaning that she was not a lunatic so found by inquisition, nor was she held in an institution of any kind: she was simply incapable of managing her property. Reference in section 116 of the Act to lunatics so found by inquisition points to the antecedents of this procedure. In the nineteenth century and before, Mrs Carr would have had to petition for a lunacy inquisition, held in public before judge and jury, for her daughter to be deemed lunatic and incapable of managing her own property. This had been changed by the 1890 Act, opening the door to a much more private process in which any kind of infirmity affecting someone's ability to manage their daily affairs could be grounds for intervention. It was also faster and cheaper, making this process accessible to many more people whose property might need protecting or controlling. The vast majority of applications were dealt with by the Master in Lunacy or one of his Assistants on the basis of written evidence alone. Mental capacity in this context was no longer something to be assessed by a jury of peers, but by a legal expert in receipt of medical evidence.

Mrs Carr's application consisted of a form detailing Jean's family and financial position, 'the circumstances giving rise to these proceedings', and proposals as to how Jean's money should be spent during her incapacity. Along with an affidavit from Jean's doctor, this was sent by the Carr family solicitors to the Master in Lunacy at the Royal Courts of Justice for consideration. The Master then drafted an Order affirming that Jean was incapable, appointing her mother as her receiver, and giving directions regarding the amount to be spent on her maintenance. Jean was formally notified, and there is no record that she raised any objections. The hearing itself was a meeting between the Carr family solicitor and the Master in the Master's office, so uneventful and brief that no record of it other than the summons remains.

What do these records tell us about the circumstances surrounding Jean's incapacity? 'The Patient has since leaving school been delicate,' Mrs Carr's application reads, 'and has lived at home and not been able or willing to take part in social affairs.'[35] She had been at The Cassel Home in Sussex, then at the family home in the care of a live-in nurse, then sent to a Dr Crouch at St Michael's, Ascot, at a cost of £39 a fortnight. Hopefully, she would soon be able to return home again with a nurse. Dr Crouch supplied the medical evidence. His patient was

> suffering from inability to concentrate on any subject for more than a few minutes at a time. e.g. she will start having a meal and forget to go on with it requiring constant urging. When spoken to on any subject she will wander on to some other in a minute or two. If about to brush her teeth will forget what she is going to do. If writing a letter will start it but is unable to continue. Will put her shoes in a cupboard and forget where they are.

Her symptoms had first manifested nearly two years ago when Jean was aged 19, and the prospects of recovery were 'Doubtful', despite some recent improvement. The cause? 'Functional disorder of nervous system'.[36]

Here is a snapshot of medical and familial ideas and practices regarding mental infirmity. Mrs Carr outlines the steps taken to care for Jean since she became ill: neither mental hospital nor treatment from a specialist on an outpatient basis, but care at home or in home-like environments (which did not come cheap). Mrs Carr is less forthcoming about what, exactly, was wrong. The very fact of her initiating these proceedings indicates that she was significantly concerned about something; this process may have been more discreet and cheaper than its nineteenth-century iterations, but it was nonetheless a substantial legal intervention into private affairs which would not be undertaken lightly. Mrs Carr's statement was probably drafted or finalised by solicitors, who may have advised that she focus on the practical side of Jean's finances and living situation, leaving the medical aspect to the medical expert. Mrs Carr could avoid saying too much about her daughter's health without jeopardising the application, but her reference to delicacy and a lack of experience or interest in social life is suggestive. Avoiding any direct reference to illness (and certainly avoiding any implication of 'lunacy' or insanity), Mrs Carr presents a picture of a timid and isolated young woman who, by implication, would not be able to cope with the management of her inheritance. Perhaps most suggestive of all is the phrase 'not able *or willing*' to engage in social life (my emphasis). There is uncertainty here: was Jean ill and therefore unable, or was she eccentric, badly behaved, or unsympathetic to social and parental pressures, and therefore unwilling? This phrase could be a glimmer of maternal impatience or legal incredulity, suggesting that Jean's diagnosis did not meet with universal acceptance.

Dr Crouch provides this diagnosis and is much more specific, as was required by the questions on the form he had to complete. He perceived Jean's primary symptom rather differently from her mother: in his view, the main problem was an inability to concentrate. His examples, taken from everyday life, are well chosen to portray her limitations in even the simplest practical matters. His diagnosis and prognosis are themselves interesting, indicating the terminology used to denote milder forms of mental illness, and a degree of pessimism regarding cure. This pessimism may not have been entirely straightforward, though. The court was reluctant to intervene and to appoint a receiver where recovery seemed imminent, and either the Carr family solicitors or Dr Crouch himself, as a specialist possibly involved in such applications before, may have been aware of this. Dr Crouch may have adopted a more negative view on this paperwork than he would express in other circumstances, to prospective or current patients or their families, for example. Importantly, his diagnosis and prognosis were accepted by the court without any qualms, suggesting that they were not unusual within these kinds of applications.

The archive contains various medical statements that describe Jean's treatment and recovery over the following years, as well as reports from the official Medical Visitors sent on behalf of the court to review her circumstances and state of mind. The latter reports were usually stored separately in the files of the Visitors and by law should have been destroyed once the case came to an end in 1940. The happy historical accident of their survival is itself revealing: Jean's case was atypical and became difficult from a medico-legal point of view, prompting more regular reference to the medical opinions contained in these reports, and the retention of the reports within this file. Medical and legal opinions differed, but notes of discussions between these experts suggest that Jean's character, wishes, and weaknesses were carefully weighed up. All agreed that Jean's condition was improving, but she remained nervous and reliant on others. There might be 'disastrous results', one such note records, 'if she ever got into the hands of dishonest persons'.[37] Later notes discuss whether there was a legal route to protect her property from devious suitors if she should regain full control over her money. As a wealthy young individual, and specifically a wealthy young woman, Jean's vulnerability to fraudsters and unscrupulous would-be husbands was at the forefront of the minds of the men who contemplated her future.

Although Jean's situation was not exactly run of the mill, her file offers several insights into matters of mental health policy in the mid-twentieth century, the relationship between psychiatry and law, and ideas of madness. It also documents Jean's life over a six-year period, discussing her living circumstances, medical treatment, and nursing care, as well as practical questions to do with her finances. Fragments of Jean's own views also appear, initially ventriloquised through the doctors that assessed her, and then in her own words as she set about overturning the legal finding of incapacity. The few letters from her in the file are extremely business-like, perhaps composed at least in part as informal evidence of her full recovery. Like her mother, she leaves almost all comment on her mental state to the medical experts, but her unhappiness and frustration with her family in particular shines through. Some legal sources can also offer such glimpses of the lives and views of those most directly affected by legal methods of responding to madness.

Conclusion: law and psychiatry

Legal systems have long been used to respond to suspected mental infirmity and have transformed – some might even say created – the discipline of psychiatry. To conclude, I would like to offer some brief comment on two further questions about the history of psychiatry, that legal sources suggest. Firstly, legal sources may have something to say about the movement of psychiatric ideas, not only between doctors, jurists, and the full gamut of people initiating or caught up in legal events, but also across place. Since colonists took their legal structures with them, legal proceedings concerning people and events in one part of the world might be passed to far-distant courts for final resolution. After all, the Privy Council of the United Kingdom was the Supreme Court of Appeal for the entire British Empire, and continued as such for commonwealth countries until the late twentieth century. More recently, international treaties have drawn to some extent on global expertise but have been received and implemented unevenly. How, then, has mental health law been applied and adapted in different settings? What role has the law played in the global transmission of psychiatric ideas, from colony to metropole or from regional to transnational contexts, and vice versa?

Then, there are the questions raised by paying close attention to individual cases within legal sources. This attention need not be limited to high-profile trials and well-known defendants; microhistorians have already modelled the use of legal sources for telling the stories of 'humble' or 'ordinary' lives. What was everyday life like, for someone like Mr Park or Miss Carr? Where did they call home, and who provided care for them? What role did psychiatry play in these routine decisions, and how were its interventions received? The factual flexibility of legal sources requires close and cautious reading, but this feature also lends itself to imaginative explorations of what may have been, beyond the courtroom and between the lines. Legal sources are full of personal stories, and can be used to address individual experiences and agency as well as broader medico-legal developments and related historical processes. For historians of psychiatry, legal sources are not only evidence of policies, ideas, and interdisciplinary entanglements, but also evidence of their impact on individual lives.

Notes

1 Peter Bartlett, 'Legal Madness in the Nineteenth Century', *Social History of Medicine*, 14, 1 (2001), pp. 107–31: p. 107.
2 Roger Smith, 'Legal Frameworks for Psychiatry', in German E. Berrios and Hugh Freeman (eds), *150 Years of British Psychiatry, 1841–1991* (London: Gaskell, 1991), pp. 137-51: p. 138.
3 Bartlett, 'Legal Madness'.
4 *Banks v Goodfellow* [1870] 5 Q.B. 549.
5 James Moran, *Madness on Trial: A Transatlantic History of English Civil Law and Lunacy* (Manchester: Manchester University Press, 2019).
6 Chantal Stebbings (ed.), *Law Reporting in Britain* (London: Bloomsbury, 1995).
7 Many judgements are available from the British and Irish Legal Information Institute (known as BAILII), a free online legal database of mostly British case law, legislation, Law Commission reports, and other legal material: www.bailii.org. In addition to the free resources of BAILII, subscription options that provide more comprehensive access to case law include the Westlaw and Justis databases. Legal library membership will generally provide free access to one or more of these. For guidance on how to locate English case law, see Bartlett, 'Legal Madness', pp. 113–4.
8 These reports are 'In re Park; Culross v. Park,' *The Times*, 1 Dec. 1950, p. 9, and 2 Dec. 1950, p. 5; *In the estate of Park, dec'd: Park v Park,* [1954] P.89 and [1954] P.112; *Park v Park* [1953] 3 W.L.R. 1012. *The Times* has a digital archive with Gale Primary Sources: https://www.gale.com/intl/primary-sources. This can be accessed through the British Library in London and many other academic libraries. The judgements published in 1953 and 1954 can be obtained from the Westlaw UK legal database: https://legalsolutions.thomsonreuters.co.uk/en/products-services/westlaw-uk.html (subscription required).
9 *In the estate of Park, dec'd: Park v Park,* [1954] P.89, pp. 105–6.
10 John Harrington, Lucy Series, and Alexander Ruck-Keene, 'Law and Rhetoric: Critical Possibilities', *Journal of Law and Society*, 46, 2 (2019), pp. 302–27: p. 308, pp. 322-324.
11 Claudia Verhoeven, 'Court Files', in Miriam Dobson and Benjamin Ziemann (eds), *Reading Primary Sources: The Interpretation of Texts from Nineteenth and Twentieth Century History* (New York: Routledge, 2009), pp. 90–105: p. 97.
12 James Moran, 'A Tale of Two Bureaucracies: Asylum and Lunacy Law Paperwork', *Rethinking History*, 22, 3 (2018), pp. 419–36.
13 These records are held by the National Records of Scotland in Edinburgh.
14 For more on the impact of adversarial and inquisitorial systems on the development of forensic medicine itself: Catherine Crawford and Michael Clark (eds), *Legal Medicine in History* (Cambridge: Cambridge University Press, 1994); Joel Peter Eigen, *Witnessing Insanity: Madness and Mad-Doctors in the English Court* (New Haven and London: Yale University Press, 1995), pp. 112–3; Katherine D. Watson, *Forensic Medicine in Western Society: A History* (London and New York: Routledge, 2011) esp. Ch. 1.
15 DPP and Metropolitan Police archives are held at The National Archives in London (hereafter TNA); records from other police forces are fragmented and mostly held in county or city archives.
16 For example, the university archive used in Günther Häßler and Frank Häßler, 'Infanticide in Mecklenburg and Western Pomerania: Documents from Four Centuries (1570–1842)', *History of Psychiatry*, 22, 1 (2011), pp. 75–92.
17 For example, MacDonald Critchley, *The trial of Neville George Clevely Heath* (London: William Hodge & Co, 1951).
18 Available at www.oldbaileyonline.org.
19 For example, Hilary Marland, *Dangerous Motherhood: Insanity and Childbirth in Victorian Britain* (Basingstoke: Palgrave Macmillan, 2004); Akihito Suzuki, *Madness at Home: The Psychiatrist, the Patient and the Family in England, 1820–1860* (Berkeley, CA: University of California Press, 2006). The British Library provides comprehensive access to digital, print, and microfiche newspaper archives.

20 Carolyn Steedman, *History and the Law: A Love Story* (Cambridge: Cambridge University Press, 2020), p. 232. For an insightful exploration of this question, see Shelley McSheffrey, 'Detective Fiction in the Archives: Court Records and the Uses of Law in Late Medieval England', *History Workshop Journal*, 65, 1 (2008), pp. 65–78.

21 Peter Bartlett, *The Poor Law of Lunacy: The Administration of Pauper Lunatics in Mid-Nineteenth-Century England* (London: Leicester University Press, 1999).

22 Pauline Prior, 'Mental Health Law on the Island of Ireland, 1800–2010', in Pauline Prior (ed.), *Asylums, Mental Health Care, and the Irish: Historical Studies, 1800–2010* (Dublin: Irish Academic Press, 2012), pp. 316-334.

23 Arlie Loughnan, 'The "Strange" Case of the Infanticide Doctrine', *Oxford Journal of Legal Studies*, 32, 4 (2012), pp. 685–711.

24 One recent example is the Domestic Abuse Bill of 2020 and its widely celebrated measures to prohibit the so-called 'rough sex defence' in homicide cases. It is already the case in common law that consent is not a defence where serious harm has been inflicted, except in the context of certain recognised activities such as sports or tattooing. Hannah Bows and Jonathan Herring, 'Getting Away With Murder? A Review of the "Rough Sex Defence"', *The Journal of Criminal Law*, 84, 6 (2020), pp. 525–38.

25 Nigel Walker, *Crime and Insanity in England: The Historical Perspective* (Edinburgh: Edinburgh University Press, 1968), 1; Roger Smith, *Trial by Medicine: Insanity and Responsibility in Victorian Trials* (Edinburgh: Edinburgh University Press, 1981), p. 109.

26 For example, James C. Mohr, *Doctors and the Law: Medical Jurisprudence in Nineteenth-Century America* (New York: Oxford University Press, 1993).

27 Eigen, *Witnessing Insanity*.

28 Simon A. Cole, 'From the Sexual Psychopath Statute to "Megan's Law": Psychiatric Knowledge in the Diagnosis, Treatment, and Adjudication of Sex Criminals in New Jersey, 1949–1999', *Journal of the History of Medicine and Allied Sciences*, 55, 3 (2000), pp. 292–314; Roger Davidson, 'Law, Medicine and the Treatment of Homosexual Offenders in Scotland, 1950–1980', in Imogen Goold and Catherine Kelly (eds), *Lawyers' Medicine: The Legislature, the Courts and Medical Practice, 1760–2000* (Oxford: Hart, 2009), pp. 125–42.

29 Moran, *Madness on Trial*.

30 Susanna L. Blumenthal, *Law and the Modern Mind: Consciousness and Responsibility in American Legal Culture* (Cambridge, MA: Harvard University Press, 2016); Arlie Loughnan, *Manifest Madness: Mental Incapacity in Criminal Law* (Oxford: Oxford University Press, 2012).

31 Kathleen Jones, *Lunacy, Law, and Conscience, 1744–1845* (Routledge & Kegan Paul, 1955); Kathleen Jones, *Mental Health and Social Policy, 1845–1959* (London: Routledge & Kegan Paul, 1960); Kathleen Jones, 'Law and Mental Health: Sticks or Carrots?', in Berrios and Freeman, *150 Years of British Psychiatry*, pp. 89–102.

32 Mathew Thomson, *The Problem of Mental Deficiency: Eugenics, Democracy and Social Policy in Britain, c.1870–1959* (Oxford: Clarendon, 1998); Clive Unsworth, *The Politics of Mental Health Legislation* (Oxford: Clarendon, 1987).

33 Bartlett, 'Legal Madness in the Nineteenth Century', p. 117. This article also gives a useful summary of different types of competency proceedings.

34 Records relating to Miss Jean Carr are in TNA, London, catalogue reference J92/77, 'CARR, Jean Alison, 1934–1941'. For more on the Court of Protection in general: Janet Weston, 'Managing Mental Incapacity in the 20th Century: A History of the Court of Protection of England & Wales', *International Journal of Law and Psychiatry*, 68 (2020), https://doi.org/10.1016/j.ijlp.2019.101524, accessed 16 Mar. 2021.

35 Initial application from Anita Carr, in TNA J92/77.

36 Medical affidavit dated 28 Jun. 1934, in TNA J92/77.

37 Anonymous file minute from Nov. 1936, in TNA J92/77.

Select bibliography

Bartlett, P., 'Legal Madness in the Nineteenth Century', *Social History of Medicine* 14, 2001, pp. 107–131.

Blumenthal, S.L., *Law and the Modern Mind: Consciousness and Responsibility in American Legal Culture*, Cambridge, MA: Harvard University Press, 2016.

Crawford, C. and Clark, M. (eds), *Legal Medicine in History*, Cambridge: Cambridge University Press, 1994.

Eigen, J.P., *Witnessing Insanity: Madness and Mad-Doctors in the English Court*, New Haven, CT: Yale University Press, 1995.

Loughnan, A., *Manifest Madness: Mental Incapacity in Criminal Law*, Oxford: Oxford University Press, 2012.

Moran, J., *Madness on Trial: A Transatlantic History of English Civil Law and Lunacy*, Manchester: Manchester University Press, 2019.

Steedman, C., *History and the Law: A Love Story*, Cambridge: Cambridge University Press, 2020.

Thomson, M., *The Problem of Mental Deficiency: Eugenics, Democracy and Social Policy in Britain, c.1870–1959*, Oxford: Clarendon, 1998.

Watson, K.D., *Forensic Medicine in Western Society: A History*, London: Routledge, 2011.

9

REMOVING THE 'VEIL OF SECRECY': PUBLIC INQUIRIES AS SOURCES IN THE HISTORY OF PSYCHIATRY, 1960S–1970S

Louise Hide

They were the stuff of Victorian gothic novels: bleak brooding asylums containing vast barrack-like ward blocks, isolated and remote. Built over the course of the nineteenth century, many of these institutions had reached their nadir by the mid-twentieth century, creating a very real lived sense of desolation for tens of thousands of people locked within their walls: wards were overcrowded and dilapidated; patients were absorbed into a monotonous routine that was largely devoid of meaning and purpose; staff were poorly trained, professionally isolated, and in short supply; investment and resources were strained to breaking point.

It was at this point that change began to happen. From the 1950s, psychotropic drugs offered the possibility of managing symptoms which could potentially enable people to leave hospital and live in the community. However, large numbers of patients remained on the hospital 'back wards' for years. Some were subjected to cruel and inhumane practices which had been absorbed 'unnoticed' into certain ward cultures over years. It was not until the late 1960s that these practices were brought to the attention of the public and politicians through the persistent actions of a small number of courageous whistle-blowers and the press. No longer could the appalling conditions in some psychiatric and 'mental handicap' hospitals, as they were then called, be ignored or denied. A series of major inquiries into some NHS hospital practices began, which played a significant role in bringing about the closure of these large and outdated institutions.

The inquiries left in their wake a vast repository of documentation. Files are thick with correspondence between governments of the day, local authorities, campaigning bodies, anguished staff, whistleblowers, people who had experienced neglect or abuse, their families and friends; they also contain transcripts of hearings as well as press cuttings. These sources are exceptionally interesting for historians of psychiatric institutions. They focus less on individual acts of cruelty and criminality perpetrated by 'bad apples', who were often dealt with by the police

DOI: 10.4324/9781003087694-10

and the courts, and more on the cultures, systems, and structures that allowed abusive and neglectful practices on certain wards to continue. The insights these records offer into the practices and meanings of care, as well as into broader political interests, and social and cultural mores, are both rich and expansive.

Surprisingly, they have rarely been consulted by historians. An exception is Claire Hilton whose book *Improving Psychiatric Care for Older People* (2017) charts the tireless work of campaigner Barbara Robb who battled with government and health authorities to improve care for older people, eventually influencing changes in policy as well as bringing about improvements in the inspection and regulation of psychiatric care.[1] Analyses of hospital inquiries in England and Wales have primarily been carried out by social scientists. John Martin's *Hospitals in Trouble* was published in 1984 and posed a question that still perplexes us today: 'How is it that institutions established to care for the sick and helpless can have allowed them to be neglected, treated with callousness and even deliberate cruelty?'[2] The book is an important historical source in itself. Martin includes an overview of the more significant hospital inquiries and examines in detail a complex web of inter-linking causations that span staffing, management, and political spectrums, discussing lessons learned and addressing important questions regarding ethics and morals.

In their study of how social welfare 'scandals' become constructed in certain ways at particular periods of time to serve specific interests, sociologists Ian Butler and Mark Drakeford argue that the 'chronic administrative failings, small carelessnesses and institutional brutality of the long-stay hospital' were not enough in themselves to trigger a scandal. The events are a necessary basis to a scandal but it is a particular set of constituent elements 'that transforms them into something beyond themselves',[3] sometimes through the power of the media. Nicky Stanley and Jill Manthorpe's thoughtful introduction to a volume of essays on different types of inquiry that were held during the 1990s reminds readers not to approach them uncritically, pointing out how they focused on what went wrong in institutions which raised anxieties around care. Importantly, they note how inquiries could be 'captured and controlled by the legal profession' early on, meaning that they were framed in a very specific way.[4] More recently, in 2019, a special issue of *The Political Quarterly* brings together work by a range of scholars and commentators to examine the processes, learning, and impact of 50 years of inquiries into NHS institutions and practices. The articles do not focus exclusively on psychiatric care or hospitals for people with intellectual disabilities. They do, however, collectively address important issues that relate to most inquiries: governance, leadership, and accountability; political interests and policy; the structure of inquiries and epistemological concerns; cultural issues; the role of the public and of families; and the degree to which inquiries brought about change.[5]

Historians today might well grapple with the same question that John Martin and so many others posed in the early 1980s: why had so little, if anything, been done to prevent abuses before the inquiries? We will never fully or satisfactorily uncover all the answers. However, a close and critical analysis of the inquiry documentation against sources relating to the wider socio-political context can offer some insights into the conditions, the attitudes and practices, the structures of power, and the subtle, and less subtle, inflections in mutable networks of personal and professional relationships. Together, these cultural mechanisms were in a continual process of reconstitution which allowed failures of care in their many forms to manifest and continue, above and below the radar.

In this chapter, I will provide an overview of the first run of inquiries into allegations of malpractice in some NHS psychiatric and mental handicap hospitals that began in the late 1960s and continued through much of the 1970s.[6] A summary of sources and where to find them is followed by reflections on some of the epistemological and ethical questions that need to be taken into account during the analysis and writing-up of the research, together with the potential challenges that come from working with such sensitive sources. By the end of the chapter, I will have explained the importance of these little-used sources in revealing how these large institutions functioned within a particular political and social context. Much historical focus on mid-twentieth-century psychiatry considers the effects of deinstitutionalisation and the shift of care into the community. But the large hospitals remained open until well into the 1980s.[7] The inquiry documentation can give us new insights into the micro and macro politics of long-term care.

The first NHS hospital inquiries

In 1965, Barbara Robb visited an acquaintance who had been admitted to a long-stay ward in Friern Hospital, a large psychiatric institution in North London. She was horrified by the sight of older female patients living in miserable conditions where they were dressed in institutional clothes, had few personal possessions, and little to occupy their time.[8] Galvanised to take action, Robb established the pressure group Aid for the Elderly in Government Institutions (AEGIS). Two years later, she presented, on behalf of AEGIS, a book titled *Sans Everything: A Case to Answer* which included accounts, many submitted by concerned hospital staff, of callous treatment and neglect on long-stay wards in psychiatric hospitals, particularly those for older people. The book was published in the summer of 1967 and caused a public outcry.[9]

Sans Everything exposed deplorable conditions on the back wards of certain hospitals, which had been exacerbated by NHS policies such as a two-tier system of care: one tier, which absorbed most of the resources, focused on acute care and treatment that would enable people to leave hospital and live in the community aided by the new psychotropic drugs, and the second, dismally under-funded, tier applied to the long-term care usually of people with severe learning disabilities and older people who were diagnosed with what were believed to be untreatable conditions such as senile dementia, or who were simply 'old' and had nowhere else to go. As younger patients and those with acute conditions began to move into the community, a large and mainly older group of patients was left behind on dilapidated and under-resourced hospital wards.

In addition to shifts in healthcare policy and practice, social change was also being driven, in part, by human and civil rights campaigns. During the 1960s, countercultural movements began to challenge the establishment, including psychiatry. Organisations such as AEGIS campaigned for improved care for those who were most vulnerable and unable to advocate for themselves; from the early 1970s, service users lobbied for greater rights to have a say in their own care and treatment through pressure groups such as MIND (for more on this, see Steffan Blayney's chapter in this volume).[10] Furthermore, a new generation of post-war sociologists and social psychiatrists began to study how large institutions such as mental hospitals, prisons, and residential homes affected the physical and mental health of their occupants.[11] Together, these factors made it increasingly difficult to ignore or deny abusive and neglectful practices that had been hidden from sight for decades. As the lid was lifted on malpractice and ill treatment, the age of the hospital inquiry began.

How the inquiries worked

When *Sans Everything* was published in 1967, the Minister of Health ordered each Regional Hospital Board responsible for a hospital that had been implicated in the book to investigate the allegations by setting up an inquiry. The committee for each inquiry was made up of a legally trained Chairman (all were Queen's Counsel), a doctor, a nurse, and at least one lay person with experience in hospital administration or public life, none of whom was from the region concerned.[12] While the committees roundly discredited many of the allegations, together with some of the individuals who made them,[13] momentum was gathering to expose and bring to an end some of the appalling conditions and practices in certain long-stay hospital wards.

Ely Hospital became the focus of what is generally considered to be the first modern inquiry in the NHS.[14] A run-down former Poor Law institution in Cardiff, it was classified as a psychiatric hospital but mainly provided care for people with severe intellectual disabilities, then referred to as 'sub-normal' or 'severely sub-normal'. Alarmed by the ill treatment of some patients and 'pilfering' by staff, a nursing assistant took his concerns to the *News of the World*. The newspaper forwarded his statement to the Ministry of Health and published it in August 1967 without naming the hospital or the people implicated.[15] The Minister instructed the Welsh Hospital Board to convene an inquiry into the allegations.

The Conservative politician Geoffrey Howe QC was appointed to chair the inquiry. Later, in 1999, he stated that one purpose of any type of public inquiry was 'to investigate serious allegations of improper conduct in the public service ... which requires thorough and impartial investigation and which may not be dealt with by ordinary civil or criminal processes'.[16] Sociologist Kieran Walshe has expanded on this by suggesting that inquiries were established for one or more of six reasons: to establish the facts; to learn from events; as catharsis or therapeutic exposure; to reassure; to hold people and organizations to account for the purposes of blame and retribution, or for political purposes.[17]

The terms of reference for the Ely inquiry were threefold: first, to investigate the claims made by the nursing assistant; second, 'to examine the situation in the wards', and third, to make recommendations.[18] It set a precedent by focusing not only on the egregious behaviours of certain individuals, but also on the failures of management that had allowed maltreatment, corruption, and poor standards of care to continue. Proceedings appear to have been fraught with problems. Even though the Committee had 'reasonable confidence' that it had achieved its objectives, the Report states that the investigation had 'an incoherent and disorganized quality' to it.[19] It was held in private and the Committee had 'no power to summon witnesses, to take evidence on oath' or to recommend awarding costs. Howe complained that the Committee had to 'fight all the way' to have the 'veil of secrecy decisively removed' so that they could appeal for witnesses in advance. Furthermore, pressure was put on them to 'prune and edit' the text of the final report by the Welsh Health Authority.[20]

In the year following the Ely inquiry, police were called to investigate brutal treatment by male nurses of men with severe learning disabilities at Farleigh Hospital in Bristol; of the nine nurses who were charged with cruelty, three were given prison sentences. Following the police investigation, an inquiry was launched into the administrative systems and conditions of the hospital. In 1969, a psychiatrist and a psychologist from Whittingham Hospital near Preston in Lancashire wrote directly to the Secretary of State for Social Services alleging 'ill-treatment of patients' on certain wards, as well as fraud, maladministration, and the suppression of earlier complaints from student nurses.[21] An inquiry was set up in 1971 under Section 70 of the NHS Act of 1946. The Committee had the same authority as a court to compel witnesses to give evidence which could be taken on oath.[22] It began work as soon as its members had been appointed and sat in the Masonic Hall in Preston where evidence was heard in public unless it related to specific patients. Eighty-five witnesses gave evidence on oath over 18 days between April and June 1971. Most appeared voluntarily, although some were summonsed. Oral evidence, which was documented, was given by the following: members of the Manchester Regional Hospital Board which was the local health authority; members of the Whittingham Hospital Management Committee; staff and former staff which included nurses and doctors of all ranks, social workers, and occupational and industrial therapists; and 'others' who included one member of the public, a detective superintendent, one patient, the Chairman of the League of Friends,[23] and two auditors.[24] Press attention was intense.

Two more inquiries were established soon after Whittingham: one related to Napsbury Hospital in North London and another to South Ockendon Hospital in East London. Therefore, five major inquiries into allegations of various forms of abuse in NHS hospitals took place within five years of the publication of *Sans Everything*. According to John Martin, the failures they exposed broadly related to problems of the 'old order' which could be ascribed to professionally and socially isolated institutions; custodial practices; the risk of corruption in closed societies; the suppression of criticism; and poor management, especially lay management.[25] Nevertheless, the inquiries continued throughout the 1970s. Although they were run along similar lines by committees that had been similarly constituted, each was different. Most were inquisitorial and established to ascertain 'the facts'.[26] Many left in their wake ruined careers, shamed professions, fractured and broken communities, and a deep raw pain in those who had been victims of or who had witnessed the abuses: patients, families, friends, and hospital staff. They also left a vast repository of documentation, newspaper reports, and publications.

Finding the sources

The main output of an inquiry would be a report. Produced by the committee according to the terms of reference, it usually included recommendations for improvements to working practices in the hospital concerned. The reports of major inquiries were Command Papers which were formally presented to Parliament. They are available as hard copies in the British Library and can be downloaded from the ProQuest U.K. Parliamentary Papers online service.[27] Inquiries, or the circumstances that gave rise to them, were frequently debated in Parliament and transcripts of the presentation of the reports and debates can be found on the Hansard website.[28] Many of the inquiry reports provide useful background information on the circumstances surrounding the inquiries and how they were set up, as well as summaries of findings and recommendations for improvement. Yet, they are in some respects secondary documents in that they represent an interpretation and summary of the proceedings of the inquiry. The underlying archival material which supported the report's findings can reveal far deeper insights into the politics that facilitated abusive practices, not deliberately but sometimes without due consideration.

The public inquiry documentation from the early 1970s was closed for 30 years and opened during the 2000s. Today, much of it – although not everything – can be consulted either in The National Archives (TNA) or in local archives. For example, most of the documents relating to the Whittingham Hospital Inquiry are held at TNA in the Ministry of Health (MH) collection while a few records relating to the hospital, although not necessarily the inquiry, are in the Lancashire Archives in Preston. Records relating to the Normansfield Hospital Inquiry are held in TNA and the London Metropolitan Archives. These archives provide a hugely valuable historical repository. Many contain vast amounts of correspondence between government and health officials, much of it annotated, as well as press cuttings, thousands of pages of transcripts of the hearings, witness statements, and drafts of the report which, again, are annotated.

The media played a major role in bringing allegations of ill treatment to the attention of the public, putting pressure on the government of the day to take action. Press reports and television documentaries add different perspectives when it comes to revealing poor conditions and inhumane practices. While the presence of cockroaches on some female wards at Whittingham was briefly mentioned in the Report, the *Daily Mirror* ran a story under the headline '"Cockroaches in a hospital" claim'.[29] Keenly engaged in inquiry proceedings, which were very much in the public interest, the press may have commented on events that are not recorded in the transcripts such as the affective responses of witnesses giving evidence. Did they appear fearful? Did they show shame and remorse? Did they appear to be unaffected by the proceedings?[30] *The Times* described the adjournment of the proceedings regarding South Ockendon Hospital as being due to a charge nurse who was 'under stress' under the headline 'Illness causes hospital inquiry delay';[31] while the *Birmingham Post* reported the same event under the headline 'Nurse is suicide risk, inquiry told'.[32]

Local as well as national newspapers were instrumental in bringing allegations of abuses to the attention of government ministers. The *Lancashire Evening Post* set up a 'press desk' in a local pub to gather information into allegations of cruelty at Whittingham Hospital.[33] The best way to access these reports now is through online services that provide access to digitised newspapers such as the British Newspaper Archive and newspaper databases such as *The Times* Digital Archive.[34] However, not all newspapers have been digitised or are available online; here, local libraries can be helpful as they often hold archives of local newspapers on microfiche.

From the 1960s, television was growing increasingly popular. Film and programme makers gained access to psychiatric and mental handicap institutions and transmitted the horrors of long-stay wards directly into people's living rooms. Programmes such as *Ward F13* (1968), *The Secret Hospital* (1979), and *The Silent Minority* (1981) supported many of the findings uncovered by the inquiries, presenting them through a different lens.[35] They, too, are legitimate subjects for critical academic inquiry, particularly in respect of the complex ethical dilemmas that arise out of filming and broadcasting footage of people who were unable to give informed consent.

Matters either directly or tangentially related to the inquiries and the circumstances that gave rise to them were raised and debated among health and social care professionals in professional journals such as *The Nursing Times*, *The Nursing Mirror*, the *Hospital and Health Services Review*, *Social Work Today*, the *British Journal of Psychiatry*, *The Lancet*, and *The British Medical Journal*. Some of these publications have been digitised and are online; in this volume Chris Millard's chapter offers further guidance on using such journals within the history of psychiatry. The location of most hard copy journals and books can be found through Jisc Library Hub Discover.[36] The AEGIS archives are held by the London School of Economics; the MIND archives by the Wellcome Collection; and the Royal College of Nursing has an extensive library and archival collection. The University of Warwick Modern Records Centre holds the Confederation of Health Service Employees (COHSE) archives as well as the unedited typescripts of the diaries of Richard Crossman, who was Secretary of State for Social Services when the Ely report was published. And for local perspectives, bear in mind that large hospitals were major employers and since their closure some local groups have assembled histories of their communities which include oral histories of people who were affected by inquiries. See, for example, People's Collection Wales.[37] Victoria Hoyle's chapter in this volume provides considerable insight into the considerations to be borne in mind when using oral histories in the history of psychiatry.

Working with the sources

The prospect of wading through a massive volume of papers generated by one inquiry, let alone several, can be daunting. Before you dive into the archives, make sure that you have an idea of the kind of research you want to do because not all of the documentation will be relevant. If you are interested in the political machinations behind the establishment of the inquiries and how terms of reference were established, you may want to focus more on the correspondence between the government, health authorities at local and national levels, and other key actors in this process. It can tell us, for example, the terms upon which some of the main people knew each other (personal and professional), how they rated each other, and the kind of person they wanted to serve on the committee, not only in terms of skills and experience, but character too. The Whittingham records describe one committee member as being '...liable to give offence owing to his downright views but very willing to accept criticism of his own ideas',[38] suggesting a broad awareness of the myriad sensitivities around the inquiry.

If you want to examine how attitudes and policies played out through social and professional relations (including unions), cultural forces, and hospital practices, a close textual analysis of the transcripts and written evidence can reveal complex networks of power dynamics as well as contemporaneous attitudes towards care and harm. Soon after the publication of *Sans Everything*, a group of student nurses at Whittingham Hospital put forward a list of complaints detailing 'malpractice' and cruelty towards patients. Afraid of legal action and 'victimisation' if they named people, wards, or complainants, their concerns did not see the light of day for another two years.[39] When a female member of the Hospital Management Committee (HMC) was asked during the inquiry why she had not taken the nurses' complaints further when they were first raised, she replied that 'student nurses in general have a horrible habit of complaining and doing nothing about it themselves and I was inclined to put the onus back on them'. The Chairman similarly dismissed the nurses' complaints as being of a 'vague nature'.[40] Not only were the opinions and complaints of student nurses suppressed, there were clearly tensions between Whittingham's HMC, which was made up of lay members and responsible for 'general policy', and the Medical Advisory Committee (MAC) which was responsible for the clinical running of the hospital.

In a large institution like Whittingham, technically a psychiatric hospital but which provided residential long-term 'care' for older people, one might ask how much 'psychiatry' as such was practised? Indeed, the Chairman of the HMC stated that they were considering employing a consultant geriatrician rather than a psychiatrist to join the clinical team.[41] Back wards were hybrid spaces: part clinical, part residential. They were staffed by nurses, many of whom were poorly trained, and were rarely visited by doctors. This ambiguity around the role and function of the long-term wards led, I suggest, to a blurring of boundaries between clinical and managerial responsibility and subsequent accountability. For example, implementing a policy to unlock ward doors and allow patients to move freely around the institution was broadly considered to be a therapeutic intervention and, therefore, a clinical matter. But these decisions needed management support. Given the poor communications between the MAC and the HMC, it was not always forthcoming. Whittingham's medical leadership came in for particular criticism, resulting in what the Report described as 'therapeutic inertia on long-stay wards'.[42] Undefined and ambiguous boundaries around responsibility and accountability left gaps through which malpractice and neglect could emerge.

Another productive line of investigation into the inquiry documentation is the unintended – or ill considered – consequences of shifts in NHS policy on lived experiences. What, for example, were the effects of the two-tier system and underinvestment in long-term care on the people who lived and worked on wards day in, day out? As a case in point, Whittingham's Ward 16 was severely criticised for a number of reasons including gross understaffing and 'totally inadequate washing and lavatory facilities'.[43] As a historian who is interested in ward cultures, I want to know exactly what 'totally inadequate' meant at the time. The transcripts give us more detail: Ward 16 contained over 90 patients, many of whom were doubly incontinent, and had only 2 baths, 1 on each floor. There was no lift.[44]

An important question for us all to consider is: what is the meaning of 'care' or 'treatment' in a given temporal and spatial context? In my own research, I am interested in how care of older people in long-stay wards was understood and interpreted by staff, by patients, by their families and friends, by the health authorities and politicians, and by society at large. How did meanings change? What brought about those shifts? What light can the inquiry documentation shed on these questions? We can gain some understanding, for example, of how meaning was constructed through language. When the Chairman of Whittingham's HMC was asked what he meant when he described patients on Ward 16 as '"low grade"', he responded that 'it is the type who sits around all day just doing nothing but becoming cabbages'. This description was repeated when he stated that the purpose of the rehabilitation committee was 'to stop people … being vegetables …'.[45] Whilst the Committee pressed him on his use of language asking how he could apply the term 'low grade' to 'fellow human beings', the Chairman made no attempt to ameliorate his language even in such a formal setting, suggesting that he did not see it as problematic. But the real point of concern is surely around how the perception of older people in his care as 'cabbages' or 'vegetables' – insentient beings without feelings – translated into practices of care. The earlier inquiries that investigated the allegations published in *Sans Everything* showed how the old style, task-centred nursing was prioritised over meeting the emotional and sensory needs of patients. One nurse who had submitted a complaint was criticised for wanting to spend time 'playing with and entertaining' patients and for not applying herself 'to learning elementary nursing duties'. She was described in the Report as someone who

> failed completely to understand that … the disciplined nurse who got on with her job expeditiously and efficiently was making a greater contribution to the care and welfare of the patients than the sentimental but inefficient and untrained member of staff who wished to spend her time singing to and playing with the patients.[46]

There is a great emphasis in the history of psychiatry on recovering the voices of patients who are so often absent from the records. Rarely do we hear their voices in the inquiries either. Even though patients may have been invited to give evidence, few were willing or able to do so. We can, perhaps, gain a shadowy idea of how they experienced ward conditions through the accounts of others who described or filmed small acts of agency and resistance: a refusal to eat, to remain in bed, to be tied to a commode, to be dressed in shapeless communal clothing. It was not unusual, however, for a family member who would not be silenced to instigate a series of complaints which could eventually contribute to the establishment of an inquiry such as South Ockendon. What, then, can the inquiries tell us about how certain social and cultural mechanisms facilitated pervasive systems of coercion and complicity, denial and disavowal?

Analysing the sources

Many of these questions revolve around epistemological issues relating to the construction of social reality and the 'official truth'.[47] A primary purpose of the early inquiries was to establish 'the facts', to find out what 'really' happened in an isolated and inward-looking culture where everyday abuses and neglect were seen but not seen, known but unknown. How, then, we might ask, was the inquiry documentation discursively constructed? How were 'truths' established? Whose knowledge counted? Which information was privileged, how, and by whom? For example, the first set of inquiries that investigated the allegations of cruelty and abuse reported in *Sans Everything* dismissed the claims of one nurse by stating that she was 'sentimental and sensitive … untrained and inexperienced in mental nursing'. Another Committee suggested that a social worker who complained about the conditions to which her father was subjected in one hospital was in a 'highly emotional state'.[48]

Unpicking the myriad ways in which knowledge can be constructed, reconstructed, ignored, and distorted can be a fertile line of investigation for historians, especially regarding the analysis of inquiry reports which were created at *the end* of the inquiry by the committee. They were, as Howe has demonstrated, political documents in their own right. While such reports might be regarded as both primary and secondary source material, depending on the focus of the research, bear in mind that their authors – members of the committee – will have engaged in a lengthy process of sifting, evaluating, and analysing the evidence in order to establish what they believed to be 'the facts'. They will have made judgements on what to include or exclude from the report, which will have been based on the terms of reference of the inquiry as well as the training, life experiences, and interests of the committee members.[49] In Walshe's opinion, there is little evidence that those who conducted the inquiries exercised a robustly reflexive or rigorous methodological approach, leading to a tendency towards 'the conventional narratives of powerful stakeholders … [to] shape inquiry findings and reports'. He suggests that this raised doubts about whether or not inquiries could achieve their objectives to establish the facts and learn from events.[50] Official documents may, therefore, be unreliable. This does not invalidate them. But it does need to be borne in mind during the process of analysis.

Walshe also suggested that even while the cross-examination may be sensitive 'there is very good reason to question whether such hearings enable people to give open, honest and candid accounts in their testimony'.[51] Reading the transcripts can give us a sense of how the hearings proceeded. We may detect subtle points and counter-points of fear and shame as witnesses were subjected to intimidating legal proceedings, all the time aware that their words might become newspaper headlines with the power to turn colleagues, families, and their local communities against them.[52] In 1969, just after the publication of the Ely Report, the matron of Ely Hospital complained about how 'the staff were receiving appalling treatment from people like bus crews who knew they worked at the hospital … the conductors sneered at staff who alighted at the Ely hospital bus stop'. Another nurse from Ely was reported to have visited her GP who told her that she should 'hang her head in shame'.[53]

Taking care with the sources

Because many inquiries have addressed the inhumane treatment of some of society's most vulnerable people who were unable to speak for themselves, research in this area is fraught with ethical challenges and sensitivities. When planning your project, it is an important part of the process to reflect on where you stand ethically regarding the research you want to do. For example, historian of emotions Katie Barclay urges us to consider not only how our work might contribute to historical debates, but the impact of it on those who survive. Will it, she asks, 'cause embarrassment, physical or emotional harm, damage character or reputation, or lead to legal liability, for those under discussion, or occasionally, the historian?'[54] It is not unusual to find in the inquiry files personal details relating to people who have not given their consent for us to view this information, let alone to use it in our work. Because we are unable to request consent from our subjects, we have an obligation to tread carefully as we approach, analyse, and disseminate our findings, even when those we are writing about are dead and even when our research is based on documentary evidence that is in the public domain.

In their Introduction to *Secrets and Silence in the Research Process. Feminist Reflections* (2010), Róisín Ryan-Flood and Rosalind Gill remind us of the challenges facing us as researchers who are in the constant process of making decisions around what to include and what to omit in our outputs. Who do we represent, and how?[55] Should we anonymise? Are we including identifiable information in our work? What if individuals were named by the press at the time of the inquiry? When we are confronted by these questions, do we base our responses on our own values of what should be private or public, what might be harmful, and what might be beneficial? Do we try to imagine how the individuals concerned may have felt, and the values of the historical period we are writing about?[56] We must find a balance because we are not only writing a history of inquiries and people and practices in hospitals; we are writing *our* history. Research institutions will have their own ethics processes and procedures, as well as committees who will ensure that your methodology meets rigorous standards which will almost certainly, and rightly, insist on confidentiality and anonymity. For more guidance on ethical practices see the Royal Historical Society's *Statement on Ethics* and the *Statement on Standards of Professional Conduct* (2019) published by the American Historical Society.[57]

There is an additional aspect to working with these sources that should not be ignored. Reading accounts of abuse and neglect that led to untold suffering can unlock a range of emotions within us as researchers and it can become almost impossible to disentangle our professional interests from our subjective feelings. This will inevitably influence the history we write. But it can also exact a heavy toll on our own mental health. The rationalist expectation for academics to approach their subject matter objectively has been challenged over the past couple of decades, particularly relating to qualitative research in the social sciences.[58] Less has been written about researchers' emotional engagement in the production of historical knowledge. When done with full awareness, our research can be strengthened rather than weakened. Janet Fink asserts that when we focus on the emotional landscape we produce 'richer and more complicated understandings of epistemology, methodology, reflexivity and ontology' as new spaces are opened enabling us to think more deeply and widely around our subject matter.[59] Emotions and subjectivities can, therefore, bring a positive value to our research. But we do need to build into the design of our research project processes that ensure that we have the support we need from a supervisor or peers when engaging with potentially distressing accounts on both a personal and a professional level.

Conclusion

In this chapter, I have focused on the first run of inquiries into allegations of mistreatment in some of the large NHS mental and mental handicap hospitals from the late 1960s to the 1970s. In many cases, files are open for consultation in national and local archives where they can reveal a great deal about wider social as well as clinical and political attitudes, interests, and practices of the time. They provide a rich and hitherto little-used resource for scholars interested in the histories of care, medicine, organizational structures, old age, disability, gender, race and ethnicity, the emotions and senses, politics, policy, and the media. Context is key. The terms of reference under which the inquiries were established framed what would and would not be included, what was and was not important for the purposes of the inquiry, and, at times, wider political interests. This limits historical knowledge that is based on the reports alone. But the underlying documentation provides a vast sweep of insights gathered at the time into the politics, the systems, the culture, and the people involved in mental health care from the late 1960s.

The final question, which nags away at all who work on inquiries, is how we can learn more from them to prevent future abuses. The first NHS hospital inquiries were held over 50 years ago and did lead to improvements in long-term care during the 1970s: more medical and nursing staff were employed, training was improved, a Hospital Advisory Service to regulate long-stay hospitals was created, and improvements to policy were set out in various white papers.[60] But the neglect and maltreatment of vulnerable people continues to this day even though most of the large psychiatric hospitals have been closed for decades. Research into the many dimensions across which these past inquiries reached can help us to think more widely and deeply about the myriad meanings of care and harm in particular contexts and moments in time to expand our understanding of how inquiries work in theory and practice, and most importantly how they can be improved to prevent further abuses in the future.

Notes

1 Claire Hilton, *Improving Psychiatric Care for Older People. Barbara Robb's Campaign 1965–1976* (Cham, Switzerland: Palgrave Macmillan, 2017); see also Claire Hilton, 'A Tale of Two Inquiries: *Sans Everything* and Ely', *The Political Quarterly*, 90, 2 (2019), pp. 185–93.

2 J.P. Martin with Debbie Evans, *Hospitals in Trouble* (Oxford: Basil Blackwell, 1984), p. xi.

3 Ian Butler and Mark Drakeford, *Scandal, Social Policy and Social Welfare,* 2nd edn (Basingstoke: Palgrave Macmillan, 2005), p. 1, 225.

4 Nicky Stanley and Jill Manthorpe, 'Introduction: The Inquiry as Janus' in Nicky Stanley and Jill Manthorpe (eds), *The Age of the Inquiry. Learning and Blaming in Health and Social Care* (London: Routledge, 2004), pp. 1–16: p. 10, 3.

5 '50 Years of Inquiries in the National Health Service', *The Political Quarterly*, 90, 2 (2019), pp. 180–244.

6 To read more about the hospital inquiries, see Louise Hide, 'Mental Hospitals, Social Exclusion and Public Scandals' in George Ikkos and Nick Bouras (eds), *Mind, State and Society. Social History of Psychiatry and Mental Health in Britain 1960-2010* (Cambridge, Cambridge University Press, 2021), 60-67.

7 See work by Vicky Long on psychiatric hospitals in the post-war period.

8 Hilton, *Improving Psychiatric Care for Older People*, p. 1.

9 Barbara Robb (presented on behalf of AEGIS), *Sans Everything: A Case to Answer* (London: Nelson, 1967).

10 John Turner, Rhodri Hayward, Katherine Angel, Bill Fulford, John Hall, Chris Millard, and Mathew Thomson, 'The History of Mental Health Services in Modern England: Practitioner Memories and the Direction of Future Research', *Medical History*, 59, 4 (2015), pp. 599–624: p. 608.

11 Gresham M. Sykes, *The Society of Captives. A Study of a Maximum Security Prison* (Princeton, NJ: Princeton University Press, 1958); Russell Barton, *Institutional Neurosis* (Bristol: John Wright & Sons, 1959); Erving Goffman, *Asylums: Essays on the Social Situation of Mental Patients and Other Inmates* (New York: Anchor/Doubleday, 1961); Peter Townsend, *The Last Refuge: A Survey of Residential Institutions and Homes for the Aged in England and Wales* (London: Routledge and Kegan Paul, 1962).

12 Martin, *Hospitals in Trouble*, p. 4.

13 National Health Service (NHS), *Findings and Recommendations Following Enquiries into Allegations Concerning the Care of Elderly Patients in Certain Hospitals*, Cmnd. 3687 (London: HMSO, 1968).

14 Martin Powell, 'Inquiries in the British National Health Service', *The Political Quarterly*, 90, 2 (2019), pp. 180–4: p. 180.

15 Martin, *Hospitals in Trouble*, p. 5.

16 Geoffrey Howe, 'The Management of Public Inquiries', *The Political Quarterly*, 70, 3 (1999), pp. 294–304: p. 295.

17 Kieran Walshe, *Inquiries: Learning from Failure in the NHS?* (London: The Nuffield Trust, 2003), p. 2.

18 NHS, *Report of the Committee of Inquiry into Allegations of Ill-Treatment of Patients and other Irregularities at the Ely Hospital, Cardiff*, Cmnd. 3975 (London: HMSO, Mar. 1969), para. 4.

19 NHS, *Report of the Committee of Inquiry at the Ely Hospital, Cardiff*, paras 5 and 8–10.

20 Howe, 'The Management of Public Inquiries', pp. 302–3.

21 Martin, *Hospitals in Trouble*, p. 12.

22 Ibid., p. 72; For a discussion on public versus private inquiries, see Howe, 'The Management of Public Inquiries'.

23 The League of Friends was a voluntary organisation founded after the NHS was established to improve conditions and care for patients.

24 NHS, *Report of the Committee of Inquiry into Whittingham Hospital*, Cmnd. 4861 (London: HMSO, 1972), paras 2, 3, 68, and Appendix 1, pp. 47–8.

25 Martin, *Hospitals in Trouble*, p. 27.

26 Walshe, *Inquiries*, p. 3.

27 ProQuest U.K. Parliamentary Papers, https://parlipapers.proquest.com/parlipapers.

28 Hansard, https://hansard.parliament.uk.

29 NHS, *Report of the Committee of Inquiry into Whittingham Hospital*, para. 37; Reg White, '"Cockroaches in a Hospital" Claim', *Daily Mirror*, 12 May 1971.

30 Alecia Simmonds, 'Legal Records', in Katie Barclay, Sharon Crozier-De Rosa, and Peter N. Stearns (eds), *Sources for the History of Emotions. A Guide* (London: Routledge, 2021), pp. 79–91: p. 83.

31 *The Times*, 16 Sept. 1972.

32 *Birmingham Post*, 19 Sept. 1972.

33 Butler and Drakeford, *Scandal, Social Policy and Social Welfare*, p. 118.

34 British Newspaper Archive, www.britishnewspaperarchive.co.uk.

35 *Ward F13* (World in Action, 1968); *The Secret Hospital* (Yorkshire Television broadcast on 22 May 1979); *The Silent Minority* (Nigel Evans, ATV, broadcast in June 1981).

36 Jisc Library Hub Discover, https://discover.libraryhub.jisc.ac.uk.

37 'Ely Hospital: Hidden Now Heard', People's Collection Wales, https://www.peoplescollection.wales/collections/579951, accessed 27 Mar. 2021.

38 Department of Health and Social Security (DHSS), Whittingham Hospital, Lancs, Section 70 Inquiry, Appointment of Chairman and Members, TNA MH150/421/np.

39 NHS, *Report of the Committee of Inquiry into Whittingham Hospital*, para. 21; Martin, *Hospitals in Trouble*, pp. 13–4.
40 Whittingham Hospital, Committee of Inquiry, Transcript of Evidence, TNA MH150/425, 393 and 221.
41 Whittingham, Transcript of Evidence, TNA MH150/425, 261.
42 NHS, *Report of the Committee of Inquiry into Whittingham Hospital*, para. 51.
43 Ibid., para. 31.
44 Whittingham, Transcript of Evidence, TNA MH150/425, 229.
45 Ibid., 256–7.
46 NHS, *Findings and Recommendations*, para. 9, p. 66.
47 Butler and Drakeford, *Scandal, Social Policy and Welfare*, p. 221; see esp. Ch. 10 for a useful discussion on the analysis of inquiries.
48 NHS, *Findings and Recommendations*, para. 13, p. 71; para. 20, p. 24.
49 Kieran Walshe, 'Public Inquiry Methods, Processes and Outputs: An Epistemological Critique', *The Political Quarterly*, 90, 2 (2019), pp. 210–5.
50 Ibid., p. 214.
51 Ibid., p. 213.
52 Stanley and Manthorpe, 'Introduction', p. 8.
53 From our correspondent, 'Ely Nurses' Complaint on Report', *The Times*, 29 Mar. 1969.
54 Katie Barclay, 'The Practice and Ethics of the History of Emotions' in Barclay, Crozier-De Rosa and Stearns, *Sources for the History of Emotions*, pp. 26–37: p. 31.
55 Róisín Ryan-Flood and Rosalind Gill, 'Introduction' in Róisín Ryan-Flood and Rosalind Gill (eds), *Secrets and Silence in the Research Process. Feminist Reflections* (Abingdon: Routledge, 2010), pp. 1–11: p. 2.
56 Barclay, 'Practice and Ethics', p. 31.
57 Royal Historical Society, 'RHS Statement on Ethics (originally published December 2004)', https://royalhistsoc.org/?s=ethics; American Historical Association, 'Statement on Standards of Professional Conduct (updated 2019)', https://www.historians.org/jobs-and-professional-development/statements-standards-and-guidelines-of-the-discipline/statement-on-standards-of-professional-conduct. Links accessed 27 Mar. 2021.
58 The notion of 'emotional labour', how we manage our feelings dependent on the emotional requirements of our work, was first advanced by Arlie R. Hochschild, *The Managed Heart: Commercialization of Human Feeling* (Berkeley, CA: University of California Press, 1983).
59 Janet Fink, 'Foreword', in Tracey Loughran and Dawn Mannay (eds), *Emotion and the Researcher: Sites Subjectivities, and Relationships* (Bingley: Emerald, 2018), pp. xvii–xx: p. xix.
60 These included: DHSS, *Better Services for the Mentally Handicapped*, Cmnd. 4683 (London: HMSO, 1971); DHSS, *Services for Mental Illness Related to Old Age*, HM 72 (71) (London: HMSO, 1972); and DHSS, *Better Services for the Mentally Ill*, Cmnd. 6233 (London: HMSO, 1975).

Select bibliography

Butler, I. and Drakeford, M., *Scandal, Social Policy and Social Welfare*, 2nd edn, Basingstoke: Palgrave Macmillan, 2005.
Hide, L., 'Mental Hospitals, Social Exclusion and Public Scandals' in George Ikkos and Nick Bouras (eds), Mind, State and Society. Social History of Psychiatry and Mental Health in Britain 1960–2010 (Cambridge, Cambridge University Press, 2021), 60–67.
Hilton, C., *Improving Psychiatric Care for Older People. Barbara Robb's Campaign 1965–1976*, Cham, Switzerland: Palgrave Macmillan, 2017.
Hilton, C., 'A Tale of Two Inquiries: *Sans Everything* and Ely', *The Political Quarterly* 90, 2019, 185–193.
Martin, J.P. and Evans, D., *Hospitals in Trouble*, Oxford: Basil Blackwell, 1984.

Robb, B. (presented on behalf of AEGIS), *Sans Everything: A Case to Answer*, London: Nelson, 1967.

Stanley, N. and Manthorpe, J. (eds), *The Age of the Inquiry. Learning and Blaming in Health and Social Care*, London: Routledge, 2004.

Various authors, '50 Years of Inquiries in the National Health Service', *The Political Quarterly* 90, 2019, 180–244.

10

ACTIVIST SOURCES AND THE SURVIVOR MOVEMENT

Steffan Blayney

The history of psychiatry is a history of power and discipline, but it is also one of solidarity and resistance. This chapter will explore some of the ways in which people deemed 'mad' or 'mentally ill' have organised themselves in opposition to the medical and legal structures which have governed their lives. Rather than concentrating on mainstream pressure groups and charities, whose histories are often well established, my focus here is on self-organised, grassroots initiatives among psychiatric patients, about which much less has been written and for which documentary evidence is scarcer.

The organised movement for liberation and recognition among those who have been on the receiving end of psychiatric treatment has gone by a variety of names, and the people involved have identified in different ways at different times and in different contexts. As such, this chapter will refer at various points to mental patients, Mad activists, ex-patients, service users, and consumers, as well as to the terms with which probably the larger number of activists in the UK now identify – survivors, and the survivor movement. In doing so, I do not intend to express a political preference for one term over another – all of which have been contested – but where possible to use the terminology appropriate to the material being discussed. Likewise, in making reference at times to 'mental patients', 'mad' people, or 'lunatics' – terms which have often been used pejoratively, or which today may be considered offensive – I have tried to match my own words to those used by historical actors of the relevant period.

The chapter will start by giving a brief outline of the history of mental health activism, chiefly focusing on developments in Britain, before going on to discuss the practical difficulties of finding and accessing source documents relating to the survivor movement, and the different kinds of materials that make up the activist archive. I will explore the ways in which these sources can tell us not just about the history of activist movements, but of psychiatry more broadly, opening up

DOI: 10.4324/9781003087694-11

critical new perspectives on medical histories 'from below'. Finally, I will reflect on some of the theoretical contributions made by service user activists and historians and suggest how engaging with activist sources might change the ways in which we write histories of psychiatry.

A brief history of the survivor movement

For as long as psychiatry and asylums have existed they have been objects of controversy and criticism, subject to near-constant calls for reorganisation and reform. Going back several centuries, we can also find instances of individuals who have been diagnosed or institutionalised as insane speaking out against the ways they have been treated. The emergence of organised activism among those on the receiving end of psychiatry, however, is a decidedly modern phenomenon. There is little evidence of collective and sustained action among patients before the nineteenth century, or of anything that could be called a survivor *movement* before the twentieth.

The first well-documented instance of collective campaigning among people who had been designated mad is also a somewhat anomalous one, being separated from later survivor organisations both in time and by its social composition. Formed in 1845, the Alleged Lunatics' Friend Society brought together former asylum inmates who argued that they had been wrongfully incarcerated.[1] In contrast to most later survivor groups, its members were drawn from the elite of British society, with one of its founders, John Perceval, the son of assassinated Prime Minister Spencer Perceval. Often drawing on members' personal connections, the Society lobbied for changes in lunacy laws, particularly regarding procedures for certification, and sought to draw public attention to the 'cruel and improper' treatment of patients in asylums.[2] In some ways anticipating the kinds of advocacy work that would be taken up by later organisations, the group would also take up individual cases of incarcerated lunatics, providing legal advice, and in some cases managing to secure their release. Though the group remained active into the 1860s, there seems to have been little continuity between this early example of patient-led campaigning and the activist groups that would emerge in the following century. In the intervening decades, organised demands for reform within mental health instead came from non-patient led groups, politicians, and charity organisations.

For the purposes of this chapter, we will be looking at the sources of survivor activism as it emerged (or re-emerged) in the later part of the twentieth century. In a number of western countries, the late 1960s and early 1970s saw the near-simultaneous formation of self-organised campaigns among psychiatric patients and ex-patients. This was a period characterised by a wave of 'new social movements' globally – including the black civil rights movement, anti-war campaigns, student protests, and women's and gay liberation. The counterculture of the 1960s had also seen the popularisation of radical 'anti-psychiatrists', such as

R.D. Laing and David Cooper in the UK, who challenged dominant medical models of psychiatry from within the profession.

While the relationship between anti-psychiatry and patient-led liberation movements has been the subject of considerable controversy among historians and activists, some of the groups that formed at this time did coalesce around dissident professionals, even if some would later distance themselves. In Italy, for example, the *Psichiatria Democratica* movement, led by the reforming psychiatrist Franco Basaglia, campaigned throughout the 1960s and 1970s against the asylum system, establishing co-operatives of workers and patients in several cities as an alternative to traditional institutions, and eventually winning a change in the law to bring about the closure of asylums.[3] In West Germany, patients at the psychiatric hospital of the University of Heidelberg organised around the Marxist psychiatrist Wolfgang Huber, forming a general assembly of patients to establish the Socialist Patients Collective (or SPK).[4] Around the same time in France, the Asylums Information Group, initially created by a politicised grouping of junior psychiatrists, was itself rapidly taken over by psychiatric patients, who formed alliances with the professionals to campaign against their treatment.[5] Elsewhere, however, patient groups emerged independently. In North America, the early 1970s saw a wave of autonomous activism, with the Insane Liberation Front (Portland, Oregon), the Mental Patients' Liberation Project (New York), the Mental Patients' Liberation Front (Boston), the Mental Patients' Association (Vancouver), and the Network Against Psychiatric Assault (San Francisco), all formed in the years between 1970 and 1972.[6]

The most significant group to form in Britain in this period was the Mental Patients Union (MPU), established at the Paddington Day Hospital in London in March 1973.[7] While some professionals (psychiatric social workers rather than psychiatrists) were involved in starting the Union, full membership of the organisation was limited to patients and ex-patients. The MPU's founding *Declaration of Intent* condemned 'the institution of repressive and manipulative psychiatry', and announced its intention to 'represent mental patients wherever they require to be represented'.[8] By 1974, the organisation had evolved into a national Federation of Mental Patients' Unions, with groups in a number of British towns and cities, including branches in psychiatric institutions.

This initial wave of patient activism was characterised by an ethos of self-organisation and an uncompromising rejection of medical authority. The MPU had been preceded, in 1971, by the shorter-lived Scottish Union of Mental Patients, and also by the looser network of People Not Psychiatry, started in 1969, which aimed to provide non-medical alternatives to psychiatric institutionalisation.[9] Many of the members of these groups had links to left-wing politics and embraced the counterculture of the period. Later in the 1970s, some MPU members moved into new groups such as PROMPT (Protection of the Rights of Mental Patients in Therapy), which in 1985 became CAPO (Campaign Against Psychiatric Oppression), adopting the aesthetics of the contemporary punk scene and direct-action tactics influenced by radical political groups.

At the same time, however, from the mid 1980s, a new wave of user-led organisations was emerging which attempted to build a broader base of support – engaging with professionals, mainstream mental health charities, and non-survivor 'allies'. New initiatives within mental health services to solicit patient involvement in provision, for example through the 1990 NHS and Community Care Act, paved the way for a shift in terminology from 'patients' to 'consumers' and 'service users', facilitating a proliferation of patient representation and advocacy groups. This was also the period in which the term 'survivors' came into widespread currency, with Survivors Speak Out (SSO) formed in 1986 as a national network to facilitate and coordinate action among the growing number of local groups. The United Kingdom Advocacy Network (UKAN), formed in 1990, performed a similar national coordinating function, promoting individual and collective self-advocacy for users of mental health services. There were also new groups coalescing around particular diagnoses or issues in mental health, for example around voice-hearing, self-harm, and eating disorders, as well as groups of survivors linked by identity categories relating to race and ethnicity, gender and sexuality.[10]

From the late 1990s, activists under the banner of Mad Pride have increasingly embraced madness as an identity category in itself, with its own distinctive culture and community, and which is deserving of political recognition. Taking inspiration from Gay Pride and the struggles of other marginalised groups, these activists have sought to reclaim the term 'mad', rejecting the medicalisation of so-called psychological disorders and seeking to reverse the negative connotations associated with madness.

Finally, since the financial crash of 2008, and the imposition of austerity policies in the UK by Conservative-led governments, a new wave of politicised mental health activism has developed. This has been defined by opposition to cuts to services, and an emphasis on the psychological costs of socioeconomic deprivation and inequality under neoliberal capitalism. The increasing imbrication of mental health services with the welfare system has also seen growing overlap between survivor groups and disabled people's activism, in organisations such as Disabled People Against the Cuts, the Mental Health Resistance Network, and Recovery in the Bin.

Finding the activist archive

One of the major challenges facing the historian of survivor movements is finding relevant material. Much of what is produced by activist organisations is ephemeral, with posters, flyers, and correspondence often not kept. Many of the activities undertaken by such groups – meetings, protests, and other events – do not necessarily leave an archival trace. Unlike the medical journals of psychiatrists, the minute books of professional bodies, or the administrative records of asylums, the documents of the survivor movement have not always been carefully or systematically preserved. The activist archive gets dispersed among the various groups and individuals who create and use it, often remaining hidden in private homes, unknown or inaccessible to researchers.[11] While recent years have seen some efforts to link up these scattered collections or to catalogue their contents, gaining access to many of these materials can often be a hit-and-miss process of attempting to cultivate personal connections with groups or individuals.

Much of the historiography that exists about the survivor movement has been written by activists themselves, who have often taken a keen interest in recording and documenting their own history. As will be explored later, survivors telling their own stories or testifying to their own experiences can be an activist act in itself, a means of asserting ownership over experiences which have more often been framed in the words of others. One of the richest source bases for historians of survivor activism, then, are the accounts of the movement written by campaigners. Histories written by participants can blur the distinction between primary and secondary sources, combining research with personal memory, scholarship with auto-biography, and historical description with political interpretation.

One of the first book-length accounts of the activities and philosophy of the mental health liberation movement is the American survivor activist (and later historian) Judi Chamberlin's *On Our Own: Patient-Controlled Alternatives to the Mental Health System*.[12] First published in 1978, the book describes Chamberlin's involvement in the early activities of the Mental Patients' Liberation Front in Boston, and a number of other early survivor groups in the 1970s. Her account of the movement is enriched by conversations with other activists and excerpts from the campaign literature of the period, and an appendix to the book includes a 'list of alternative facilities, organisations, and publications', predominantly in the US, but also Canada, Belgium, England, France, the Netherlands, and New Zealand.

In the UK, too, the first histories of the movement were written by activists, with Peter Campbell's 1996 essay, 'The History of the User Movement in the United Kingdom', an important early example.[13] In 2003, a larger survivor-led research project into the movement and its history was published under the title *On Our Own Terms*, drawing on surveys and interviews with over 300 people active in user-led groups.[14] In 2005, building on these survivor-led approaches, a group of survivors and activists came together to form the Survivors History Group (SHG), initially conceived of as a project 'to rescue the physical history of the mental patients' movement from the skip'.[15] Over the years, the SHG has done an enormous amount of work to record and catalogue the various private collections of archival material held by individuals involved in the movement, as well as publishing its own histories, responding to the work of other historians, and creating forums – both online and in person – to discuss 'the contribution that mental health service users/survivors have made and are making to history'.[16]

Of particular importance and value to historians is the SHG website, created and maintained by Andrew Roberts, a founding member of the MPU and one of the movement's most prominent historians and archivists.[17] A sprawling en-terprise, the site contains a vast wealth of material for the historian of survivor movements including: timelines of mental health history and of survivor move-ments; bibliographies of secondary material on user movements, and of published and unpublished works by survivors; histories of the movement in the 1970s, 1980s, and 1990s written by activists from each period; and a catalogue (in progress) of the vast collection of archival material which Roberts currently holds at his home in London. A number of previously unpublished primary documents have also been made digitally available through the site, either scanned as images or typed, further opening up the activist archive and making it accessible to new audiences. The SHG website – through Roberts – has also acted as a hub for researchers keen to make contact with those active in the movement, or to make use of their personal archives.

Despite the lack of public collections dedicated to survivor activism in the UK, it is still possible to trace the history of the movement through traditional archives and libraries. While many of the more ephemeral publications have not been preserved, survivor activism has occasionally attracted wider attention and has left traces in less immediately obvious places. Often, this has been in archives associated with other radical or countercultural movements. Hannah Proctor, for example, has drawn on the archive of the socialist organisation Big Flame, held at the May Day Rooms in London, to uncover the story of Red Therapy, a leaderless self-help group started by left-wing activists in London in the late 1970s, while Sarah Crook has traced the development of similar groups within the Women's Liberation Movement through the feminist press.[18] For historians looking to follow stories of activism in radical publications, specialist archives like the Bishopsgate Institute and the Feminist Library in London, or the Working Class Movement Library in Salford, can provide a wealth of sources, as can the extensive collections of the British Library. The early history of the MPU, for example, can be traced sporadically through titles including *Time Out*, *Socialist Worker*, *Peace News*, and *People's News Service*, as well as in some of the smaller papers associated with radical psychology, such as *Red Rat* and *Humpty Dumpty*. More occasionally, survivor activism – and protests in particular – have caught the attention of the mainstream press, with local newspapers and local authority archives a good route for tracking the activities of smaller groups.

One of the few British publications relating to the survivor movement to be archived in its entirety is *Asylum: A Magazine for Democratic Psychiatry*, which has been published near-continuously since 1986. The complete back catalogue is now held at the Wellcome Library in London. While initially created by radical professionals – taking inspiration from the Italian *Psichiatria Democratica* movement – *Asylum* has from its earliest editions been an important and welcoming outlet for service users, and in recent years has given increasing precedence to survivor voices. A current project by Helen Spandler – a member of the magazine's editorial collective – has, among other things, shed light on *Asylum*'s longstanding coverage of service user activism and its links to the movement.[19] Early issues dedicated features to Survivors Speak Out and CAPO, while more recently editorial control has been given over to activist groups, such as the Mad Hatters of Bath, who presented a Mad Pride special issue in 2011.[20]

Spandler's work on *Asylum* also reminds us that the sources of survivor activism are not just textual. As she notes in a recent chapter, survivors have made effective use of visual 'styles of contestation', in particular cartoons and comic strips, as a means of conveying political messages in concise and accessible ways, with activists often deploying humour as a 'form of covert resistance'.[21] In survivor activism, jokes, cartoons, illustrations, and other creative forms have featured prominently. Some of the radical groups of the 1980s had strong links to London's alternative music scene, and would often combine protest with performance, a tradition continued in later decades through Mad Pride's 'celebration of mad culture'.[22] Frank Bangay, an activist with PROMPT and CAPO, has also been a key figure in the Survivors' Poetry movement, seeing poetry as a way 'to help change attitudes and break barriers down'.[23] His 1999 collection, *Naked Songs and Rhythms of Hope*, combines poetry and drawing with annotations on his experiences of psychiatric treatment and his involvement in activism.[24] When read alongside other activist sources, such documents can provide a valuable personal or emotional perspective often missing from more directly political publications.

As well as the written and visual records that we can discover in these diverse activist archives, historians of the survivor movement have also made use of oral history interviews. The comparatively recent development of survivor activism as a phenomenon means that talking to people directly involved even in the early years of the movement's history is often still possible, and the relative scarcity of easily accessible documentary sources has made this an attractive option for historians and other researchers.[25] The particular challenges of oral history are covered in Victoria Hoyle's chapter in this volume.

As we approach the present day, the archive of survivor activism is increasingly being created online. The internet has made possible resources like the SHG website, the uploading and sharing of documents, photographs, and videos which might previously have languished in attics, and the forging of new connections between activists and historians. At the same time, for groups active today, the internet is increasingly a site of activism in its own right, and social media pages in particular are becoming an immediate repository for the archives of contemporary social movements.[26]

In some ways, these social and technological developments promise an abundance of source material for historians of activism, with a range of new media and visual formats, such as memes, requiring researchers' scrutiny.[27] At the same time, however, the accelerated pace of production and consumption of activist content online, and the dependence for its preservation on private companies whose approaches to the collection and use of data are often extremely opaque, in some ways make this new kind of archive even more precarious and ephemeral than the physical documents of earlier groups. In addition, while social media promises a wealth of new source material, the repurposing by researchers of posts made online from personal accounts – particularly when they discuss an individual's medical history or their political activity – raises difficult questions around anonymity and informed consent. How researchers should manage or engage with the vast amounts of data created daily online is a methodological and ethical problem which has only recently begun to be theorised, but it is one that historians of survivor activism will increasingly need to pay attention to.[28]

Activist sources and the history of psychiatry

Beyond the important task of reconstructing the history of the survivor movement itself, activist sources can also be a valuable resource for historians of psychiatry more broadly. Since the 1980s, the discipline has been increasingly concerned with writing histories 'from below'. Rather than approaching the history of psychiatry from the perspective of the medical profession – looking at the evolution of diagnoses or particular treatments, for example – this kind of history instead privileges, as an influential 1985 essay by Roy Porter put it, 'the patient's view'.[29]

Building on Porter's work, Anne Rogers and David Pilgrim suggested in a 1990 article, built around interviews with activists, that research on the mental health service user movement could provide an 'alternative perspective' to professional and academic discourses which tend towards depicting the patient 'as existing as a by-product of a particular clinical gaze'. Rather than viewing those in psychiatric care as 'passive victims of government policy', or as a mere effect of 'economic and social structures' beyond their control, this type of work could emphasise the agency of psychiatric patients, and their collective role in establishing new agendas in the field of mental health.[30] However, with a few notable exceptions (often from survivor researchers), activist material has remained a significantly underused resource among even those historians of medicine who have attempted to foreground patient voices.

Psychiatric histories from below have often relied on memoirs, autobiographies, diaries, and other forms of first person life-writing – often written by middle- or upper-class patients. Rather than a fundamental reorientation of the historical perspective, critics have argued, the result has been an accumulation of individual cases, which remain 'enclosed in their singularity', and which are heavily determined both by the social positionality of the author and by the narrative conventions of published memoirs.[31] Moreover, in taking Porter's lead and focusing on the 'medical encounter' between patient and doctor, historians have often ended up reproducing a narrow understanding of the patient only insofar as they have been constructed through their interaction with medicine. Few have taken up Rogers and Pilgrim's call for a greater understanding of 'the wider collective role of consumers as a group within civil society', or even as a 'movement'.[32]

In contrast to the individual memoir, activist sources can often provide historians with a more collective approach to survivor testimony. The 1986 film *We're Not Mad, We're Angry*, for example, originally broadcast on Channel 4's *Eleventh Hour* programme (and currently available on YouTube), was created collaboratively by patients and activists, with full editorial control of the production.[33] The hour-long film is composed mostly of direct-to-camera interviews, with survivors detailing their experiences of mental illness and the psychiatric system, both in hospital and in the community. Participants describe being sectioned under the Mental Health Act, and living with the stigma attached to psychiatric diagnoses. They discuss their experiences of psychiatric medication, occupational therapy, and forced treatment including electroconvulsive therapy (ECT). They describe abuse and humiliation at the hands of staff, and institutional racism, sexism, and homophobia. In a series of short narrative segments, written by Peter Campbell and performed by fellow survivors, the 'patient's view' is literalised through the camera, as the viewer is placed in the shoes of 'Alice', adopting her perspective via long, continuous point-of-view shots, as we follow her through the psychiatric system.

One objection to drawing on activist sources of this kind as a source for understanding the psychiatric system might be that activists are not 'typical' service users, or representative of the wider patient experience. It might be argued that most people who are diagnosed with a mental health condition, or who use mental health services, do not become activists, and the negative portrayals of psychiatry within activist sources are therefore unlikely to be reflective of wider currents of opinion. On closer inspection, though, such arguments are difficult to sustain. Throughout the history of the survivor movement, activists have been dismissed in similar terms, and not just by historians. As the authors of *On Our Own Terms* put it:

> Many of us have been accused of not being typical users. We are told we are too articulate and educated, or too angry and radical, too well, too ill, or in some way different from the majority of 'ordinary' service users. Most often that accusation comes from professionals, but sometimes it comes from other service users/survivors. It can leave us rather confused. Who are the 'ordinary' service users? Are they the ones with the most severe and acute problems, which leave them too vulnerable to cope with involvement? Or are they people who are being made better by their treatment and don't wish to complain?[34]

As activists have often been the first to point out, there is no such thing as the 'typical' patient, or a single, uncomplicated survivor 'experience'. Neither are survivor activists themselves a homogenous 'community'. User groups have encompassed a wide range of ideological viewpoints, tactical strategies, and positions with respect to controversial issues such as diagnosis, medication, and the role of non-survivor 'allies'. As the survivor activist and academic Diana Rose has demonstrated, 'there is a difference between being "representative" and striving to "represent" a collective discourse of contention, collaboration and change'.[35] Precisely because activists do speak out – arguably insofar as they *are* unrepresentative in this sense – their contributions are of use to historians seeking to understand how the mental health care system operates in practice, disturbing easy narratives of medical hegemony and psychiatric progress.

Because the politics of mental health liberation are so often grounded in people's experiences of psychiatric systems, activist materials can provide us with important information about how these systems have worked in practice that is unlikely to be recorded in official sources. In forming the Scottish Union of Mental Patients, for example, patients at Hartwood Hospital produced a list of 'tabulated grievances and some suggested remedies', which they presented to visiting Mental Welfare Commissioners in 1971. The document, held in the private SHG archive but also summarised and quoted on the website, contains accounts of specific injustices committed against individual patients, as well as more general complaints about conditions, with demands ranging from the abolition of the parole system and the stratification of patients to improving the quality of food in the hospital canteen.[36] A little under two years later, the MPU produced their own *Declaration of Intent*, following a meeting of over 100 patients from across the UK. In the document (the full text of which is also available on the SHG website), activists highlight censorship of communications by hospital authorities, confiscation of patients' clothing and personal belongings, the forcible detention of 'voluntary' patients, the exploitation of patients' labour through occupational therapy, lack of informed consent in treatment, the use of 'treatments' as punishments, and the use of solitary confinement for resistant or difficult patients.[37]

Frequently, groups have attempted to canvass the wider population of service users to gather information on their experiences and opinions of psychiatric treatment. One of the first projects of the MPU, for example, was to design a questionnaire to be distributed to members and in hospitals, inviting respondents to detail their own medical history, their experiences of psychiatric treatment, and their concerns and complaints. The returned forms provide a snapshot of psychiatry in the early 1970s, with a diverse collection of views from patients from a range of types of institution. Together, they help us to build a picture of some of the ways in which individuals were able to negotiate institutionalisation and treatment, or to understand or influence their own situations. One woman describes a two-year involuntary stay at a Welsh psychiatric institution and her fears of readmission: 'I am afraid to be myself in case I find myself back in hospital. I am acting a part and sometimes I get desperately tired of it.' In hospital she finds herself 'having to exercise an iron self control in case display of feeling got me a "bad mark"'. Another respondent from a London hospital recalls: 'The staff was all right if you dident [*sic*] bother them with your problems.'[38]

Service user groups have also produced practical materials to help people navigate the psychiatric system, often explicitly promoted as alternatives to information provided through official channels. In 1975, MPU activists in London researched and published *A Directory of the Side Effects of Psychiatric Drugs*, a ten-page pamphlet aimed at helping patients understand the risks associated with common medications, now held in the SHG's private collection.[39] In Manchester, the local MPU branch published *Your Rights in Mental Hospital*, outlining the provisions of the Mental Health Act as they pertained to patients, and their operations in practice. 'The law gives power over you to your nearest relative, your social worker, your GP, your psychiatrist, the hospital, the Home Secretary and the police', wrote the authors of the latter pamphlet. 'We think that part of getting better is taking some of that power back. To do this ... you need to understand the situation you're in.'[40] In the same vein, from the 1980s onwards, with the rise of 'user participation' in mental health care, survivor groups produced or contributed to a variety of practical guides to patient representation and self-advocacy.

With the emergence of Mad Pride over the last two decades, and its celebration and promotion of Mad culture, historians can now draw upon a whole range of activist sources that take us beyond the medical encounter and the hospital, expanding beyond conventional narratives of illness, treatment, and recovery to embrace a range of genres, topics, and styles. The movement has emphasised, as the editors of an eclectic 2003 *Mad Pride* writing collection put it, 'that "madness" is as much to do with sex, drugs and rock 'n' roll [as] with the "long echoing corridors" described repeatedly by survivor poets'.[41] Perhaps the creative and experimental output of writers and artists associated with Mad Pride can help historians of psychiatry find our way out of our own narrow asylum corridors, to begin to approach survivor subjectivities and cultures in a fuller and more expansive light.

Activism and the practice of history

As we have seen, survivor activists have often been deeply invested in writing the history of their own movement. Mental health activism and historiography have often been intimately intertwined, with history-writing a key means by which survivors have been able to assert their status as political actors and agents of change, challenging the passive status too often ascribed to them by both the medical establishment and conventional histories of psychiatry. 'Like other liberation struggles of oppressed people,' Judi Chamberlin wrote in 1990, 'the activism of former psychiatric patients has been frequently ignored or discredited. Only when a group begins to emerge from subjugation can it begin to reclaim its own history.'[42] More recently Jayasree Kalathil has emphasised the importance of documenting developments within the survivor movement (in this context as they relate to the involvement of Black and ethnic minority service users) as a means to 'learn from our experiences, celebrate our achievements and create our own history'.[43] Establishing the long-term continuity of survivor activism has helped to provide a 'usable past' for campaigners, who have been able to draw on the history of the movement for encouragement, inspiration, and models of action.[44]

Beyond the movement's own history, survivor activism has also contested mainstream histories of psychiatry more broadly, and in doing so, poses important challenges to the practice of historians in the field. These critiques have centred broadly on three interrelated questions: the place of survivor stories within the history of psychiatry, the subject-position of the person telling these stories, and what counts as legitimate historical evidence or source material.

These debates were spectacularly dramatised in 1997, when the Bethlem and Maudsley NHS Trust announced plans to 'celebrate' the 750th anniversary of the notorious Bethlem Royal Hospital with a series of public events, and an exhibition at the Museum of London. Despite plans for a single 'user's day' to be included within the programme of events, there had been no consultation with current or ex-patients and, crucially, the stories of survivors were excluded from the version of history espoused by the Trust. Many of those involved in user activism saw nothing to celebrate in 'a history that from its earliest days reveals a familiar catalogue of inquiries, scandals, abuse and inhumanity', and challenged the exhibition's presentation of medical history 'in classic modernist terms of centuries of progress, culminating in modern psychiatry and the Maudsley Hospital'.[45]

In response, the Reclaim Bedlam campaign, started by Pete Shaughnessy – a former Maudsley patient active in local user groups – sought to challenge both the exclusion of survivors inherent in the anniversary events and to present an alternative narrative to that promoted by the hospital: a 'commemoration' of the lives of those who had suffered, and continued to suffer, under psychiatry's regime, as opposed to a 'celebration' of medical progress.[46] Protestors held a carnival 'picnic' – 'Raving in the Park' – at the former Bethlem site at the Imperial War Museum, and picketed an anniversary 'thanksgiving' service at St Paul's Cathedral, holding a minute's silence 'for people who have died of distress or at the hands of the mental health system over 750 years'.[47]

Reclaiming psychiatry's history for survivors has meant contesting the narratives that are presented and used by historians, the medical profession, and other non-survivor organisations. Events and projects organised by activist groups – such as the Health Through History writing collective run by Tower Hamlets African and Caribbean Mental Health Organisation, the Oor Mad History initiative among survivor groups in Lothian, Scotland, or the Pageant of Survivor History organised by F.E.E.L. (Friends of East London Loonies) in 2011 – have decentred professional knowledge and celebrated survivor histories. At the same time, campaigns like Reclaim Bedlam have also been about challenging who can legitimately tell such histories in the present, about what kinds of evidence or knowledge should be privileged in the telling, and the political implications that different kinds of histories entail. Writing a year after the Bedlam anniversary, the activist and academic Peter Beresford argued that 'if mental health service users/ survivors are to take charge of our future', then it was essential also to take back control of a past, which, 'at both individual and collective levels, has been largely appropriated, denied, controlled and reinterpreted by other powerful interests'.[48]

Adopting the imperative of 'nothing about us without us' developed within the wider disability rights movement, activists in recent years have asserted the need for research in mental health to include not only the perspectives but the active participation of those on the receiving end of psychiatric treatment, 'balancing the overwhelming majority of material written about those who are labelled mad by those who do the labelling and those who study them'.[49] Participatory forms of research have championed the value of previously marginalised 'experiential' knowledge, challenging positivist and professional-centred approaches to mental health and advocating constructive dialogue between researcher and researched.[50]

While these conversations have so far largely taken place in relation to health research and the design of services, recent activist interventions, particularly in the burgeoning field of Mad Studies, remind us that not only medical professionals, but also historians can be counted among 'those who study those who are labelled mad', and have often been complicit – even as 'allies' – in the exclusions, co-options, and unequal power relationships that survivors have sought to challenge.[51] As the Survivors History Group have argued, whereas 'the academic historian/sociologist may only be concerned to find some rough fit between theoretical models and data ... the detail of history matters to us because it bears on our lives and our heritage'.[52] Foundational to the SHG project is the principle that 'service users own their history'.[53]

For historians of psychiatry – particularly those who are not mental health service users or survivors themselves – the challenges posed by these interventions are substantial, but taking them seriously can enrich our practice. We might think, for example, about how models of 'co-production' pioneered in survivor research might be applied to the work of history, bearing in mind the historian Katie Barclay's observation that 'all encounters with others, but not least through writing, involve at least two people'.[54] This would mean handling survivor source material – whether an interview with a living person sitting in front of you, or an anonymous scrap of writing in an archive – with an attitude of openness and collaboration; seeing service users not simply 'as a source of experiential data', as Peter Beresford and Jan Wallcraft put it, but 'as creators of our own analysis and theory'.[55]

In this chapter I have tried to emphasise the value of activist sources not just as a narrow window onto the history of the survivor movement, critical though such histories are, but as a diverse body of work which can provide new perspectives on the history of psychiatry more broadly. In setting out the range of activist materials available for research, I have hopefully suggested some promising leads for other historians to pursue. The sources referred to here give only a glimpse of the range of groups, activities, and political orientations which have characterised the survivor movement in recent history, and – largely due to my own research limitations – have been drawn almost exclusively from the British movement. As new research into the global dimensions of the survivor movement is demonstrating, there are many more unexplored source bases for historians to investigate, and with the activist archive being added to daily online and on the streets, there will be plenty of opportunities for new histories to be written.[56]

Notes

1 Nicholas Hervey, 'Advocacy or Folly: The Alleged Lunatics' Friend Society, 1845–63', *Medical History*, 30, 3 (1986), pp. 245–75.

2 Alleged Lunatics' Friend Society pamphlet (1846), quoted in Sarah Wise, *Inconvenient People: Lunacy, Liberty, and the Mad-Doctors in England* (Berkeley, CA: Counterpoint, 2013), p. 79.

3 John Foot, *The Man Who Closed the Asylums: Franco Basaglia and the Revolution in Mental Health Care* (London: Verso, 2015).

4 Helen Spandler, 'To Make an Army out of Illness: A History of the Socialist Patients' Collective Heidelberg 1970–2', *Asylum*, 6, 4 (1992), pp. 5–12.

5 Jacques Lagrange, 'Course Context', in Michel Foucault, *Psychiatric Power: Lectures at the Collège de France, 1973–1974*, ed. Jacques Lagrange, trans. Graham Burchell (New York: Picador, 2008), p. 353.

6 Judi Chamberlin, 'The Ex-Patients' Movement: Where We've Been and Where We're Going', *Journal of Mind and Behaviour*, 11, 3 (1990), pp. 326–7.

7 Helen Spandler, *Asylum to Action: Paddington Day Hospital, Therapeutic Communities and Beyond* (London: Jessica Kingsley Publishers, 2006), pp. 52–67.

8 Survivors History Group Archive (SHG), Mental Patients' Union, *Declaration of Intent* (1973).

9 Mark Gallagher, 'From Asylum to Action in Scotland: The Emergence of the Scottish Union of Mental Patients, 1971–2', *History of Psychiatry*, 28, 1 (2017), pp. 101–14; Michael Barnett, *People Not Psychiatry* (London: Allen & Unwin, 1973).

10 For examples see Adam James, *Raising Our Voices: An Account of the Hearing Voices Movement* (Gloucester: Handsell Publishing, 2001); Mark Cresswell and Tom Brock, 'Social Movements, Historical Absence and the Problematization of Self-Harm in the UK, 1980–2000', *Journal of Critical Realism*, 16, 1 (2017), pp. 7–25; Jayasree Kalathil, *Dancing to Our Own Tunes: Reassessing Black and Minority Ethnic Mental Health Service User Involvement* (National Survivor User Network in collaboration with Catch-a-Fiya, 2008).

11 Sarah Chaney, 'Where Is the Survivor Archive?,' *Wellcome Library* (blog), 15 Dec. 2016, http://blog.wellcomelibrary.org/2016/12/where-is-the-survivor-archive, last accessed 5 Dec. 2020.

12 Judi Chamberlin, *On Our Own: Patient-Controlled Alternatives to the Mental Health System* (New York: McGraw-Hill, 1979).

13 Peter Campbell, 'The History of the User Movement in the United Kingdom', in Tom Heller, Jill Reynolds, Roger Gomm, Rosemary Mustin, and Stephen Pattison (eds), *Mental Health Matters: A Reader* (Basingstoke: Macmillan, 1996), pp. 218–25.

14 Jan Wallcraft, Jim Read, and Angela Sweeney, *On Our Own Terms: Users and Survivors of Mental Health Services Working Together for Support and Change* (London: The Sainsbury Centre for Mental Health, 2003).

15 Andrew Roberts, 'History as Research Method: The Survivors History Group,' *Andrew Roberts' Home Page*, 2010, http://studymore.org.uk/hisnot.htm, last accessed 5 Dec. 2020.

16 Survivors History Group, 'Survivors History – Mental Health and Survivors' Movements and Context,' *Andrew Roberts' Home Page*, 2005, http://studymore.org.uk/MPU.HTM, accessed 5 Dec. 2020.

17 Ibid.

18 Hannah Proctor, 'Lost Minds: Sedgwick, Laing and the Politics of Mental Illness', *Radical Philosophy*, 197 (2016), pp. 45–6; Sarah Crook, 'The Women's Liberation Movement, Activism and Therapy at the Grassroots, 1968–1985', *Women's History Review*, 27, 7 (2018), pp. 1152–68.

19 Helen Spandler, '*Asylum*: A Magazine for Democratic Psychiatry in England', in Tom Burns and John Foot (eds), *Basaglia's International Legacy: From Asylum to Community* (Oxford: Oxford University Press, 2020), pp. 205–26.

20 'Survivors Speak Out Conference in September '87,' *Asylum*, 2, 1 (1987), p. 5; 'The CAPO Interview', *Asylum*, 3, 3 (1989), pp. 5–8; *Asylum*, 18, 1 (The Mad Hatters of Bath Take Over the Asylum) (2011).

21 Helen Spandler, 'Crafting Psychiatric Contention through Single-Panel Cartoons,' in Susan Merrill Squier and Irmela Marei Krüger-Fürhoff (eds), *PathoGraphics: Narrative, Aesthetics, Contention, Community* (University Park: Penn State University Press, 2020), pp. 115–34.

22 Robert Dellar, Ted Curtis, and Esther Leslie (eds), *Mad Pride: A Celebration of Mad Culture* (London: Chipmunka, 2003). See also Robert Dellar, *Splitting in Two: Mad Pride and Punk Rock Oblivion* (London: Unkant Publishers, 2014).

23 Frank Bangay, 'An Uphill Struggle, but It's Been Worth It,' in Dellar et al., *Mad Pride*, pp. 101–4: p. 101.

24 Frank Bangay, *Naked Songs and Rhythms of Hope: An Illustrated Collection of Poems from 1974 to 1999* (London: Spare Change Books, 1999).

25 See for example, Anne Rogers and David Pilgrim, '"Pulling down Churches": Accounting for the British Mental Health Users' Movement', *Sociology of Health & Illness*, 13, 2 (1991), pp. 129–48; Spandler, *Asylum to Action*; Nick Crossley, *Contesting Psychiatry: Social Movements in Mental Health* (Abingdon: Routledge, 2006).

26 Cayce Myers and James F. Hamilton, 'Social Media as Primary Source: The Narrativization of Twenty-First-Century Social Movements', *Media History*, 20, 4 (2014), pp. 431–44.

27 Lucy Johnson, '#Relatable: An Ethnography of Mental Health Memes on Instagram', MSc dissertation, University of Glasgow, 2018.

28 For discussions of some of these problems see Jack Dougherty and Kristen Nawrotzki (eds), *Writing History in the Digital Age* (Ann Arbor, MI: University of Michigan Press, 2013); Kandy Woodfield (ed.), *The Ethics of Online Research* (Bingley: Emerald Publishing, 2018).

29 Roy Porter, 'The Patient's View: Doing Medical History from Below', *Theory and Society*, 14, 2 (1985), pp. 175–98.

30 Rogers and Pilgrim, '"Pulling down Churches"', pp. 129–30.

31 Alexandra Bacopoulos-Viau and Aude Fauvel, 'The Patient's Turn Roy Porter and Psychiatry's Tales, Thirty Years On', *Medical History*, 60, 1 (2016), pp. 1–18: p. 12. See Flurin Condrau, 'The Patient's View Meets the Clinical Gaze', *Social History of Medicine* 20, 3 (2007), pp. 525–40.

32 Rogers and Pilgrim, '"Pulling down Churches"', p. 130.

33 *We're Not Mad, We're Angry* (Albany Videos, 1986), https://www.youtube.com/watch?v=qD36m1mveoY, accessed 22 Oct. 2020.

34 Wallcraft, Read, and Sweeney, *On Our Own Terms*, p. 32.

35 Diana Rose, 'A Hidden Activism and Its Changing Contemporary Forms: Mental Health Service Users/Survivors Mobilising', *Journal of Social and Political Psychology* 6, 2 (2018), pp. 728–44: p. 736.

36 Survivors History Group Archive, Scottish Union of Mental Patients, 'Tabulated Grievances and Some Suggested Remedies – These are for the Attention of the Mental Welfare Commissioners' (1971). See http://studymore.org.uk/MPU.HTM#SUMPbox, accessed 15 Mar. 2021.

37 Mental Patients' Union, *Declaration of Intent*. See http://studymore.org.uk/MPU.HTM#MPUDeclaration, accessed 15 Mar. 2021.

38 Survivors History Group Archive, MPU Questionnaire Answers (1973).

39 Survivors History Group Archive, Chris Hill, Joan Martin, and Andrew Roberts, *A Directory of the Side Effects of Psychiatric Drugs* (Oct. 1975).

40 Private collection (Terry Simpson, Leeds), Manchester Mental Patients' Union, *Your Rights in Mental Hospital* (c.1977), p. 1. A copy of this is also held at the British Library.

41 Robert Dellar, Ted Curtis, and Esther Leslie, 'Introduction', in Dellar et al., *Mad Pride*, pp. 7–8: p. 8.

42 Chamberlin, 'The Ex-Patients' Movement', p. 323.

43 Kalathil, *Dancing to Our Own Tunes*, p. 5.

44 Nick Crossley, 'Working Utopias and Social Movements: An Investigation Using Case Study Materials from Radical Mental Health Movements in Britain', *Sociology*, 33, 4 (1999), pp. 809–30.

45 Peter Beresford, 'Past Tense. On the Need for a Survivor-Controlled Museum of Madness', *OpenMind* (May/Jun. 1998), http://studymore.org.uk/mpuhist.htm, accessed 15 Mar. 2021.

46 Pete Shaughnessy, 'Into the Deep End', in Dellar et al., *Mad Pride*, pp. 20–22.

47 Crossley, *Contesting Psychiatry*, p. 205. Even for such relatively recent events as these, few documents have been kept, with those that survive mostly in private collections. Researchers such as Crossley have relied on interviews with participants, as well as the brief reports that appeared in some contemporary newspapers.

48 Beresford, 'Past Tense'.

49 David Crepaz-Keay and Jayasree Kalathil, 'Introduction', in Jayasree Kalathil (ed.), *Personal Narratives of Madness* (Oxford: Oxford University Press, 2013), https://global. oup.com/booksites/content/9780199579563/narratives/, accessed 15 Mar. 2021.

50 Alison Faulkner, 'Survivor Research and Mad Studies: The Role and Value of Experiential Knowledge in Mental Health Research', *Disability & Society*, 32, 4 (2017), pp. 500–20.

51 Jasna Russo and Peter Beresford, 'Between Exclusion and Colonisation: Seeking a Place for Mad People's Knowledge in Academia', *Disability & Society*, 30, 1 (2015), pp. 153–7.

52 Survivors History Group, 'Survivors History Group Takes a Critical Look at Historians', in Marian Barnes and Phil Cotterell (eds), *Critical Perspectives on User Involvement* (Bristol: Policy, 2012), pp. 7–18: p. 17.

53 Roberts, 'History as Research Method'.

54 Katie Barclay, 'Falling in Love with the Dead', *Rethinking History*, 22, 4 (2018), pp. 459–73: p. 465.

55 Peter Beresford and Jan Wallcraft, 'Psychiatric System Survivors and Emancipatory Research: Issues, Overlaps and Differences', in Colin Barnes and Geof Mercer (eds), *Doing Disability Research* (Leeds: The Disability Press, 1997), pp. 66–87: p. 73.

56 See, for example, the Wellcome Trust and King's College London's EURIKHA initiative, 'a global research project looking at the emergence of social movements which privilege the rights and perspectives of people who experience severe mental distress.' 'Who Are We, and Why Are We Here?,' EURIKHA, 19 Feb. 2018, https://www. eurikha.org/blog/who-are-we-and-why-are-we-here/, accessed 15 Mar. 2021.

Select bibliography

Barnes, M. and Cotterell, P. (eds), *Critical Perspectives on User Involvement*, Bristol: Policy, 2012.

Chamberlin, J., 'The Ex-Patients' Movement: Where We've Been and Where We're Going', *Journal of Mind and Behaviour* 11, 1990, pp. 326–327.

Crossley, N., *Contesting Psychiatry: Social Movements in Mental Health*, Abingdon: Routledge, 2006.

Dellar, R., Curtis, T., & Leslie, E. (eds), *Mad Pride: A Celebration of Mad Culture*, London: Chipmunka, 2003.

Gallagher, M., 'From Asylum to Action in Scotland: The Emergence of the Scottish Union of Mental Patients, 1971–2', *History of Psychiatry* 28, 2017, pp. 101–114.

Hervey, N., 'Advocacy or Folly: The Alleged Lunatics' Friend Society, 1845–63', *Medical History* 30, 1986, pp. 245–275.

Kalathil, J. (ed.), *Personal Narratives of Madness*, Oxford: Oxford University Press, 2013.

Rose, D., 'A Hidden Activism and Its Changing Contemporary Forms: Mental Health Service Users/Survivors Mobilising', *Journal of Social and Political Psychology* 6, 2018, pp. 728–744.

Russo, J. & Beresford, P., 'Between Exclusion and Colonisation: Seeking a Place for Mad People's Knowledge in Academia', *Disability & Society* 30, 2015, pp. 153–7.

Spandler, H., '*Asylum*: A Magazine for Democratic Psychiatry in England', in T. Burns and J. Foot (eds), *Basaglia's International Legacy: From Asylum to Community*, Oxford: Oxford University Press, 2020, pp. 205–226.

11

PATIENTS, PRACTITIONERS, AND PROTESTORS: FEMINIST SOURCES AND APPROACHES IN THE HISTORY OF PSYCHIATRY

Sarah Crook

One of the most famous images of psychiatry in action is also one of the most provocative – or useful – to feminist historians of psychiatry. In the picture (see Figure 12.3 in Chapter 12 of this volume, p. 203), Jean-Martin Charcot (1825–1893), a French neurologist and advocate of the use of hypnosis to investigate hysteria, stands close to a young woman. Her white blouse slips down her exposed shoulders and décolleté; her neck and arms drape backwards; she is supported by a male attendant. Charcot's gaze is not on her – although with her exposed skin and vulnerable dress she draws the eye of the viewer – but on his male audience. To the left of the picture is a group of smartly dressed men, apparently appreciatively listening to Charcot's enunciation of his expertise. Several are writing, others lean forwards in their interest. The men are fully dressed; the young female hysteric is exposed. The seated men look to the male expert; the female patient alone looks outwards towards the viewer. Her gaze does not unambiguously meet ours, though: her eyes may be closing. Two female attendants stand on the right periphery of the picture, one leaning towards the patient. The picture, from 1887, intends to depict Charcot demonstrating hysteria at the Parisian hospital, the Salpêtrière. What it depicts to those attentive to the gendered dimensions of the history of psychiatry, however, is something else: the gendered dimensions of the location of expertise, authority, and psychiatric power. The young female patient, Blanche Wittman, is at the mercy of the male authority figure. The men listen to the pronouncements of the male expert. Female healthcare workers are relegated to a peripheral, ancillary role.

This is, of course, an interpretation of a painting that can only show a partial snapshot of the practice of mental health care at a particular historical moment. For example, in the 1970s the French feminist Hélène Cixous evoked ways that hysteria, could be mobilised by women as a mode of socially acceptable rebellion at a point where there were few such outlets.[1] Perhaps the young woman is not a

DOI: 10.4324/9781003087694-12

victim of patriarchal medicine but is rather subverting its power for her own ends. This interpretation, in turn, was challenged by other scholars, who pointed to hysteria's limited efficacy as a mode of revolt. Other historians have looked at how hysteria, as a gendered diagnosis, was used to uphold the exclusion of women from the political and public realm at a time of increasing political agitation and rapid social change. Others have pointed to the racial and racist implications of hysteria in nineteenth-century psychiatry; hysteria, it has been argued, was a diagnosis that was associated with white women, whose nervous 'over-civilisation' was contrasted with the robust, fertile bodies of Black women.[2] Regardless of interpretative frame, the picture, like other sources feminist historians use in the history of psychiatry, raises questions of power, authority, and expertise, and how these have been shaped by gender in the long history of the mind sciences.

This chapter has three aims: first, it seeks to establish the types of sources that historians can use to understand women's experiences as both patients and practitioners in the history of psychiatry; second, it seeks to set out how sources can be used to examine the history of psychiatry from a feminist angle; third, it seeks to chart the development of the feminist historiography of psychiatry. Feminist perspectives on the history of the psy professions are not homogenous in their approaches and goals. Sources for feminist histories of psychiatry are not restricted to materials produced by feminists, or even women. Instead, they are sources that have the potential to be used to expose how psychiatry has shaped, and been shaped by, ideas about gender and power. Feminist research might seek to draw women's contributions to the intellectual development of a set of ideas to the fore, for example, or it might focus on the mechanisms by which psychiatry has played a role in the oppression and subjugation of women, or it might examine how women have organised to dispute and challenge psychiatric orthodoxies. Put another way, the questions that feminist studies of the history of the psy professions might ask range from, for example, 'what have women contributed to the development of psychoanalytic theory?' to 'how did the diagnosis of hysteria enforce gender norms in Victorian Britain?' to 'why did American women's movements contest psychiatric power?'

Feminist approaches to the history of psychiatry, then, can draw upon intellectual history, cultural history, social history, political history, and histories of activism, to name just a few. What feminist perspectives in this area generally have in common, however, is their attentiveness to the location and utilisation of power in psychiatric practice and how this acts upon gendered lines; a critical approach to how psychiatric thought has played a role in delineating male- and female-associated roles and qualities in line with the view that these qualities are cultural constructions, and are thus historically contingent; and an interest in the ways that ideas about mental health have shaped women's experiences in the world. Feminist approaches to the history of psychiatry tend to focus on women and the construction of femininity – and it is this that this chapter emphasises – but feminist ideas have played a formative role in enabling a broader gendered critique of psychiatry and how it shaped ideas about masculinity and sexuality, too.

The emphasis on how gender has acted as an important vector in the history of psychiatry does not, however, mean that feminist approaches to the history of psychiatry can or should ignore other axes of difference. In 1989 legal scholar Kimberlé Crenshaw influentially articulated the idea that structures around gender and race interact, particularly in the lives of Black women, terming such a frame 'intersectionality'.[3] This intersectional position – that studies of race need to be alive to the power structures around gender, and that studies of gender need to be attentive to the effects of racial discrimination and privilege – has come to be essential to feminist work. Another mode of difference that is critical to the history of psychiatry is class. Historians have shown that certain diagnoses have been associated with social privilege (for example, neurasthenia, an illness manifesting in a diffuse set of symptoms attributed to a depletion of mental energy) while, as Louise Hide's work has shown, class shaped patients' experiences in English asylums.[4] While this chapter focuses on British and American sources and approaches, it is important to acknowledge the rich work that explores the gendered dimensions of colonial psychiatry and the ways that race and psychiatry interacted in colonial and racist regimes.[5]

The history of feminist critiques of psychiatry

While doing a feminist history of psychiatry does not rely upon using sources created by feminists, women, or women activists, critiques of psychiatric power were rife during the wave of feminist activism that swelled between the 1960s and the 1980s. This period was formative in developing strands of criticism that remain influential in contemporary feminist work. It is useful, therefore, to set out the origins of the British Women's Liberation Movement and post-war American women's movements, their trajectories, and their relationship with those who claimed psychiatric expertise.

In 1963 Betty Friedan (1921–2006), an American psychology graduate, journalist, housewife, and mother, published *The Feminine Mystique*. There was a 'problem with no name', Friedan wrote, 'shared by countless women in America'.[6] These women, Friedan claimed, felt bereft. Living in a culture that hailed the (white) suburban housewife as the apotheosis of feminine achievement, that acclaimed their responsibilities for childrearing and domesticity as the very culmination of womanhood, these women felt a quiet, low-level despair. Sometimes their feelings brought them to an analyst's couch, sometimes they manifested in somatic symptoms that brought them to their physician's offices, and other times it just brought them to tears, she said. The problem, Friedan proposed, was not the women themselves or their failure to adjust to the 'feminine role'; the problem was a culture that stultified women's professional and intellectual promise by sequestering them in unfulfilling domesticity. Friedan placed the blame for this sociocultural phenomenon partially on Freud. Freud's theories rendered women subservient to men and dependent upon them. The oppression of women, then, did not manifest in the same way as it had in the past – for example, through denying them the vote – but had taken on another pernicious form: the oppression of women was now manifested through psychological means and was spread through psychoanalytic ideas about healthy behaviour.[7] The first paperback run of *The Feminine Mystique* sold 1.4 million copies. It spent six weeks on *The New York Times'* bestseller list. It was a phenomenon: 'second wave' feminism had arrived, and patriarchal values espoused by the psy sciences were in its sights.

The rise of women's movements in America emerged alongside and were informed by other social movements of the 1960s, including the anti-war movement and the civil rights movement. The women's movements of the 1960s to 1970s aimed to transform social and cultural life as well as secure further legal and political rights. Feminists took issue with women's subordination across the board: in the home, in the workplace, in healthcare settings, through sexual oppression, and in popular culture. The movement operated at the grassroots, without formal leadership, and women came together in 'consciousness-raising' groups to explore their personal experience. Feminists and activists established women's studies courses in universities and poured new energy into investigating women's histories. As Nancy Tomes has demonstrated, these sites enabled the development of sophisticated, diverse, and extensive historiographies of psychiatry and analytical work on women's place in psychological medicine.[8] This literature now occupies a curious position for historians: it is both a body of historiography and can also be used as a primary source. The arguments, priorities, and critiques expressed by women's movements tell us about the movement itself and the climate of the era. So how should they be approached, and how does the feminist critique of psychiatry fit into the broader field of activism in this period?

Feminist goals and activities were bound together by the conviction that social attitudes, cultural norms, and political legislation enforced the disempowerment of women. Psychiatry, and the psy sciences more widely, were seen by some activists to be a part of the patriarchal infrastructure that administered this. The disproportionate prescription of mood-enhancing drugs was pointed to as evidence that psychopharmacological interventions aimed to reconcile women to their individualised discontent, rather than allowing women to see their discontent as widely shared, and symptomatic of the need for social change.[9] Thus Friedan was not the only American feminist who set her sights on the psy professions. Naomi Weisstein wrote an influential paper in 1968 arguing that 'Psychology has nothing to say about what women are really like, what they need and what they want, especially because psychology does not know'.[10] Others saw the mind sciences as being part of the machinations that oppressed women.[11] This did not necessitate that the entire intellectual legacy of the psy professions be jettisoned, however. Consciousness-raising groups made use of the ideas established in the mind sciences, and women activists developed alternative models of psychiatric support that embodied feminist ideas, while others argued that theories put forward by

Freud could be modified. More broadly, health and women's self-knowledge became an important area for activism: the Boston Women's Health Book Collective was founded in 1969 and published its handbook, *Our Bodies, Ourselves* in 1971, selling 250,000 copies.[12] The wave of activism that took place in America following the early 1960s had fallen into division during the 1980s, at which point the 'sex wars' proved to reveal foundational disagreements.

The British Women's Liberation Movement is widely seen to have begun in earnest with the inaugural National Women's Liberation Conference at Ruskin College, Oxford, in 1970. Like their American counterparts, the British Women's Liberation Movement centred its politics on the maxim that the 'personal is political' (a phrase popularised by American liberationist Carol Hanisch in 1969).[13] The British Women's Liberation Movement was influenced by the student protests of the 1960s and informed by female activists' often dispiriting involvement in the socialist and New Left movements of the period. Similar to their American peers, the British movement was diffuse and organised in local groups. As with the American movement, defining an 'end' date for a diffuse social movement is a contentious issue – not least because closing this period of activism in 1978, with the final National Women's Liberation Conference in Britain, obscures Black women's activism in the 1980s.[14] It also, as I have argued elsewhere, distracts attention from the activism and institutions that continued at a local level, including around psychiatry and mental health. For example, the Women's Therapy Centre in London was established by Luise Eichenbaum and Susie Orbach in 1976, while the Bristol Women and Mental Health Network was founded in the 1980s, as was the Islington Women and Mental Health Project.[15] These institutions modelled new feminist practices around psychiatry. Like these institutions, some of the key trends and schisms in the feminist historiography of psychiatry developed within the energy of the women's movements of this period; like grassroots feminist practices, they continued to hold influence past the formal 'end' of the Women's Liberation Movement.

Members of the Women's Liberation Movement pioneered new fields of criticism, developing bodies of research into women's history and theories about the structural forces that enabled the oppression of women in Britain. Psychiatry was seen by some to be a critical part of these oppressive structural forces. Some of these ideas were shaped by the anti-psychiatry theories put forward by David Cooper and R.D. Laing;[16] unlike Laing and Cooper, however, women's liberationists not only saw psychiatry as a profession that enforced social norms and questioned the legitimacy of psychiatric authority, but argued that patriarchal psychiatric norms imposed particularly punitive strictures on women. Some believed that psychiatry and its attendant practices could be subverted, with women's liberation magazines providing spaces for debate: *Spare Rib*, the most prominent of the women's liberationist magazines, ran a forum on 'Therapy: Reform or Revolution' in April 1978.[17] Some of these issues were discussed at the first Women and Mental Health conference, held in London in October 1977, coverage of which was published in *Spare Rib*.[18]

Feminist magazines, including *Spare Rib* (1972–1993), *Shrew* (1969–1974), *Trouble & Strife* (1983–2002), and *Women's Voice* (1972–1982) are increasingly digitally available and form an important resource for historians. Each of these magazines had a different editorial perspective and set of priorities. To use these most profitably, you should examine questions about their production and perspective. Who edited the magazine? Where was it published? What was its circulation and readership? Was it a radical, Marxist, or socialist feminist magazine? Looking at the editorials can be useful for this sort of framing. While digitisation has fantastic advantages, including the ability to search by keyword, it is also worth looking at the context of the article that you are using. Historians can get a more holistic understanding of source material by looking at the articles it is adjacent to, and the types of advertisement, cartoon, or commentary it features alongside. Letters to the editor are a useful way of accessing how articles were received by readers – although, of course, they can only provide a fragmentary insight, as the letters published will show a tiny sample of reader responses. There is an increasingly rich historiography of 'second wave' feminist magazines, and it is worth drawing upon the work of scholars including Laurel Forster, Angela Smith, and Joanne Hollows to provide context when using these sources.[19]

Recently the British Women's Liberation Movement has seen a concerted attempt to archive its materials and record the experiences of its participants.[20] The largest-scale oral history project was conducted by the British Library as part of its Sisterhood and After project; several of these interviews explore themes relevant to the history of psychiatry.[21] Oral history has encouraged a particularly reflexive body of work: in keeping with this, the curators of Sisterhood and After have published useful reflective articles about the process of creating the archive.[22] The Black Cultural Archives in London hold an oral history of the Black Women's Movement. Feminist ephemera, including newsletters, magazines, and pamphlets, is held by archives across Britain, not least by the Women's Library, the Feminist Library, the Bishopsgate Institute (all in London), Feminist Archive North (Leeds), Feminist Archive South (Bristol), Glasgow Women's Library, and Women's Archive Wales. There has also been an expansion of historiographical interest in feminist approaches to psychiatry: as well as monographs and articles exploring class, race, and geography, historians have studied consciousness-raising, attitudes to selfhood and therapy, and the establishment of grassroots feminist mental health organisations.[23]

Sources from the American women's movement are also being made digitally available. There are too many to comprehensively cover here, but a few that are readily accessible, and particularly noteworthy, are worth flagging. *Notes from the Second Year* published Kathie Sarachild's article on consciousness-raising, presented at the first National Women's Liberation Conference outside Chicago in November 1968. This set out some of the key ideas that underpinned consciousness-raising, a practice that provided the opportunity for women to politicise what had previously been relegated to the private, emotional realm. Consciousness-raising, often conducted in women's homes, and always in small groups, allowed women to speak about their personal experiences and to derive theory and political action from them. 'In our groups, let's share our feelings and pool them', Sarachild wrote, 'Let's let ourselves go and see where our feelings lead us. Our feelings will lead us to ideas and to actions.'[24]

Newsletters provided a mechanism through which ideas could be shared amongst feminist activists. *Off Our Backs* was first published in Washington DC in February 1970 as 'a paper for all women who are fighting for the liberation of their lives'.[25] The paper occasionally covered conferences and issues around psychiatry and psychosurgery.[26] A selection of pamphlets have been digitised on the Redstockings website,[27] including an edition of *The Radical Therapist*'s special edition on women from August 1970. Written and edited exclusively by women, this edition of the journal argued that 'Women's oppression is an objective condition in women's lives which a wholesided therapeutic approach must recognise as *the* central cause of female "impairment." Blaming women for their suffering and trying to teach them to blame themselves and each other has been a prime practice of therapy.' Moreover: 'Psychology took over where the church left off in fostering self-blame rather than collective struggle.'[28] The second edition of *Woman's World*, published in New York between April 1971 and September 1972, ran an article by Carol Hanisch arguing that the language of psychology around sex roles continued to oppress women.[29] The website 'Psychology's Feminist Voices' provides a useful starting point for biographies and resources.[30]

Feminist and institutional repositories, for example at Duke, Barnard, and Harvard universities, hold archival materials that can be used to explore feminist writings on psychiatry. The establishment of women's studies and women's history within universities also enabled the creation and collection of a body of sources that can be used by historians. Scholarly journals that were established as part of the influx of feminist thought into the academy can be used to explore feminist academic thinking. See, for example, *Feminist Review* (established 1979), *Feminist Studies* (established 1972), and *Signs* (established 1975). These scholarly journals can be used to examine the development of ideas and to assess the influence of particular concepts. Who do articles cite in their footnotes? Who do articles agree and disagree with? Who do authors thank in their acknowledgements? Are there themed special editions that show that there was a particular interest in an area at a distinct moment? As with feminist magazines, it is also worth looking at the context of the journal's production. To this end, it can be helpful to examine what the editorial statement – usually made in the first edition of the journal – says about the journal's aims and scope.

Doing a feminist critique of the history of psychiatry

Feminist critiques of the history of psychiatry can be undertaken in a variety of ways. The first choice is perhaps between focusing on women as patients or practitioners. The former would prompt questions about treatment, diagnosis, and representation; the latter might prompt questions around how women have developed ideas within the psy disciplines. This second approach might also encourage investigations into the interventions of reformers. For example, Dorothea

Dix (1802–1887), an American who provoked reforms in the treatment of the mentally ill. Or this approach might facilitate investigations into the contributions of female psychoanalysts, including Anna Freud (1895–1982), Karen Horney (1885–1952), or Melanie Klein (1882–1960); it might also look at how women's research has shaped political and social change. Here we might consider the work of Mamie Phipps Clark (1917–1983), a Black woman whose work was cited by the Supreme Court in the Brown v Board of Education decision that outlawed the racial segregation of public schools in 1954, or Inez Beverly Prosser (1895–1934) the first African American woman to complete a doctorate in Psychology in the United States.[31] Further, this lens animates investigations into grassroots alternative psychiatric and psychological support established by feminists, opening up avenues of research into the theories, ideas, and practices that underpin such enterprises. Such historical studies make new understandings of psychiatry's past possible and facilitate an analysis of feminist ideas about what constitutes psychological health for women. However, it is the first approach – that which examines the history of women as the patients and subjects of psychiatric practice – that has ignited some of the most productive and fiercely argued debates in the feminist historiography of psychiatry.

One debate is whether mental illness is a social construct that polices women's behaviours in differentiated ways or if women's mental illness is a result of their oppression in a patriarchal society. As Joan Busfield frames it, in the latter 'the emphasis … is less on mental illness as a social construct than on mental illness as a social product'.[32] The former was most famously put forward by Phyllis Chesler. In *Women and Madness* (1972) Chesler suggests that:

> women who fully act out the conditioned female role are clinically viewed as 'neurotic' or 'psychotic' … women who reject or are more ambivalent about the female role frighten both themselves and society… such women are assured of a psychiatric label and, if they are hospitalized, it is for less 'female' behaviours, such as 'schizophrenia', 'lesbianism,' or 'promiscuity'.[33]

She pointed to evidence that women were not only more liable to psychiatric diagnosis but were also more likely to be prescribed psychopharmaceuticals and were vulnerable to being sexually abused by their psychiatrists. Chesler argues that women's sex role is socially constructed in such a way as to make it pathological in the eyes of psychiatry. A landmark text when it was published, *Women and Madness* was widely reviewed and sold prolifically.[34] These reviews can be used to examine the book's significance and reception. It is now an example of a text that established ways of critiquing the history of psychiatry but can also be used as a historical text in and of itself. Put another way, we can both use its ideas to look at the history of psychiatry and use it as a text that tells us about the historical moment – nearly 50 years ago – in which it was created. Moreover, in her introduction to the 2005 edition Chesler discusses areas in which her understanding has changed, reminding historians that while texts stand as products of their moment of creation, the minds that produce them change.[35]

The arguments put forward in a feminist text were rarely accepted without broader discussion or debate. The content of this debate now provides a critical toolkit for historians and can also be used to construct a genealogy of feminist debates in the history of psychiatry. Again: discussions that put forward divergent views of psychiatry can be both primary and secondary sources. For example, the social product approach – put forward by Friedan in the early 1960s – explains women's mental illness as arising from the toxic environment of a patriarchal culture. 'From this perspective it is the sexism of society rather than of psychiatry that is fundamental to any understanding of women's mental disturbance', Busfield suggests, and the role of psychiatry is 'to ameliorate the suffering that is brought about by the inequities and discrimination faced by women in their daily lives'.[36] This approach gained ascendency in the later 1970s and 1980s – a trend Busfield attributes to the decline of anti-psychiatry and labelling theory, to this mode of critique's general acceptability to psychiatrists, its convergence with feminists' critique of domesticity, and its apparent recognition of the reality of women's psychological suffering.[37] Both constructivist and social product perspectives are useful for taking an intersectional approach: normative behaviours and the psychologically unhealthy environment created by oppression are exacerbated and differentiated by racism.

The basis of these arguments – that women have been disproportionately affected by the definition, diagnosis, and treatment of mental illness in the past – has also been subject to debate. In 1985 Elaine Showalter argued that women were not only preponderant in the statistics around psychiatric illness in Britain, but that madness was itself represented as a female complaint in literary and visual cultures.[38] This argument was criticised by Busfield, who argued that:

> Rather than being *a* or *the* female malady, madness took on many forms, some of which were strongly linked to women and femininity, others far less so… some were linked to men and masculinity, and it is the complex interrelation of *gender* and madness, not just of women and madness in isolation, that needs to be examined.[39]

Feminist historians of the mind sciences have also been attentive to the particular ways that psychiatric thought has shaped ideas about the life course. For example, we might consider the ways that psychoanalysis has shaped ideas about women's sexuality. Freud's proposals about the importance of penis envy and femininity were fiercely contested by some feminists – not least because Freud's treatment of some of his female patients, for example Dora, was highly problematic. Nonetheless, the case of Dora has proved productive for feminist arguments about sexuality.[40] Psychiatry has also shaped sexuality by establishing behavioural norms and using coercive, and often violent, approaches to policing them. For example, homosexuality was classified as a mental disorder within the first edition of the 'bible' of American psychiatry, the *Diagnostic and Statistical Manual of Mental Disorders* (DSM-I), issued in 1952, and was only removed as a disorder in 1973.[41]

To this end successive editions of the *DSM* can themselves be used as a source. Historians have productively traced changing terminology and diagnostic criteria as a way of highlighting shifting ideas about psychiatric illnesses across time.[42]

Motherhood is another area that has attracted interest from the psy sciences and from feminist historians of psychiatry. This interest has a long history: in 1858 Louis Victor Marcé (1828–1864) published a treatise on puerperal mental illness.[43] Historians have used parenting guides, medical textbooks, diagnostic criteria, and psychiatric articles to explore how motherhood was constructed over time, and to look at how reactions to mothering that were considered to be psychiatrically aberrant were described and treated by the medical professions.[44] These types of sources tell us more about how disordered motherhood was perceived and re-presented than how it was experienced. However, they can also be used as sources to understand the climate in which women mothered and about how ideas about the family circulated through society. These types of sources have informed recent work by Hilary Marland, who has explored puerperal insanity in Victorian Britain, and Nancy Theriot, who has argued that puerperal insanity offended nineteenth-century physicians' sensibilities about appropriate maternal behaviour in America.[45] Feminist writers have done much to complicate the often sanitised images of mothering that have circulated in the public sphere: their writings form a source for the study of how women themselves have articulated experiences of mothering and its social context.[46] For example, sociologist Ann Oakley has written about her own experience of mothering and postnatal depression, while also pioneering fields of academic study around mothering.[47]

A third area that has proved particularly rich for feminist analysis has been women's relationships with their bodies and food. Perhaps the most important source for this is *Fat is a Feminist Issue* (1978) by Susie Orbach. 'Fat is a social disease, and fat is a feminist issue,' Orbach wrote. 'Fat is *not* about a lack of self-control or lack of will power. Fat *is* about protection, sex, nurturance, strength, boundaries, mothering, substance, assertion and rage. It is a response to the in-equality of the sexes.'[48] Other feminist texts, published by feminist publishing houses, also turned their attention to the issue.[49] Historians have recently estab-lished how bookshops and publishing houses, including Virago (founded 1973), The Women's Press (1978), Sheba Feminist Press (1980), and Onlywomen Press (1974), disseminated ideas within the Women's Liberation Movement.[50] It is therefore not only the book itself that is important: students should also be mindful of the context of production. This might entail looking at who the author was and if a book was published by a feminist publishing house.

Cultural sources for the feminist history of psychiatry

The sources that historians have used to conduct these analyses are diverse and reflective of the heterogeneous approaches to feminist history that have flourished across recent decades. The digitisation of historical sources has made them in-creasingly accessible to scholars and to students in the field. This is particularly true of projects that are open access: here, the Wellcome Library is a particularly useful resource. For historians interested in visual sources including portraits, paintings, and sketches the materials the Wellcome library have made available online are invaluable, although their physical archives (in London) offer an abundance of materials that span medical history. Medical journals, asylum records, and medical textbooks all form sources that can be used to explore the gendered history of psychiatry.

Useful sources for the study of psychiatry from a feminist perspective are not, however, restricted to those formally labelled as part of the 'history of medicine'. Films, for example, offer insights into the ways that the psyche, its experts, and patients were represented in the past – and such a resource can hardly escape a gendered analysis. The film *Gaslight*, made in Britain in 1940 (and remade in America in 1944), shows a wife being manipulated into thinking that she is losing her mind by her husband (and has entered the popular vernacular with the term 'gaslighting'). *The Snake Pit* (1948) depicts a woman – played by Olivia de Havilland – receiving treatment in an asylum. Such a film might be compared to *Girl, Interrupted* (1999), in which 18-year-old Susanna Kaysen is consigned to a psychiatric hospital. The use of films to construct a cultural history of psychiatry offers rich potential (for more on film see Katie Joice's chapter in this volume) but you should have some critical questions in mind. Who wrote the film's script or story, and what was their background? What was the climate of film production at the time? How was the film received, and how can we know what audiences thought of it? This final question can be particularly tricky: it can be difficult for historians to gauge reactions to films, but film reviews in newspapers and magazines can provide some idea as to their critical reception. Universities usually have subscriptions to a handful of newspaper archives, for example through Nexis, *The Times* Archive, or ProQuest US Newsstream; local libraries often also hold subscriptions to digitised newspaper collections. Searching these collections for the source you are interested in can be productive.

Women's writing about mental illness provides another source base for historians interested in the representation and experience of distress. *Girl, Interrupted* was initially published as a memoir in 1993 and attained widespread acclaim: it was on *The New York Times* bestseller list as a hardback for 11 weeks and for 23 weeks in paperback. It was followed a year later by the similarly successful *Prozac Nation: Young and Depressed in America* by Elizabeth Wurtzel. These were not the first memoirs of mental illness by women, however: in 1990 Kate Millett, author of *Sexual Politics*, published *The Looney Bin Trip* about her experience of manic depression and prescription of lithium. Women's writings on their experiences of mental illness go still yet deeper: some of the best-known accounts are Sylvia Plath's *The Bell Jar* (1963), Janet Frame's *Faces in the Water* (1961), and Penelope Mortimer's *The Pumpkin Eater* (1962), while *The Yellow Wallpaper* (1892) by Charlotte Perkins Gilman is still in print. These are just a few of the memoirs and novels written by women. Historians should be wary of using these sources to extrapolate too far about women's distress, or to draw universalising conclusions from them. For example, when approaching these sources you should ask questions about the positionality of the author. Might their class or race have shaped their access to and experience of psychiatric expertise? How might the form that the source takes – for example, the difference between a memoir and a work of fiction – shape the way that illness is represented? As with films, book reviews in newspapers and magazines can be used to examine critical reception. Male authors and playwriters have also mobilised the image of the distressed woman; perhaps the most iconic of these – represented thousands of times on stage and in art – is Shakespeare's Ophelia, although his Lady Macbeth offers another famous vision of women's mental illness. Shifting trends in how these characters were represented can tell us about cultural attitudes to women's distress.

Conclusion

Since the 1960s feminist critiques of psychiatry have flourished and feminist analyses of the history of the mind sciences have thrived. These feminist critiques have done more than merely establish a new body of scholarly work: they have fundamentally reshaped the lens through which historians consider the practice of psychiatry in the past. This chapter has set out some of the critical areas and themes that shape feminist research into the history of psychiatry. It has established that sources do not need to have been written by feminists to be subjected to a feminist critique; that sources can be used to construct a feminist cultural, social, intellectual, or political history of psychiatry; and that feminist studies should be alive to intersectional oppression. I have also set out how critiques of psychiatry that were developed by the Women's Liberation Movement now have a dual use: they both provide an explanatory model of psychiatry's past and are historical artefacts in themselves. As such, they should be seen as products of the debates, anxieties, and preoccupations of their time, much like contemporary historians' work on the history of psychiatry will come to be seen as products of ours.

Notes

1 Hélène Cixous and Catherine Clement, *The Newly-Born Woman*, trans. Betsy Wing (Minneapolis, MN: University of Minnesota Press, 1986 [1975]). For a discussion see Elaine Showalter, 'Hysteria, Feminism, and Gender', in Sander L. Gilman, Helen King, Roy Porter, G.S. Rousseau, and Elaine Showalter, *Hysteria Beyond Freud* (Berkeley, CA: University of California Press, 1993), pp. 286–344.
2 For histories of hysteria and for more on these perspectives, see Andrew Scull, *Hysteria: The Disturbing History* (Oxford: Oxford University Press, 2011); Laura Briggs, 'The Race of Hysteria: 'Overcivilization' and the 'Savage' Woman in Late Nineteenth-Century Obstetrics and Gynecology,' *American Quarterly*, 52, 2 (2000), pp. 246–73; Asti Hustvedt, *Hysteria in Nineteenth-Century Paris* (London: Bloomsbury, 2012); Carroll Smith Rosenberg, 'The Hysterical Woman: Sex Roles and Role Conflict in Nineteenth Century America,' *Social Research*, 39, 4 (1972), pp. 652–78; Elaine Showalter, *The Female Malady: Women, Madness, and English Culture, 1830–1980* (New York: Pantheon, 1985); Joan Busfield, *Men, Women and Madness: Understanding Gender and Mental Disorder* (London: Macmillan, 1996); Anne Digby, 'Women's

Biological Straitjacket', in Susan Mendes and Jane Rendall (eds), *Sexuality and Subordination: Interdisciplinary Studies of Gender in the Nineteenth* Century (London and New York: Routledge, 1989), pp. 192–220; Mark S. Micale, *Approaching Hysteria: Disease and Its Interpretations* (Princeton, NJ: Princeton University Press, 1995); Mark S. Micale, 'Hysteria Male/Hysteria Female: Reflections on Comparative Gender Construction in Nineteenth-Century France and Britain', in Marina Benjamin (ed.), *Science and Sensibility: Gender and Scientific Enquiry, 1780–1945* (Oxford: Basil Blackwell, 1991), pp. 200–39. For perspectives on masculinity and hysteria, see Mark S. Micale, 'Charcot and the Idea of Hysteria in the Male: Gender, Mental Science, and Mental Diagnosis in Late Nineteenth-Century France', *Medical History*, 34, 4 (1990), pp. 363–411; Mark S. Micale, *Hysterical Men: The Hidden History of Male Nervous Illness* (Cambridge, MA: Harvard University Press, 2008); Jan Goldstein, 'The Uses of Male Hysteria: Medical and Literary Discourse in Nineteenth-Century France', *Representations*, 34 (1991), pp. 134–65; John Starrett Hughes, 'The Madness of Separate Spheres: Insanity and Masculinity in Victorian Alabama', in Mark C. Carnes and Clyde Griffen (eds), *Meanings for Manhood: Constructions of Masculinity in Victorian America* (Chicago, IL: University of Chicago Press, 1990), pp. 53–66.

3 Kimberlé Crenshaw, 'Demarginalizing the Intersection of Race and Sex: A Black Feminist Critique of Antidiscrimination Doctrine, Feminist Theory and Antiracist Politics', *University of Chicago Legal Forum*, 1, 8 (1989), pp. 139–67.

4 Louise Hide, *Gender and Class in English Asylums, 1890–1914* (Basingstoke: Palgrave Macmillan, 2014). For more on gender and class, see Jonathan Andrews and Anne Digby (eds), *Sex and Seclusion, Class and Custody: Perspectives on Gender and Class in the History of British and Irish Psychiatry* (Amsterdam and New York: Rodopi, 2004).

5 See for example, Waltraud Ernst, 'European Madness and Gender in Nineteenth-Century British India', *Social History of Medicine*, 9, 3 (1996), pp. 357–82; Sally Swartz, 'Lost Lives: Gender, History and Mental Illness in the Cape, 1891–1910', *Feminism and Psychology*, 9, 2 (1999), pp. 152–8; Jacqueline Leckie, 'Unsettled Minds: Gender and Settling Madness in Fiji', in Sloan Mahone and Megan Vaughan (eds), *Psychiatry and Empire* (Basingstoke: Palgrave Macmillan, 2007), pp. 99–123; Catharine Coleborne, *Reading 'Madness': Gender and Difference in the Colonial Asylum in Victoria, Australia, 1848–1888* (Perth: Network Books, 2007); Tiffany Fawn Jones, *Psychiatry, Mental Institutions, and the Mad in Apartheid South Africa* (New York: Routledge, 2012). On sources on colonialism and the history of psychiatry see Sloan Mahone's chapter in this volume.

6 Betty Friedan, *The Feminine Mystique* (New York: W.W. Norton, 1963), p. 20.

7 Ibid. For more on feminism and psychoanalysis, see Mari Jo Buhle, *Feminism and its Discontents: A Century of Struggle with Psychoanalysis* (Cambridge, MA: Harvard University Press, 1998).

8 Nancy Tomes, 'Feminist Histories of Psychiatry', in Mark S. Micale and Roy Porter (eds), *Discovering the History of Psychiatry* (Oxford: Oxford University Press, 2014), pp. 348–83. This is an excellent and useful text.

9 For example, 'Health: Victims of Valium Usually Women', *New Women's Times*, 6, 8 (1980), p. 4; Maureen McKaen, 'Prescriptions: Legal Drug Abuse', *Pandora*, 3, 18 (1973), p. 5.

10 Naomi Weisstein, *Kinder, Kuche, Kirche as scientific law: Psychology constructs the female*, revised and expanded edn (Boston, MA: New England Free Press, 1968).

11 See Kate Millett, *Sexual Politics* (New York: Doubleday, 1970); Shulamith Firestone, *The Dialectic of Sex: The Case for Feminist Revolution* (London: Cape, 1971).

12 The first incarnation of *Our Bodies, Ourselves* was *Women and Their Bodies: A Course*, first published in 1970. This has been digitised and is available here: https://www. ourbodiesourselves.org/cms/assets/uploads/2014/04/Women-and-Their-Bodies-1970. pdf, accessed 16 Mar. 2021. The Schlesinger Library at Harvard University holds the archives of the collective: https://guides.library.harvard.edu/c.php?g=310923&p= 2081805.

13 Carol Hanisch, 'The Personal is Political', in Shulamith Firestone and Anne Koedt (eds), *Notes from the Second Year: Women's Liberation: Major Writings of the Radical Feminists* (New York: Radical Feminism, 1970). The full pamphlet is available through Duke University at https://repository.duke.edu/dc/wlmpc/wlmms01039, accessed 16 Mar. 2021; a physical copy is held at the Bishopsgate Institute archive in London (as well as elsewhere).

14 See Natalie Thomlinson, *Race, Ethnicity and the Women's Movement in England, 1968–1993* (Basingstoke: Palgrave Macmillan, 2016).

15 See Sarah Crook, 'The Women's Liberation Movement, Activism and Therapy at the Grassroots, 1968–1985', *Women's History Review*, 27, 7 (2018), pp. 1152–68. Susie Orbach has discussed establishing the Women's Therapy Centre as part of the Sisterhood and After project: https://www.bl.uk/collection-items/susie-orbach-the-womens-therapy-centre, accessed 16 Mar. 2021.

16 On anti-psychiatry, R.D. Laing and David Cooper, see Nick Crossley, 'R.D. Laing and British Anti-Psychiatry: A Socio-Cultural Historical Analysis', *Social Science and Medicine* 47, 7 (1998), pp. 877–89; Digby Tantam, 'The Anti-Psychiatry Movement', in German E. Berrios and Hugh Freeman (eds), *150 Years of British Psychiatry, 1841–1991* (London: Gaskell, 1991), pp. 333–47. See also R.D. Laing, *The Divided Self* (London: Penguin, 1990 [1960]).

17 'Therapy: Reform or Revolution', *Spare Rib*, 69 (1978), pp. 20–1.

18 Ruth Wallsgrove, 'Choosing to Fit In … Or Not Fit In', *Spare Rib*, 65 (1977), p. 13.

19 See Laurel Forster, 'Spreading the Word: Feminist Print Cultures and the Women's Liberation Movement', *Women's History Review*, 25, 5 (2016), pp. 812–31; Laurel Forster, *Magazine Movements: Women's Culture, Feminisms and Media Form* (London: Bloomsbury, 2015); Joanne Hollows, '*Spare Rib*, Second-Wave Feminism and the Politics of Consumption', *Feminist Media Studies*, 13, 2 (2013), pp. 268–87; Angela Smith (ed.), *Re-Reading Spare Rib* (Basingstoke: Palgrave Macmillan, 2017).

20 *Shrew*, British Library (hereafter BL) General Reference Collection P.2000/1413; *Spare Rib*, https://www.bl.uk/spare-rib; *Trouble & Strife*, https://www.troubleandstrife.org/; *Red Rag*, http://banmarchive.org.uk/collections/redrag/index_frame.htm. All links last accessed 16 Mar. 2021.

21 Clips are available online and the full collection is held by the BL.

22 Margaretta Jolly, 'Recognising Place, Space and Nation in Researching Women's Movements: Sisterhood and After', *Women's Studies International Forum*, 35, 3 (2012), pp. 144–6; Polly Russell, 'Using Biographical Narrative and Life Story Methods to Research Women's Movements: Sisterhood and After', *Women's Studies International Forum*, 35, 3 (2012), pp. 132–4; Rachel Beth Cohen, 'Researching Difference and Diversity within Women's Movements: Sisterhood and After', *Women's Studies International Forum*, 35, 3 (2012), pp. 138–40; Margaretta Jolly, 'Assessing the Impact of Women's Movements: Sisterhood and After', *Women's Studies International Forum*, 35, 3 (2012), pp. 150–2.

23 See Crook, 'The Women's Liberation Movement, Activism and Therapy'; Mathew Thomson, *Psychological Subjects: Identity, Culture, and Health in Twentieth-Century Britain* (Oxford: Oxford University Press, 2006); Sue Bruley, 'Consciousness Raising in Clapham: Women's Liberation as "Lived Experience" in South London in the 1970s', *Women's History Review*, 22, 5 (2013), pp. 717–38; Kate Mahoney, 'The Political, the Emotional and the Therapeutic: Narratives of Consciousness-Raising and Authenticity in the English Women's Liberation Movement', in Joachim C. Häberlen, Mark Keck-Szajbel, and Kate Mahoney (eds), *The Politics of Authenticity: Countercultures and Radical Movements across the Iron Curtain, 1968–1989* (New York: Berghahn Books, 2018), pp. 65–88; Kate Mahoney, '"Finding Our Own Solutions": The Women's Movement and Mental Health Activism in Late Twentieth-Century England.' Doctoral thesis, University of Warwick, 2017; George Stephenson, *The Women's Liberation Movement and the Politics of Class in Britain* (London and New York: Bloomsbury Academic, 2019),

Thomlinson, *Race, Ethnicity and the Women's Movement*; Sarah Browne, *The Women's Liberation Movement in Scotland* (Manchester: Manchester University Press, 2014).

24 Kathie Sarachild, 'A Program for Feminist "Consciousness Raising"', in Firestone and Koedt, *Notes from the Second Year*, pp. 78–80: p. 78. See also Kathie Sarachild, 'Consciousness-Raising: A Radical Weapon', in Kathie Sarachild (ed.), *Feminist Revolution* (New York: Random House, 1978), pp. 144–50.

25 'Editorial', *Off Our Backs*, 1, 1 (1970), p. 2.

26 See 'Mind Control', *Off Our Backs*, 3, 5 (1973), pp. 2–3.

27 Redstockings, https://www.redstockings.org/.

28 Judith Brown, 'Editorial', *The Radical Therapist*, 3 (Aug. 1970), p. 2.

29 Carol Hanisch, 'Male Psychology: A Myth to Keep Women in Their Place', *Woman's World*, 1, 2 (1971), p. 2.

30 See www.feministvoices.com.

31 An oral history with Mamie Phipps Clark is available here: https://oralhistoryportal. library.columbia.edu/document.php?id=ldpd_4074144 and see also http://www. columbia.edu/cu/lweb/digital/collections/nny/clarkm/introduction.html. Some primary sources on Inez Beverly Prosser are held at the University of Akron Cummings Center for the History of Psychology. See also Ludy T. Benjamin Jr, Keisha D. Henry, and Lance R. Mcmahon, 'Inez Beverly Prosser and the Education of African Americans', *Journal of the History of the Behavioral Sciences*, 41, 1 (2005), pp. 43–62. See also http://www.feministvoices.com/inez-beverly-prosser/. All links last accessed 16 Mar. 2021.

32 Joan Busfield, 'Sexism and Psychiatry', *Sociology*, 23, 3 (1989), pp. 343–64: p. 344.

33 Phyllis Chesler, *Women and Madness* (New York: Doubleday, 1972), p. 56. For a discussion of Chesler's argument, see Busfield, *Men, Women and Madness*, pp. 98–118. Chesler's papers are held at Duke University: https://library.duke.edu/rubenstein/findingaids/chesler/, accessed 16 Mar. 2021.

34 See for example Adrienne Rich, 'Women and Madness', *New York Times*, 31 Dec. 1972.

35 Phyllis Chesler, *Women and Madness* (Chicago: Lawrence Hill Books, 2005), p. 2, 40.

36 Busfield, 'Sexism and Psychiatry', p. 345.

37 Ibid., pp. 345–6.

38 Elaine Showalter, *The Female Malady: Women, Madness, and English Culture, 1830–1980* (New York: Pantheon, 1985).

39 Joan Busfield, 'The Female Malady? Men, Women and Madness in Nineteenth-Century Britain', *Sociology*, 28, 1 (1994), pp. 259–77.

40 See for example, Toril Moi, 'Representation of Patriarchy: Sexuality and Epistemology in Freud's Dora', *Feminist Review*, 9 (1981), pp. 60–74.

41 See 'The APA Ruling on Homosexuality', *New York Times*, 23 Dec. 1973, p. 109 for press coverage.

42 See for example, Katherine Angel, 'Contested Psychiatric Ontology and Feminist Critique: 'Female Sexual Dysfunction' and the *Diagnostic and Statistical Manual*', *History of the Human Sciences*, 25, 4 (2012), pp. 3–24.

43 For discussion, see Katharina Trede, Ross J. Baldessarini, Adele C. Viguera, and Alain Bottero, 'Treatise on Insanity in Pregnant, Postpartum, and Lactating Women (1858) by Louis-Victor Marcé: A Commentary', *Harvard Review of Psychiatry*, 17, 2 (2009), pp. 157–65.

44 See Barbara Ehrenreich and Deirdre English, *For Her Own Good: 150 Years of the Experts' Advice to Women* (New York: Anchor Books, 1979); Julia Grant, *Raising Baby By the Book: The Education of American Mothers* (New Haven and London: Yale University Press, 1998).

45 Hilary Marland, *Dangerous Motherhood: Insanity and Childbirth in Victorian Britain* (Basingstoke: Palgrave Macmillan, 2004); Nancy Theriot, 'Diagnosing Unnatural Motherhood: Nineteenth-Century Physicians and 'Puerperal Insanity'', *American Studies*, 30, 2 (1989), pp. 69–88.

46 Adrienne Rich, *Of Woman Born: Motherhood as Experience and Institution* (New York and London: W.W. Norton & Company, 1986 [1976]); Stephanie Dowrick and Sibyl Grundberg, *Why Children?* (London: Women's Press, 1980); Nancy Chodorow, *The Reproduction of Mothering: Psychoanalysis and the Sociology of Gender* (Los Angeles, CA: University of California Press, 1979); Elisabeth Badinter, *Mother Love: Myth and Reality, Motherhood in Modern History* (New York: Macmillan, 1981).
47 Ann Oakley, *Taking it Like a Woman* (London: Jonathan Cape, 1984). See also Ann Oakley, *Becoming a Mother* (New York: Schocken Books, 1980)
48 Susie Orbach, *Fat is a Feminist Issue* (London: Hamlyn, 1978), p. 18.
49 See 'Introduction' in Marilyn Lawrence (ed.), *Fed Up and Hungry: Women, Oppression & Food* (London: Women's Press, 1987), pp. 8–14.
50 See Lucy Delap, 'Feminist Bookshops, Reading Cultures and the Women's Liberation Movement in Great Britain, c. 1974–2000', *History Workshop Journal*, 81, 1 (2016), pp. 171–96; Catherine Riley, *The Virago Story: Assessing the Impact of a Feminist Publishing Phenomenon* (London: Berghahn, 2018).

Select bibliography

Andrews, J. and Digby, A. (eds), *Sex and Seclusion, Class and Custody: Perspectives on Gender and Class in the History of British and Irish Psychiatry*, Amsterdam and New York: Rodopi, 2004.
Bruley, S., 'Consciousness Raising in Clapham: Women's Liberation as "Lived Experience" in South London in the 1970s', *Women's History Review* 22, 2013, pp. 717–738.
Buhle, M.J., *Feminism and its Discontents: A Century of Struggle with Psychoanalysis*, Cambridge, MA: Harvard University Press, 1998.
Busfield, J., *Men, Women and Madness: Understanding Gender and Mental Disorder*, London: Macmillan, 1996.
Chesler, P., *Women and Madness*, Chicago, IL: Lawrence Hill Books, 2005.
Coleborne, C., *Reading 'Madness': Gender and Difference in the Colonial Asylum in Victoria, Australia, 1848–1888*, Perth: Network Books, 2007.
Digby, A., 'Women's Biological Straitjacket', in S. Mendes and J. Rendall (eds), *Sexuality and Subordination: Interdisciplinary Studies of Gender in the Nineteenth Century*, London and New York: Routledge, 1989, pp. 192–220.
Jones, T.F., *Psychiatry, Mental Institutions, and the Mad in Apartheid South Africa*, New York: Routledge, 2012.
Showalter, E., *The Female Malady: Women, Madness, and English Culture, 1830–1980*, New York: Pantheon, 1985.
Tomes, N., 'Feminist Histories of Psychiatry', in M.S. Micale and R. Porter (eds), *Discovering the History of Psychiatry*, Oxford: Oxford University Press, 2014, pp. 348–383.

12

USING ART IN THE HISTORY OF PSYCHIATRY

Nicholas Tromans

A prominent British asylum physician claimed in the 1920s that there was a 'formidable array of evidence of degeneration in those who are acknowledged to be geniuses in art'.[1] If art, in the form of paintings, sculptures, or drawings, has meant – at least in the west – a special form of commodity expressive of an individual's unique aesthetic, then it is easy to see how art might come under suspicion from those concerned with distinguishing psychological 'normality' and 'deviance'. Art and psychiatry have indeed had a rather tempestuous relationship. At various points in this relationship it was assumed that each might offer a direct portal to the inner meaning of the other. This idea now seems to belong strictly to the twentieth century. Today, a visit to the headquarters of the Royal College of Psychiatrists, near London's Tower Bridge, suggests a profession sceptical of images and perhaps of any cult of the eccentric individual. In the lobby area are portraits, all in more or less sober styles, of past presidents of the College. With a bit of searching you can also locate a nineteenth-century marble bust of John Conolly, who legendarily forbade the use of physical restraints at the Middlesex County Asylum at Hanwell in west London from 1839.[2] The College itself was founded just a couple of years later as the Association of Medical Officers of Asylums and Hospitals for the Insane, so Conolly stands as a kind of adopted founder by virtue of the compassionate professionalism he was seen to embody. As for the website of the Royal College, this shows recent photographs of people attending relaxed meetings as if the entire realm of the extraordinary, and therefore of art, is something the profession would now rather leave to others. Bearing in mind these hints of modern psychiatry's attitude towards images of individuals, in this chapter we will ask how historians of psychiatry might go about using artworks. We will look at three instances where art and psychiatry appear to have had especially close encounters: the founding of the modern profession as celebrated in painting; the visual representation of asylum patients for diagnostic purposes; and the collecting and interpretation of artworks created by people under psychiatric care.

DOI: 10.4324/9781003087694-13

Heroic imagery in the history of psychiatry

First, then, the founding of modern psychiatry. In Britain, as we have seen, the adopted founding father of the profession of psychiatry was Conolly. Other countries had comparable narratives in which brave men placed themselves between the sick person and an uncomprehending public, symbolising the creation both of the psychiatric patient and of the alienist or psychiatrist. A contender for the title of Europe's first psychiatric hospital is the Hospital dels Innocents, founded in Valencia in Spain early in the fifteenth century. Joan Gilabert Jofré was a notable local preacher primarily concerned with redeeming Christian captives and hostages in neighbouring Muslim territories. But in 1409, according to the story, he underwent a charitable epiphany closer to home when he encountered a group of boys taunting an ill man in the street. In the 1880s the scene was painted in oils by a young Valencian artist, Joaquín Sorolla, when on a scholarship in Italy funded by the regional authority who now own and display the work (*Father Jofré Protecting a Madman*, oil on canvas, 1887, Palau de la Generalitat, Valencia).

Sorolla, who went on to become Spain's most celebrated modern painter, positions Jofré as the mediator between the two parties, demonstrating the fundamental idea of the asylum as it was understood by the nineteenth century. With its local colour and historical costumes, the painting conforms to the standards of popular salon art of its age, to which we might contrast the harrowing Realist painting, *The Idiot*, made a few years later by the Belgian artist Evert Larock (oil on canvas, 1892, Royal Museum of Fine Arts, Antwerp). Realist, or Naturalist, painting took its energy from the vacuum left by traditional art's dereliction of reality, especially unpleasant, ugly reality, using the shock of recognition to address the public. Here, more boys threaten a vulnerable homeless man, but the horror of the image lies precisely in the absence of a doctor: there is no one to intervene to prevent the abuse that seems about to take place.

It is hard to imagine Larock's disturbing painting being on view anywhere other than in an art gallery, whereas Sorolla's picture, not proposing any startling new style or technique, is shown in the main civic building of Valencia, effectively as a monument to a local hero. They are pictures with different purposes and different kinds of audience. Those historians working with images today will not necessarily be specialist art historians, but scholars learning from a range of sources, artworks among them, interested in how similar images might be used in varying or even conflicting ways. For example, it is not difficult to show that the stories of these wise, kind men put forward as the founders of modern psychiatry were not always entirely accurate, and that the legendary moments at which they intervened do not comprise the whole story. In a 1994 paper, Schoeneman et al. showed how textbooks still used such heroic imagery, to the detriment of a more nuanced history of psychiatry.[3] Yet, this tendency to hark back to foundation myths is an important theme for any profession or institution, as we see even in the self-consciously modernised foyer of the Royal College of Psychiatrists. This is where art has a special role to play in the history of psychiatry and many other disciplines – in fixing images of founders and their acts, and giving concrete form to those images such that they might play a further role in the making of professional spaces.

The most familiar and powerful legend of the founding fathers of psychiatry was that of the physician Philippe Pinel who, during the French Revolution, is supposed to have commanded restraining irons to be removed from the insane inmates of the great hospitals of Paris. In the 1790s – so the story goes – Pinel threw off, in sight of more senior political authorities, the manacles from the insane at the Salpêtrière Hospital (mainly for indigent, infirm, or sick women and girls) and Bicêtre Hospital (for men). The story commits modern psychiatry to assuming the principle of institutional asylum; to aspiring to treat, and not simply contain, those suffering from mental illness; to having fundamental Enlightenment values aligned with the Revolution; and – crucially for grasping the novelty of the story – to being ready to account for its actions to the public and the state. Admirers of Pinel echoed his call for this new branch of medicine to operate a 'frank and open system of conduct'.[4] Such principles, however, were not so easily publicly promoted during the first half of the nineteenth century, for most of which France was again ruled by a series of kings. It was only with the arrival of the Second Republic in 1848 that *le geste de Pinel* (Pinel's gesture) was commemorated in a major public artwork (Figure 12.1).

This was a painting by Charles-Louis Müller, commissioned by the Ministry of the Interior for the new home of the Académie Nationale de Médecine (previously the Académie Royale). In a former chapel adapted for teaching, a pair of large paintings by Müller were placed high up where the walls met the interior of the dome. One showed the famous surgeon Dominique-Jean Larrey operating under fire during the Revolutionary wars, the other Pinel at the Bicêtre. Both subjects suited the new national political order which, as a Republic, revived the rhetoric of the Revolution. Generally, paintings were created without a specific destination in mind, and so the spaces they represented were typically imagined as existing on the same level as the viewer. But because Müller would have known

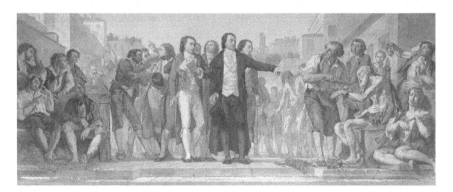

FIGURE 12.1   Charles-Louis Müller, *Pinel Has the Irons Removed from the Insane of the Bicêtre*, oil (with wax?) on canvas, 1850, Académie Nationale de Médecine, Paris. © Archives Charmet/Bridgeman Images

the elevated position his picture was to occupy, he adopted a perspectival scheme that assumed the viewer looking steeply upwards towards the figures. And because of the formal architectural setting of the work, the arrangement of the figures is itself structural, symmetrical, and rigidly explicit. The dancing limbs of some of the inmates suggest harmless derangement of the senses, while the elderly man having his irons removed looks like a philosopher fallen on hard times. To the left of Pinel, ready to take down the details of each case, is the young Jean-Etienne-Dominique Esquirol, Pinel's heir and a legendary compiler of asylum statistics.

How should we approach this picture as historians? Scholars have been able to show that the precise details of Pinel's 'liberation' of the insane were, unsurprisingly, not quite those of the legend. Michel Foucault famously saw in Pinel's gesture – whether historical or fictive – the opening up not of imprisoned lives but of a newly confident disciplinary regime.[5] But what about Müller's picture itself? As a bespoke commission for a specific location within a medical institution, the picture has never entered the art world. No reproductive engraving was made, it has not been lent to exhibitions about nineteenth-century French art, and its custodians have not felt it a priority to research as an object. Indeed, especially since its removal to a foyer in the Académie's current premises early in the twentieth century, it has evidently proven impossible to obtain a decent photograph of the work, thereby restricting its circulation and consequent use as an historical source. To research it, we need to see the painting as part of its original milieu, as an aspect of the visual rhetoric of the Académie Nationale de Médecine, as George Weisz successfully did in his history of the Académie, *The Medical Mandarins* (1995). We can go further by looking up articles published at the time of the inauguration of the Académie's new premises. While specialist art publications might be the obvious starting point, more general journalism may give a better sense of a work's public significance, while the dry records of the institutions that commissioned works such as Müller's may throw up significant evidence unobtainable elsewhere.[6] In such sources we learn, for example, that Müller's picture was painted 'à la cire', that is, using wax instead of (or more likely mixed with) the standard oil, suggesting Müller sought to make the picture look more like a mural by introducing a material associated with architectural painting. This is only a detail, but a basic one when considering a physical artwork. The fact that it has been forgotten suggests that works that have lived in medical institutions, as opposed to museums and galleries, are relatively under-researched and might prove a fertile body of source material for historians in the future. Elemental details of medical art collections are often available online, offering a place to start. Müller's picture and other works of art owned by the Académie Nationale de Médecine can be browsed on their library's website.[7] In the UK, the charity Art UK offers an ever-expanding online listing of works in public collections of all kinds, including the portraits in the Royal College of Psychiatrists mentioned above.[8] A great many works formerly in hospitals have been acquired in recent decades by the Wellcome Collection in London.[9]

The picture of Pinel by Tony Robert-Fleury, commissioned by the state for the Salpêtrière itself in 1876, the fiftieth anniversary of the death of Pinel (and just a few

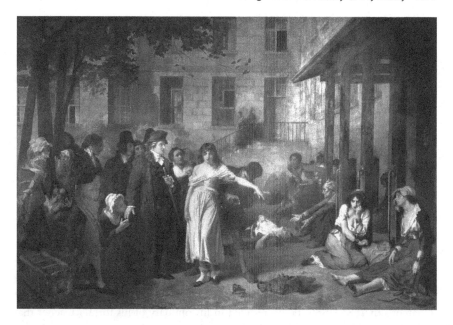

FIGURE 12.2   Tony Robert-Fleury, *Pinel, Médecin en Chef of the Salpêtrière, in 1795.* Oil on canvas, 1876. Hôpital universitaire la Pitié-Salpêtrière, Paris. Credit: Public domain, via Wikimedia Commons

years after the founding of a Third Republic), remains at the hospital (Figure 12.2). Relatively few art historians have seen the painting in the flesh, but it is nevertheless very well known due to the high-quality contemporary photographic reproduction of the painting issued by the leading dealers and publishers Goupil. Such reproductions could be framed and glazed for display in any study or consulting room. In Robert-Fleury's composition, the loosely extended arm of an inmate becomes the image's focal point, replacing the imperiously gesturing arm of Pinel himself in Müller's picture. The woman's arm is being held up by an attendant as he removes from her a restraining iron belt of the type still being worn by the seated women on the right. Pinel's intervention is restricted to his verbal commands, other than to allow another woman to kiss his hand in gratitude. He is a philosopher-physician who works with words and ideas. Using his social and political authority he decrees that these inmates (inconvenient prisoners) shall henceforth be patients (beneficiaries of medical science).

As several historians have observed, Robert-Fleury's account of the patient-doctor relationship was surely informed by the star Salpêtrière doctor of his own day, Jean-Martin Charcot, general physician to the hospital since 1862.[10] Charcot's international fame as a classifier of neuroses dates from the 1880s but by the 1870s he was already busy recording the alleged symptoms of hysteria and many other conditions among the population of the Salpêtrière: the *Iconographie photographique de la Salpêtrière* (*Photographic Portraits from the Salpêtrière*) commenced publication in 1876 (for more on this, and photographs in psychiatry more generally, see Beatriz Pichel's chapter in this volume). Charcot's notoriously showman-like clinical demonstrations were commemorated a decade later by the painter André Brouillet in *Une leçon clinique à la Salpêtrière* (1887, Musée de l'Histoire de la Médecine, Université de Paris: see Figure 12.3 for a print after this painting). Here the neurologist is shown hypnotising patient Blanche Witman as his eager students look on. The spatial relationships of physician, assistant, and patient – not to mention the posture and vulnerably *déshabillée* appearance of Witman – clearly echo Robert-Fleury's picture. That picture was in fact hung in the Salpêtrière lecture theatre shown in Brouillet's composition, thereby suggesting that Charcot's neurological dramatics had an immediate pedigree in a humane founding moment of modern mental health care.

This is a good example of what we referred to earlier as the uses of pictures. Once created, they do not stay put (unless they are frescoes or murals) and may become multiplied if reproduced as prints. If we think about the presence of Robert-Fleury's image of Pinel in Charcot's lecture room, we can see how the former helped legitimise what risked appearing outlandish experiments on the part of the latter. To be sure, it is not easy to document such shifting relationships, but in this instance we have no less a witness than Sigmund Freud, a student of Charcot's in 1885–1886. Freud recalled in his obituary of his former teacher that

> In the hall in which he gave his lectures there hung a picture which showed "citizen" Pinel having the chains taken off the poor madpeople at the Salpêtrière. The Salpêtrière, which had witnessed so many horrors during the Revolution, had also been the scene of this most humane of all revolutions.[11]

For Freud, the visual rhetoric worked and the lesson was learned: the study of the mind might overcome the trauma of history. Freud acquired a print after Brouillet's painting of Charcot (Figure 12.3) which to this day hangs over his famed consulting couch in the Freud Museum in London, self-consciously forming a series of links, provided by images, from Revolutionary Paris all the way to 1930s London.[12] The student is well advised to look for evidence to be garnered from artworks outside of art galleries, considering where these works were placed and who put them there. A great many fascinating pictures, prints, and sculptures were generated by and for the medical professions and are best understood in their original social and architectural environments. Reconstructing those environments is precisely the work of the historian.

Patient portraits

The pictures we have considered so far were public works of art to at least some extent. The images of Pinel by Müller and Robert-Fleury were two-dimensional rhetorical monuments around which a sense of professional identity might coalesce. But they also aspired to project that identity to a broader public, albeit a limited one. I would now like to turn to a type of image which was used primarily within the psychiatric profession: representations of its patients.

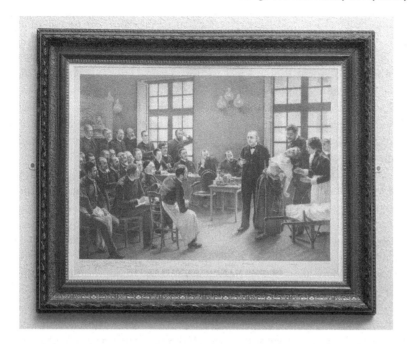

FIGURE 12.3   "Une leçon clinique du Dr. Charcot à la Salpêtrière" (A Clinical Lesson at the Salpêtrière), lithograph by Eugène Louis Pirodon (1888) after painting by André Brouillet (1887). Source © Freud Museum London

The nineteenth-century iconography of the insane has become familiar, not least thanks to Sander Gilman's compendious survey of the subject, *Seeing the Insane*, first published in 1982. This imagery, when it later circulated to those outside the psychiatric profession, added to the scepticism with which psychiatry has often been met. Here surely was evidence of medicine collecting mugshots of patients as if they were criminals, defining both through pseudo-anatomical classifications which elided all too easily with eugenics and, later, state murder. Schooled by Foucault, we feel we recognise ideology masquerading as objective data-gathering when we see it. And yet, from the start of modern psychiatry, we find too an unapologetically romanticised pleasure in the appearance of madness. Here is Esquirol, kingpin of the French psychiatric profession in the wake of Pinel, opening his definition of 'Folie' in 1816:

> What food for thought awaits the philosopher, who, slipping away from the tumult of the world, makes a tour of a lunatic asylum! He finds there the same ideas, the same errors, the same passions, the same misfortunes: it is the same world; but in such a place, the features are more pronounced, its shades more marked, its colours more vivid, its effects more striking, because man there displays himself in all his nakedness, because he does not dissimulate his thinking, because he does not conceal his defects, because he never lends to his passions any seductive charm, nor to his vices deceitful appearances.[13]

At this time Esquirol was busy, alongside his many other forms of asylum-based enquiry, collecting evidence of the physical characteristics of patients. When the Scottish alienist Alexander Morison (later a Visiting Physician to Bethlem Hospital among other roles) visited Esquirol in Paris for the first time in 1818, Morison noted that 'he has near 200 plaster of paris Casts of the faces of insane persons and 60 skulls', the latter retained from the post-mortems that were *de rigueur* during this most physicalist phase of French psychiatry (on post-mortems in psychiatry, see Jennifer Wallis's chapter in this volume).[14] Esquirol lent Morison examples from his collection, especially more portable drawings, to illustrate Morison's *Outlines of Lectures on Mental Diseases* of 1826, this being just one way in which alienists around the world borrowed from Esquirol's compounding of 'big data' from the French asylum system. Looking through the plates in Morison's book, engraved by the Edinburgh printmaker William Home Lizars after originals by unnamed artists, is now somewhat disturbing. The figures are presented in what seems a deliberately grotesque way, that is, to suggest their deviance from an aesthetic norm of human beauty, their 'defects' – Esquirol's word – shown as their defining characteristics. It seems likely that Lizars, who after all was not answerable to the artists whose works he was copying (as he would have been were he engraving an important oil painting for a commercial publisher), further exaggerated the expressiveness of the heads, in pursuit of what Morison termed '*moveable* physiognomy', that is, habitual but not anatomically-fixed facial expression.

One example of Morison's borrowing from Esquirol in his 1826 *Lectures* is the image of a patient suffering from lypemania (literally grief-madness), a diagnosis invented by Esquirol to allow depression to become one of the new monomanias – psychological disturbances fixed around one event or idea.[15] The young woman in Morison's plate is given the label 'Monomania with Depression', her malady said to have been caused by grief 'occasioned by the loss of a brother'. In Esquirol's own account of this case (1820; republished in 1838 in his *Des Maladies mentales*) we learn that the woman's grief was provoked by the death, not of a brother, but of her childhood friend the duc d'Enghien who was cruelly executed in 1804 for alleged royalist conspiracies.[16] Esquirol describes more fully her habits, which included remaining huddled up in bed, her eyes upon a fixed point, entirely uncommunicative. The plate in Esquirol's book (Figure 12.4) – by the distinguished engraver Ambroise Tardieu after the still unattributed original drawing – shows the anonymous patient in this position, suggesting a fuller case history than could be communicated through the head alone, as in Lizars' cropped version. She was picked out by reviewers of Esquirol's volume, one of whom wrote that 'we can scarcely imagine anything more touching than the fixed and hopeless expression of the lady' whose case was just one of many 'commentaries, afforded by the madhouse, on the crimes of those reputed sane'.[17]

The patient portraits in books by Esquirol, Morison, and other nineteenth-century alienists offer a wealth of opportunities for historians of psychiatry. They are, after all, a fascinating art-historical novelty in that non-elite people did not

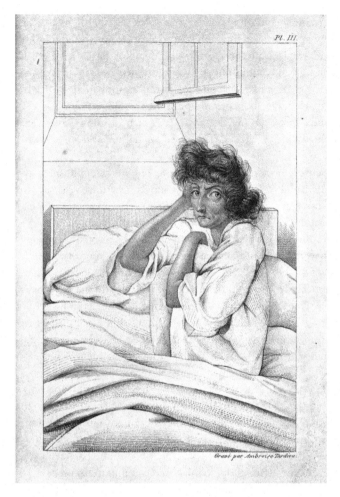

FIGURE 12.4   Lypémaniaque (portrait of an unidentified early nineteenth-century patient). Engraving by Ambroise Tardieu after unidentified artist in Jean-Etienne-Dominique Esquirol, *Des Maladies mentales considérées sous les rapports médical, hygiénique et médico-légal*, 1838. Credit: Wellcome Collection

traditionally have their portraits painted or drawn. Who were these patients, these individuals made to stand as types or cases? Following the publication of his *Lectures*, Morison progressed to commissioning his own portraits of asylum patients, some 249 of which survive in the archives of the Royal College of Physicians of Edinburgh. Many of these were reproduced in Morison's *Physiognomy of Mental Diseases* of 1838 and in the fourth, much expanded edition of his *Lectures* in 1848. Allan Beveridge has painstakingly related the original drawings to the published plates, revealing the identities of some of the sitters and much about Morison's attitudes towards them, a project of biographical recovery that it would be valuable to emulate in other cases.[18] Beveridge also asks about the artists involved, their training and approach to the work set for them by the physicians. Again, many such fundamental art-historical problems, paying attention to the graphic, sculptural, printmaking, and photographic processes used in recording, sharing, editing, and publishing patient portraits, remain to be addressed. More interpretive problems surround the clinical use of patient portraits. Did doctors really compare new patients to the portraits in volumes by Morison, Esquirol, and others, and allow such imagery to inform their diagnoses? Or were these images fundamentally visual rhetoric deployed to bolster a given writer's preferred classificatory system?

A further subtle question is at stake regarding the politics of these pictorial repertoires or atlases of madness. To us they may appear reactionary, a cast of mythic stereotypes of use only in producing content for the discipline of psychiatry, not in understanding or helping patients. But we must recall that the aspiration to coordinate nosologies with visible physiological signs was originally perceived as dangerously politically progressive because of its apparent materialism (as had been the claims of the phrenologists who asserted identifiable localisation of brain function). This appeared a threat to religion on one hand and the law's basis in volition on the other. Esquirol and the confident young members of his circle were seen to be elbowing out not only the Church but also the legal profession with their diagnoses of monomanias, *idées fixes* that crippled the will but left the intellect otherwise sound, and which might, furthermore, be transient. The 'discovery' of the monomanias therefore seemed to risk allowing insanity to become an explanation for almost anything involving a passing irrational obsession. Monomania also meant that the countenance of madness became harder to identify, implying a register of facial diagnosis somewhere between the passions (the passing emotional responses to actual events which young artists were traditionally trained to depict) and physiognomy (the art of reading character from the shapes of the facial features). Each monomaniac face was unique, expressive of obscure inner psychic currents but retaining fixed traces of those repeated expressions. Only the most sensitive observer could read them. At the same time, Esquirol was at pains to point out how traumatic public events were frequently bound up with cases of mental illness, especially as the foci of lypemania. The recent history of France provided all too many examples.[19] So the portrait of a person suffering mental anguish might provide, in compellingly distilled fashion, a picture of humanity confronting the dramas of its age. Might then patient portraits become great works of art? Among the most famous portraits of the entire Romantic age are Théodore Géricault's series of paintings of sufferers from different forms of monomania, made for Esquirol's pupil Etienne-Jean Georget in the early 1820s.[20] One of these, the enigmatic *Portrait of a Kleptomaniac*, appeared on the cover of Jan Goldstein's *Console and Classify: The French Psychiatric Profession in the Nineteenth Century* (1987). This now classic book offers an exemplary history of the profession in France in this period, yet the role of images in that larger cultural and political history remains to be written.

Patient art

Our third and final topic is the collecting and interpretation of artworks created by people under psychiatric care. An obscure link between insanity and originality was accepted as an ancient tradition. But if madness was now being subjected to scientific analysis, might it fall to psychiatrists to reveal the secrets of artistic creativity that previously had seemed so hard to explain? One popular hypothesis, or guess, about the mysterious commissioning of Géricault's monomania portraits is that the artist's own battles with depression recommended him as a perspicacious interpreter of others' mental suffering. Artists and the insane were both imagined by the Romantics as post-Enlightenment visionaries, able to see into the deeper truths of the human condition and having a special affinity for one another. Art, it came to be believed, could reach those parts of the distressed mind that other interventions could not. One of the artists regularly employed by Morison to take portraits of asylum patients, Charles Gow, told the story of drawing an utterly raving patient who, as it were, stepped out of his role of lunatic while his portrait was being worked on and even 'made some just and sensible remarks upon it' before reverting to type the moment the artist left him. Later the patient, fully recovered, greeted Gow at a Royal Academy *soirée*.[21] An equivalent story was told of photography by Hugh Welch Diamond who pioneered the use of the technique in asylums. In an 1856 paper Diamond claimed the first step to recovery of a patient believing herself to be a queen was her being shown a series of photographic portraits of several other people all under comparable delusions of royal status.[22]

This notion of an image as a tool with which to somehow triangulate the patient back into society – to use an artwork as a link between self and others – led to the invention of art therapy. The modern profession of art therapy emerged around the time of the Second World War, but a century earlier William Browne reported that at the private Crichton Royal Institution outside Dumfries, of which he had been appointed founding Superintendent in 1838, 'Drawing has been prescribed as medicine'.[23] The Crichton specialised in well-to-do patients and 'refinement' is a key term in the discussion of art there. Pictures on easels and on walls were among the welcome signs of restored gentility. Instruction was on hand from both experienced patients and external tutors, the latter engaged 'to guide hands, recently familiar with destruction, or with daubing paper grotesquely, by the principles of perspective, and to fix wandering and wayward minds upon the relations of forms'.[24] Pressing upon patients their existing relationships, beyond their own selves, with other people and things was, for Browne, an extension of the tradition of moral therapy (working upon the morale and sense of duty of the patient). As such, it was an alternative to the lazy prescription of cannabis – which he intriguingly implies was prevalent elsewhere – to induce solipsistic 'happy and hilarious visions'.[25] Art-making thereby assumed a modernising aspect, rejecting the coercion and cruelty of former times. An emblem of this could be seen in the picture gallery at Crichton: a painting by a patient (only recorded as 'W.C.') of *The Taking of the Bastille* which was framed, not in conventional gilt wood, but in 'a massive hoop of iron, worn smooth, or ruddy with rust, adapted for the waist, with corresponding hoops for the hands, and which was used as a means of restraint within the last thirty years'.[26] Naturally the patient-artists were put to useful work within Crichton, for example copying the plates of physiognomies in Esquirol and Morison to illustrate Browne's lectures on alienation. One patient, William Bartholomew (of the distinguished Bartholomew family of map publishers), became something of a specialist in this line. Browne later claimed that the use of Bartholomew's portraits of his fellow patients in lectures, alongside full case histories of the sitters, made them more significant as scientific contributions than those images published by Morison, despite enjoying nothing like their degree of circulation.[27]

The story of Browne and his patients at Crichton was only recovered in recent years thanks to the research of Maureen Park in the archives of the NHS health board which eventually succeeded the Crichton and its sibling county (public) hospital next door. As the state took firmer control of the British asylum system during the early Victorian age, record-keeping became a more formal affair, and when – from the later twentieth century – the large asylums were closed, their papers often came to rest in county record offices. These are not places regularly haunted by art historians, but there is much visual material to be uncovered in those patient files that are old enough to be made accessible to researchers under Freedom of Information legislation. For example, in the Surrey History Centre (formerly the Surrey Record Office) at Woking are drawings and papers relating to the so-called genius of Earlswood (the Asylum for Idiots in Surrey), James Henry Pullen, who created astonishing drawings and models of boats, some of them reductions of actual vessels, others the products of his imagination. These sources have only very recently been made use of by Kirsten Tambling in her reconstruction of Pullen's career, a good example of how far it is possible to bring institutionalised artists back into the historical record.[28] Such feats of modern scholarship have been necessary when the work of asylum artists was originally considered an essentially private, more or less therapeutic affair. But from around 1900 some psychiatrists had themselves begun to use their patients' artworks as an element in their own public polemics, either in defence of particular medical theories or, just as often, as a means of establishing a stronger cultural presence for psychiatry itself.

John MacGregor's 1989 book *The Discovery of the Art of the Insane* is a fine-grained history of the individuals – doctors, artists, collectors – whose stories support the idea of a special relationship between art and madness. That idea is, to be sure, perennial in Western history. It was given new impetus, as we have seen, in the Romantic period, and then again late in the nineteenth century as many professional artists sought to distance themselves from established academies with their traditional teaching syllabuses and bourgeois cultural norms. This 'secession' movement – closely allied to the Naturalist impulse – was the seedbed of the avant-garde styles that so shocked mainstream commentators, and which gave 'modern art' the compromised public reputation it has endured ever since. The fascination with the art of the insane evolved in dialogue with the anxiety that modern culture itself was, if not mad, then degenerate, neurotic, or at the very least unhealthily self-obsessed. The image of the artist as madman (very rarely madwoman) was meanwhile embraced by some of the radicals themselves as a fitting representation of their outsider status.

MacGregor identifies the first formal exhibition of the art of psychiatric patients as the one held at Bethlem in London in 1900, assembled by the hospital's Superintendent, Theo Hyslop, whose claim for the correlation between modern art and degeneration opens this chapter. This display, although very substantial (comprising some 600 items), was only nominally public, and only remembered by a few specialists, although these included Auguste Marie (a pupil of Charcot) who himself established a *Musée de la folie* (Museum of Madness) including patient art at the Villejuif asylum outside Paris in 1905.[29] Hyslop's pioneering exhibition was followed in 1913 by a sequel that had massively more impact, occurring as it did in the immediate wake of the first significant exhibition in London of recent avant-garde French painting from Gauguin to Picasso. Hyslop had denounced the whole 'borderland' of such artists and their supporters as degenerates and hinted that some form of incarceration or even euthanasia was their fate.[30] The press eagerly took up the supposed parallels between Hyslop's patient art and the 'Post-Impressionists' (as modern European art was labelled in Britain), and Hyslop was accepted as the expert in judging the relationship between the two. He had little patience with either. He may have spoken of '[t]he crude, barbarous splendour of the insane artist's production', but this was, however, 'often due to optical illusions'. He saw the mad artist as a true aesthete – 'his efforts are mostly for art's sake alone' – yet ultimately their work was of no immediate scientific value, only really functioning as a control against which to measure the art of the fashionable galleries, establishments of which Hyslop took to making 'sanitary inspections'.[31]

Central to Hyslop's case was that modern art was only pretending to be mad. He liked to quote his anonymous patient who saw in Post-Impressionism 'shamming degeneration'.[32] Hyslop also liked to cite Max Nordau, the prominent denouncer of modern European degeneration, to the effect that pretending to membership of a superior social caste through superficial emotionalism – as Hyslop claimed avant-garde intellectuals did – was a sign of mental disease.[33] Many of the Modernists did indeed seek, or affect to seek, the bedrock of humanity that madness was romantically believed to lay bare. The psychiatrist-philosopher Karl Jaspers felt this on visiting Germany's revelatory 1912 Post-Impressionist exhibition. Vincent van Gogh was, he wrote, the only 'unwilling madman among so many who wished to be insane but were, in fact, all too healthy'.[34] Soon after the First World War, Bauhaus master Oscar Schlemmer warned that this dalliance with madness was 'a dangerous game of the moderns'.[35] At this point appeared the landmark studies of Walter Morgenthaler (1921) and Hans Prinzhorn (1922), putting well-illustrated flesh on the bones of the beautiful idea of a pure and authentic asylum art, a degree zero of human image-making comprising only what *must* be set out to survive.[36] Prinzhorn's sumptuously produced *Bildnerei der Geisteskranken*, based on the archive of works he assembled at the University of Heidelberg, became a textbook for the French Surrealists, but what was psychiatry supposed to do with these artworks? Prinzhorn himself was to find no career in the German medical profession and from the 1930s 'degenerate art' was suppressed there, and psychiatric patients murdered. Among the latter was Franz Karl Bühler, for Prinzhorn the paramount genius among asylum artists, who was put to death in 1940 at the Grafeneck Euthanasia Centre.

This heroic, sometimes tragic, version of psychiatric art is now firmly part of the museum world. The French artist Jean Dubuffet gave it a label in 1945: *Art Brut*, or raw art, a category that often extended beyond patient art to embrace the extra-cultural more generally. Dubuffet's own huge collection was eventually opened as a museum in Lausanne in 1976. The Prinzhorn Collection has had a dedicated building open to the public in Heidelberg since 2001. In 2015 the Museum of the Mind opened in a former administrative building at Bethlem's south London site. These institutions and comparable museums around the world offer researchers rich opportunities to uncover the lives and works of artists living under extraordinary circumstances, and to relate those works to artists in the mainstream professional world. The Prinzhorn Collection, for example, has undertaken an impressive programme of exhibitions and research relating to its collections, while at the smaller Museum of the Mind, the remains of Hyslop's collection are preserved, awaiting historians ready to revisit the ambiguous pioneer of the 'discovery of the art of the insane'. Yet the very success of Art Brut, or Outsider Art as it later came to be known in English, as a kind of existentialist art-world 'ism', soon carried it well away from professional psychiatry. Outsiderdom need not be confined to asylums, but might include anyone marginalised from the professional art world. In recent years the category has been extended to embrace, for example, some African-American artists isolated by poverty and racism rather than illness.[37] The historian may feel this classification was in some way gradually appropriated from psychiatry by the art market – but equally they may want to argue that such a legacy to non-medical culture was precisely the aspiration of many psychiatrists of previous generations.

For patient art to become Outsider Art and thereby enter the museum and the art market, it had to be authentic, spontaneous, expressive of something urgent. Those defending this Art Brut tradition have therefore been sceptical of any artist aided and abetted in their self-expression. MacGregor, for example, felt that art classes had no meaningful place in psychiatric contexts. The patient was either an artist or they weren't. But in recent years historians have looked again at continued efforts, in the twentieth century, to achieve psychiatric findings – facts about mental illnesses *per se* – through patients' art. For example, Eilís Kempley has studied the projects of the circle of researchers at the Maudsley Hospital in London, among them Eric Guttmann and Francis Reitman, who sought insights into schizophrenia by giving mescaline to Surrealists and asking them to draw the results. It was hoped that this would give rise to visual expressions equivalent to the hallucinations of patients who, untrained in art, were unable to fix on paper what they had seen (an intriguing realisation of the 'shamming' which psychiatry had previously seen in modern art).[38] Connor Cummings, meanwhile, has followed Reitman's career to the Surrey County Asylum at Netherne.[39] There, from the later 1940s, Reitman led a team seeking to return to Prinzhorn's methods but with a sterner clinical eye, aiming to gather international examples of what Reitman termed 'psychotic art' and to identify spontaneous schizophrenic characteristics therein. The very limited results have not impressed. For example, the Netherne researchers published papers announcing discoveries such as that schizophrenics had a penchant for 'mauvish-red'. Reitman and his colleagues made much of the allegedly insane combination of writing and image-making, although the briefest reflection should have led to the realisation that this has been the historical norm outside of western Fine Art traditions.[40] Reitman himself was very taken with an example of psychotic art, sent to him by a doctor in Cairo, which seemed to fit his schema, but he was unable to recognise what now seems obvious, namely that the patient-artist (a medical student) had been strongly influenced by the lively Egyptian Surrealist movement of the period.[41]

Assisting Reitman and his colleague Eric Cunningham Dax at Netherne was the Art Master, Edward Adamson. Instructed only to facilitate patient art, never to guide it, let alone interpret it, Adamson supplied the psychiatrists with the graphic data upon which their publications depended (compare Morison and his initially anonymous artists).[42] Reitman was aloof in his attitude towards that data: it was rarely proper art, and of little or no benefit as a treatment; it was useful only as evidence.[43] But Reitman failed, as others before him had failed, to convince the scientific world of any coherent objective criteria for psychotic art, and today most would accept that 'It is necessary to drop stereotypes about "the mentally ill artist"', as two writers on the Victorian asylum artist Richard Dadd concluded in 1999 when seeking in vain to diagnose his illness from his work.[44]

The long quest to quantify madness using art may have been, thankfully, abandoned by researchers. But the supposed special relationship between artistic genius and madness remains a credo of general culture. Dadd's reputation increasingly eclipses that of his mainstream Victorian contemporaries because his story is so compelling. Equally, the work of Yayoi Kusama – a strong candidate for the title of the world's most popular living artist – is always linked by commentators to her life under long-term (voluntary) psychiatric care in Japan. In this chapter we have traced the ancestry of these enthusiasms to nineteenth-century psychiatry. The role of psychiatry in helping to define the modern artist as an heroic outsider has been much explored. But far less frequently asked is: what did art do for psychiatry? To answer that question historians need to revisit and re-imagine the specific places where psychiatry took place, and to ask how the visual and spatial rhetoric of artworks helped create those spaces. If you have found this chapter interesting, I hope you will explore the art collections of hospitals, medical museums, and galleries showing Outsider Art. Look again at old prints and photographs of psychiatric hospitals and clinics and try to identify any paintings, prints, or sculptures in the background. Pay attention to the pictures in old psychiatry books: who made the images, how, and at whose request? Finally, combine your study of visual material with other sources. Think of pictures not just as illustrations underlining certain passages in a text; think of them rather as forms of communication resorted to when words were not enough.

Notes

1 Theo B. Hyslop, *Mental Handicaps in Art* (London: Baillière, Tindall & Cox, 1927), p. 87.
2 The bust, by Giovanni Maria Benzoni, is on loan from the Royal College of Physicians.
3 T.J. Schoeneman, S. Brooks, C. Gibson, J. Routbort, and D. Jacobs, 'Seeing the Insane in Textbooks of Abnormal Psychology: The Uses of Art in Histories of Mental Illness', *Journal for the Theory of Social Behaviour*, 24, 2 (1994), pp. 111–41.
4 Samuel Tuke, *Description of The Retreat* (York: Alexander, 1813), pp. ix–x.
5 Dora B. Weiner, '*Le geste de Pinel*: The History of a Psychiatric Myth', in Mark S. Micale and Roy Porter (eds), *Discovering the History of Psychiatry* (Oxford: Oxford University Press, 1994), pp. 232–47.
6 George Weisz, *The Medical Mandarins: The French Academy of Medicine in the Nineteenth and Early Twentieth Centuries* (Oxford: Oxford University Press, 1995), pp. 118–9; Isidore Bricheteau, 'Inauguration de la nouvelle salle', *Bulletin de l'Académie Nationale de Médecine*, 14 (1849–1850), pp. 1080–90; *L'Illustration*, 27 Sept. 1850, pp. 203–4.
7 Académie Nationale de Médecine, http://bibliotheque.academie-medecine.fr/estampes-oeuvres-dart-objets/, accessed 28 Mar. 2021.
8 Art UK, https://artuk.org/, accessed 28 Mar. 2021.
9 You can search for images in the Wellcome catalogue at https://wellcomecollection.org/collections, accessed 28 Mar. 2021.
10 Jonathan W. Marshall, *Performing Neurology: The Dramaturgy of Dr Jean-Martin Charcot* (New York: Palgrave Macmillan, 2016), pp. 49–50.
11 Sigmund Freud, *Complete Psychological Works*, ed. and trans. James Strachey, vol. 3 (London: Hogarth Press, 1962), pp. 17–18 (I have emended Strachey's 'madmen').
12 Wesley G. Morgan, 'Freud's Lithograph of Charcot: A Historical Note', *Bulletin of the History of Medicine*, 63, 2 (1989), pp. 268–72.
13 Reprinted in Jean-Etienne-Dominique Esquirol, *Des Maladies mentales*, 2 vols and *Atlas de 27 planches,* vol. 1 (Paris: Baillière, 1838), p. 1 (my translation).
14 Allan Beveridge, 'Sir Alexander Morison and *The Physiognomy of Mental Diseases*', *Journal of the Royal College of Physicians of Edinburgh*, 48 (2018), pp. 272–83, 352–67: p. 275; Jan Goldstein, *Console and Classify: The French Psychiatric Profession in the Nineteenth Century* (Cambridge: Cambridge University Press, 1987), Ch. 7.
15 Alexander Morison, *Outlines of Lectures on Mental Diseases*, 2nd edn (London: Longman, 1826), p. 126, 138, and plate 7.
16 Esquirol, *Maladies*, vol. 1, pp. 409–11 and *Atlas*, plate 3.
17 Anon., 'Analytical and Critical Reviews', *British and Foreign Medical Review*, 7, 13 (1839), pp. 1–55: p. 46.
18 Beveridge, 'Sir Alexander Morison'.
19 Esquirol, *Maladies*, vol. 1, pp. 401–2.
20 These are oil paintings and therefore anomalous within the general history of clinical portraiture, if that is where they should be situated. Since the announcement of their rediscovery in the 1860s by Viardot there has arguably only been a single publication to throw significant light on their production (Miller, 1941–1942) – a dearth that has added to their mystery. Louis Viardot, 'Cinq études d'aliénés par Géricault', *Chronique des Arts et de la Curiosité*, 46 (1864), pp. 3–5; Margaret Miller, 'Géricault's Paintings of the Insane', *Journal of the Warburg and Courtauld Institutes*, 4, 3–4 (1941–1942), pp. 151–63.
21 William Powell Frith, *My Autobiography and Reminiscences*, vol. 3 (London: Bentley, 1888), pp. 93–5.
22 Sander Gilman, *The Face of Madness: Hugh W. Diamond and the Origin of Psychiatric Photography* (New York: Brunner, Mazel, 1976), p. 23.
23 Maureen Park, *Art in Madness: Dr W.A.F. Browne's Collection of Patient Art at Crichton Royal Institution* (Dumfries: Dumfries and Galloway Health Board, 2010), p. 33 (1847).
24 Ibid. (1853).

25 W.A.F. Browne, *Moral Treatment of the Insane: A Lecture* (London: Adlard, 1864), p. 6.

26 Park, *Art in Madness*, p. 37 (1851).

27 W.A.F. Browne, 'Mad Artists', *Journal of Psychological Medicine*, 6 (1880), pp. 33–75: pp. 33–4; Park, *Art in Madness*, Appendix.

28 Kirsten Tambling, 'The Idiot as Artist: The Fantasy Boats of James Henry Pullen', *Art History*, 43, 5 (2020), pp. 928–52.

29 This collection has been reconstructed by Allison Morehead, 'The Musée de la folie: Collecting and Exhibiting *chez les fous*', *Journal of the History of Collections*, 23, 1 (2011), pp. 101–26.

30 Theo B. Hyslop, 'Post-Illusionism and Art in the Insane', *The Nineteenth Century and After*, 69 (1911), pp. 270–81: p. 281.

31 Ibid., p. 274, 270; Theo B. Hyslop, *The Borderland: Some of the Problems of Insanity* (New York: Doran, 1925), p. 133.

32 Hyslop, 'Post-Illusionism', p. 270.

33 Ibid., p. 281.

34 John MacGregor, *The Discovery of the Art of the Insane* (Princeton, NJ: Princeton University Press, 1989), p. 222.

35 Thomas Röske, 'Expressionism and Insanity', *Raw Vision*, 45 (2003), pp. 32–9: p. 38.

36 Walter Morgenthaler, *Ein Geisteskranker als Künstler* (Bern: Bircher, 1921); Hans Prinzhorn, *Bildnerei der Geisteskranken: ein Beitrag zur Psychologie und Psychopathologie der Gestaltung* (Berlin: Springer, 1922).

37 See for example *Outsider Art*, Christie's auction, New York, 17 Jan. 2020.

38 Eilís Kempley, 'Julian Trevelyan, Walter Maclay and Eric Guttmann: Drawing the Boundary between Psychiatry and Art at the Maudsley Hospital', *British Journal for the History of Science*, 52, 4 (2019), pp. 617–43.

39 Connor Cummings, 'The Science of Therapeutic Images: Francis Reitman, Schizophrenia and Postwar Psychiatric Art at the Maudsley and Netherne Hospitals', *History of the Human Sciences*, 30, 2 (2017), pp. 69–87.

40 J.P.S. Robertson, 'The Use of Colour in the Paintings of Psychotics', *Journal of Mental Science*, 98 (1952), pp. 174–84: p. 174; J.P.S. Robertson, 'Mixture of Writing with Drawing as a Psychotic Behavior', *Journal of General Psychology*, 54 (1956), pp. 127–31. Robertson was Senior Psychologist in the Research Department at the Netherne.

41 Francis Reitman, *Insanity, Art, and Culture* (Bristol: Wright, 1954), pp. 31–2 and plate 2.

42 Adamson's sensitive drawing out of visual expression among patients helped give purpose to the emerging field of Art Therapy, initially a form of occupational therapy in the tradition of Browne at Crichton, but which, as it became professionalised, was later informed by psychoanalysis. See Susan Hogan, *Healing Arts: The History of Art Therapy* (London: Kingsley, 2001), Ch. 7.

43 Francis Reitman, *Psychotic Art* (London: Routledge & Kegan Paul, 1950), p. 163, 166.

44 Jonathan C. Motley and Robert Sommer, 'A Content Analysis of Richard Dadd's Art', *The Arts in Psychotherapy*, 26, 5 (1999), pp. 295–301: p. 299. On Dadd, also see Nicholas Tromans, *Richard Dadd: The Artist and the Asylum* (London: Tate, 2011).

Select bibliography

Beveridge, A., 'Sir Alexander Morison and The Physiognomy of Mental Diseases', *Journal of the Royal College of Physicians of Edinburgh* 48, 2018, pp. 272–283, 352–367.

Cummings, C., 'The Science of Therapeutic Images: Francis Reitman, Schizophrenia and Postwar Psychiatric Art at the Maudsley and Netherne Hospitals', *History of the Human Sciences* 30, 2017, pp. 69–87.

Hogan, S., *Healing Arts. The History of Art Therapy*, London: Kingsley, 2001.

Kempley, E., 'Julian Trevelyan, Walter Maclay and Eric Guttmann: Drawing the boundary between psychiatry and art at the Maudsley Hospital', *British Journal for the History of Science* 52, 2019, pp. 617–643.

MacGregor, J., *The Discovery of the Art of the Insane*, Princeton, NJ: Princeton University Press, 1989.

Park, M., *Art in Madness: Dr W. A. F. Browne's Collection of Patient Art at Crichton Royal Institution*, Dumfries: Dumfries and Galloway Health Board, 2010.

Tambling, K., 'The Idiot as Artist: The Fantasy Boats of James Henry Pullen', *Art History* 43, 2020, pp. 928–952.

Tromans, N., *Richard Dadd: The Artist and the Asylum*, London: Tate, 2011.

13

USING FILM IN THE HISTORY OF PSYCHIATRY

Katie Joice

Introduction

In 1951, American anthropologists Margaret Mead and Gregory Bateson released a film called *Trance and Dance in Bali*, based on footage of the ritual Kris dance shot during the 1930s, in the Balinese village of Pangoetan. The dance enacts a conflict between a pestilence-spreading witch, who throws her enemies into a state of trance, and the king's emissary, disguised as a dragon, who revives them. As the villagers drift in and out of the witch's spell, they turn their krisses (carved daggers) against their own breasts, yet mysteriously inflict no wounds. The film ends with close-ups of the local priest restoring the last swooning participants to their ordinary selves, administering holy water, incense, and meat from a sacrificial bird. 'The play is over,' concludes Mead's commentary, over the noise of the temple bells, 'but it will be given again and again, as the Balinese re-enact the struggle between fear and death on the one hand, and life-protecting ritual on the other.'

As the opening credits note, this film, and the fieldwork from which it emerged, was funded by the Committee for Research in Dementia Praecox (Emil Kraepelin's original description for what we now call schizophrenia). The Committee was founded in 1935 by a group of influential American psychiatrists who were concerned by rising rates of schizophrenic diagnosis in the US, a failure on the part of their own profession to find effective treatments, and the economic costs of long-term institutionalisation. But what did a film about Balinese dance have to do with the problem of psychotic illness? Bateson and Mead argued, both in their original grant application to the Committee, and in subsequent publications such as *Balinese Character* (1942) and *Growth and Culture* (1951), that the Balinese often displayed the same flat affect, waxy flexible limbs, and disassociated eyes as catatonic schizophrenics. States of disassociation seemed to permeate Balinese society, from religious trances to eating habits. Through close examination of their footage of village life,

DOI: 10.4324/9781003087694-14

they traced this strange demeanour to the child-rearing style of its women, which was teasing and provocative, but rejected any form of emotional climax. Their controversial claim was that Balinese culture was schizoid, meeting anxiety and desire with laughter or sleep. Bateson worked up these observations into his theory of 'the double bind', in which psychosis was recast as a communicative disorder brought about by contradictory or squashed signals from mother to infant. He and Mead concluded that in Bali these contradictions were experienced collectively in religious ritual, and repeatedly dissolved in the looping, ahistorical drama of the Kris dance. In the West, in contrast, mental crises caused by unfeeling or inconsistent parenting were privatised and hidden from sight. We may reject Mead and Bateson's peculiar brand of orientalism, but as a historical document, *Trance and Dance* stands as important evidence for mid-century theories of the cultural origins of mental illness. It is also a cinematic touchstone for the performance and documentation of un-reason, or the cinema of altered states. The film's ambiguous power lay in the fact that despite being commissioned by a group of psychiatrists, it pointed *away* from psychiatric categories altogether, to a world in which non-psychological under-standings of mind and self held sway.

I begin with this unlikely example of 'psychiatric' film to challenge your as-sumptions about where the boundaries of our topic might be drawn. Over the course of the twentieth century, films were made by the psychological professions in a wide range of settings. These included footage of asylums and clinics, but also of anthropological fieldwork, monkey laboratories, the staff meetings of ther-apeutic communities, children's homes, and interviews with the unemployed. The history of filmmaking as a psychiatric practice has a particular shape, and its net was cast widest in the middle of the century, in the decades between 1930 and the end of the 1970s. This essay will touch on films made before and after this period, but its main focus will be film sources from the post-war era. This archival 'bulge' can be explained by the coincidence of two historical developments, one material, the other theoretical. Nitrate film stock, used between the 1890s and the 1930s, was highly unstable, and only a very small number of scientific films made during this era survived fire or disintegration. Film became more portable during the 1920s, when the gradual replacement of nitrate film with non-flammable acetate led to the development of smaller, fully mechanised, 16mm cameras and projectors. During the 1930s and forties, these cameras were marketed particularly at academic and amateur researchers who wished to make documentary films 'in the field'. The 16mm camera quickly developed into an essential tool of analysis for many social scientists, a means of capturing human behaviour in new, re-plicable detail.

The historian Alison Winter has discussed the ways in which a 'rising realist epistemology' became attached to film at this time. The indefatigable cine-camera promised to disclose truths about human nature that the naked eye failed to register. The psychological professions in particular, felt an acute urgency to fix the 'ineffable qualities' of mental states by visual means.[1] As Lorraine Daston and Peter Galison have shown in their seminal account of the rise of mechanical objectivity as 'epistemic virtue', the camera promised to provide a non-interventionist account of nature (or human nature), purged of the observer's will or desires.[2] After the Second World War, a new interest in the environmental and interactionist, rather than genetic and hereditary, causes of mental illness led psychiatrists to study the non-clinical settings where madness might originate, as well as their own experiments in therapeutic community. In terms of psychiatry's history, this was a period of reinvention and rebellion, in which the foundations of the discipline eventually came under attack. Film – as emotive force, and analytic tool – was central to these critiques. The post-war era produced not only an intriguing, if disparate, collection of film sources for historians of psychiatry to work with, but also the critical eye upon which we rely for our analyses of visual sources within the discipline as a whole. The 'flowering' of psychiatric, and anti-psychiatric, filmmaking arguably came to an end in the 1980s, when genetic and neuroscientific models for mental illness gained ascendancy once more, and the primary causes of mental illness were sought in the brain, rather than in the familial or social environment.

During the last decade, the use of film technology within 'psy' science has become a new topic of interest to historians. This is partly a consequence of greater interdisciplinarity within academia, as well as the ongoing shift towards the study of practice, rather than disembodied theory, in the history of the natural and human sciences. We live in a culture saturated with digital media, which has made us all savvier and more confident viewers (and creators) of the moving image. Nevertheless, there has been no systematic attempt to catalogue or classify film sources relevant to psychiatry since the 1970s.[3] Historians seeking an overview of the topic have needed to be like magpies, drawing their evidence from archives and websites relating to medicine, anthropology, family research, film history, or 1960s counterculture. If the evidence is scattered, so theoretical reflections on the relationship between psychiatry and film have not yet been gathered together in one place. Recent research on this topic has clustered around four areas – war neuroses, cybernetics, attachment theory, and anti-psychiatry – and scholars have tended to focus on close analyses of individual films, or the work of single practitioners.[4] Important though this work has been in integrating the history of the psychological sciences with the methods of media history and visual studies, we lack more ambitious studies on the epistemological role that film has played in shaping categories such as schizophrenia, autism, child development, or institutionalisation. Films made in the service of the 'psy' sciences also have much to tell us about social history, the history of emotions and the body, and material culture. My aim in this chapter is to encourage you to draw connections across these historiographies and to approach film sources with the conviction that they are constitutive, rather than merely illustrative, of psychiatry's past.

From the earliest neurological films on movement disorders, to the confessional vlogs of the survivor's movement,[5] film has served many overlapping functions. It has been used both diagnostically and curatively, as documentary proof, teaching aid, provocation, and exposé. Some films, like *Trance and Dance in Bali*, or Eric

Duviver's films about psychosis for Sandoz Pharmaceuticals, offered immersive and aesthetic experiences for their viewers which exceeded any interpretive claims. Yet, however they are framed, these films all claim to be indexical, in that they point to something 'out there' that we call mind or madness. For this reason, I have excluded fictional films from our discussion, though I encourage interested readers to follow up references in the notes on this topic.[6] Many feature films about mental illness and its treatment have played an important role in public perceptions of the profession: Anatole Litvak's *The Snake Pit* (1948), Ken Loach's *Family Life* (1971), and Miloš Forman's *One Flew Over the Cuckoo's Nest* (1975) are well known examples. The boundaries between film and fiction are sometimes fuzzy: Loach used real psychiatric patients as extras to enhance his film's au-thenticity, and Duvivier's films are surrealist concoctions, despite being funded by a psycho-pharmaceutical giant. It is difficult to know to what extent the presence of the camera distorts behaviour, encouraging a fantasised performance of nor-mality, insanity, or even probity on the part of psychiatrists themselves. Nevertheless, my emphasis is on film as disciplinary intervention or method, on the unique ways in which film produces and disseminates knowledge, and how we might approach these documentary films as a distinctive type of historical evi-dence. Throughout the essay I will be suggesting questions that you can ask of your own sources.

All the films I discuss here were produced by American and western European psychiatrists or their associates. Although I am aware of a small number of post-war mental health documentaries made in the Soviet Union, Czechoslovakia, and Japan, my knowledge ends at these familiar geographical borders – the edges of what has been described as 'the cognitive empire'.[7] The references provide a framework upon which the known canon of film sources in psychiatry might expand, to include audio-visual sources made, for example, in Eastern Europe, China, Africa, and Latin America. It would be fruitful if insights drawn from transnational and postcolonial psychiatry could be brought to bear more fully on the epistemologies of film, and vice versa.

Psychiatry and the epistemological value of film

What kinds of knowledge were psychiatrists in search of when they made or commissioned a film? And how, in turn, might we read film sources in order to broaden our historical understanding of psychiatric practice? Influential discussions of this topic by Sander Gilman and Andreas Killen have grouped photography and film under the general rubric of 'visual culture'.[8] The first issue to think about, then, is how uses of the moving image overlap with, or depart from, uses of the photograph. There are three dimensions of experience that film alone is able to document, in a directly analogical way: movement, time, and relationship (or the 'behavioural field'). We shall look at their importance for one area of psychiatry below. However, film did not simply supplant photography as documentary method at a particular point, despite having distinct analytic advantages for psychiatrists. The moving image always remained in tension with the still image; whether those stills were quantifiable 'behaviour units' or emblematic moments of psychological transformation or decline. Both photography and film have enabled 'psy' professionals to sidestep problems of verbal description and observer reliability, and to stabilise, and immortalise, patients' expressions, gestures, and gait. Hugh Diamond's mid nineteenth-century psychiatric portraits and the 1938 hospital film *Symptoms of Schizophrenia*, which documents patients' mannerisms and tics, are both specimen collections in this sense. Photography and film are means of exploring the embodiment of mental illness: the relationship between fugitive surface phenomena, and what lies beneath, whether these are hidden physical or psychic structures. This gap between surface and depth, or symptom and cause, is the space in which psychiatric theory operates. In order to have a true epistemological value, still and moving images need to be described and re-described, to be yoked repeatedly to texts, voiceovers, or inter-titles. As historians interested in visual evidence, we must learn to translate between picture and word, and to evaluate the translations of others. However, films are made not only in dialogue with texts, but also with other films and images. It is important to think visually as well as discursively: seeking out aesthetic and formal connections both within psychiatry's filmmaking history and wider cinematic culture.

We should also bear in mind that making a film was an unusual intervention on the part of a psychiatrist or researcher, a privileged form of evidence-gathering that required funding, technical expertise, and an explicit intellectual agenda. We can therefore usually assume that if a film was made in a psychiatric setting, it documents a turning point or controversy in psychiatric practice. Useful questions to ask at an early stage of your research are: what is the status of the psychiatric disorder, or psychiatric treatment, being described in the film, at this historical moment? Is it new or under critique? Why is constructing visual evidence (rather than just written accounts) of this particular symptomatology or treatment important to the filmmaker? Who is the intended audience (and what groups of people ended up seeing it and commenting on it)? What is the observational stance of the clinician, cameraman, and other participants? How might you map these relationships spatially, and what can this tell you about how psychiatric practice was changing at that time and in that place?

In order to think in more detail about the epistemological value of film in psychiatry, I have adapted Scott Curtis's classification of medical films, whose functions he outlines as experimental, documentary, and educational. These functions are dynamic, with individual pieces of footage 'circulating' from one category to another over time.[9] I will draw from examples in the field of infant and child psychiatry, where film and video research has been (and continues to be) extensive. This was an area of enquiry which exploded after the Second World War, when the origins of mental illness began to be sought in the experiences of early childhood. Both psychoanalysts and cyberneticians, like Gregory Bateson, became interested in how babies' everyday interactions with their mothers, particularly mothers' feeding styles, might be constitutive of personality and later pathology. Film provided a way to identify and quantify mothers' fleeting

movements and expressions, from which typologies of good or pathogenic mothering could be constructed. Our opening example, *Trance and Dance in Bali*, was
a riot of movement, whose shape and tempo Bateson and Mead mapped onto
other observable behaviours, including child-rearing practices. On returning to
the US, Bateson inspired many other researchers to study non-verbal communication, particularly within families, and its implications for psychiatry. The
camera was used here as a technology of suspicion, an exploratory device which
could break behaviour into between 6 and 24 units per second. Frame analysis, or
microanalysis as it came to be known, exposed a more complex and disturbing
reality than could be perceived in natural conditions. In this case, slow-motion
playback of apparently competent mothering revealed a failure to make proper eye
contact with their babies, or care that was judged to be mechanical or inconsistent.
This was the realm of 'the optical unconscious', or what film critic Hollis
Frampton described as 'the monsters cunningly concealed within time'.[10] Infant
psychiatry claimed to be a preventative science, which used the camera to identify
micro-traumas *as they were being inflicted*, rather than their effects in adolescence or
adulthood.

A good example of film's experimental function can be seen in the 1967 film
Mother-Infant Interaction, made by American child psychologist Sylvia Brody, and
now available to download from the US National Library of Medicine website.[11]
Brody presents numerous case studies of mothers feeding their babies, descending
the typological ladder from the highest, Type I ("highly empathic and in control
throughout the feeding") to the most damaging, Type VII ("withdrawn, detached
and protected by routine"). This classification scheme was constructed from slow-
motion analysis of footage she took in her New York clinic during the 1960s,
measuring the quantity and quality of actions such as feeding, cleaning, moving,
touching, offering objects, and speaking. Although we do not have access to her
unedited film reels, we can reconstruct her methodology from the teaching film (see
Fig. 13.1) – in which an ever-present clock splices the action – and her accompanying publications, which describe the translation of this visual evidence into
statistical analysis. From these typologies she was able to make prognoses about the
children's future propensity to mental illness. 'Movie analysis' of this footage involved a number of investigators watching the reels in slow-motion, ratifying each
other's observations, and dividing the action up into behaviour units ('a single event
with patent beginning and end').[12] The finished film pre-categorises these mothers
for the viewer, but it is likely that Brody also used the uncategorised footage more
ambiguously, to test both students' reactions and the validity of her own classification scheme. A close examination of the editing process, and its effects, is central
to our analysis of the filmmaker's narrative control.

In Brody's work, and that of many other infant psychologists and psychiatrists,
the archival or documentary function of film preceded its experimental or diagnostic use. The first task of many infant psychiatrists was to collect a great quantity
of case studies, an extensive library of images of babies' movements at various ages,
from which a graph of normal, and deviant, development could later be plotted.

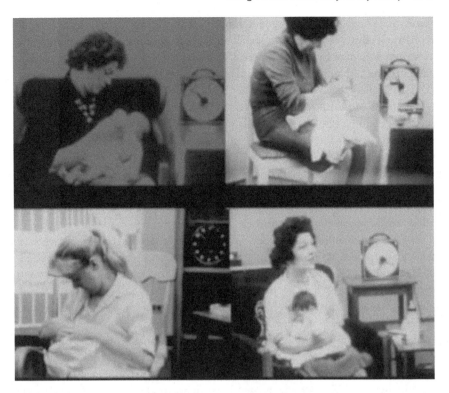

FIGURE 13.1 Composite stills from *Mother-Infant Interaction* (1967). U.S. National Library of Medicine

This method was pioneered by psychologist Arnold Gesell, who created the concept of 'developmental milestones' by filming over 100 babies in the first year of life, and selecting frames which reflected average physical and psychological growth at three months, six months, and so on. These he gathered into an atlas of film stills which he described as 'biopsies' and 'dissections', likening the film camera to the scalpel and the microscope.[13] Post-war infant psychiatrists more concerned with abnormal psychological development, such as Hungarian émigrés Margaret Mahler and René Spitz, cross-examined their own archives of mother-baby interaction (or in Spitz's case, institutionalised babies) in order to identify 'sensitive periods' and 'critical thresholds', rather than plot a smooth temporal curve.[14] These cinematic archives seek to define the borderline between normal and abnormal behaviour within the wider population. The relationship of the individual shown in the film to the illness he or she is exhibiting (a typical, in-conclusive, or ground-breaking case), and the perceived prevalence of this dis-order, therefore merits our careful consideration.

The educational function of these studies was more problematic in psychiatry than it was for general medicine, where clinicians created films which taught diagnostic or surgical technique within established disease categories. In the case of

René Spitz and his English contemporary, psychiatric social worker James Robertson, film was a means of shocking both professionals and the public into awareness of a new category of mental illness, and a new category of psychiatric patient. Spitz's film *Grief* (1947), and Robertson's *A Two Year Old Goes to Hospital* (1952) travelled the world during the 1950s, purportedly exhibiting the devastating effects of institutional life and maternal deprivation to doctors, nurses, directors of children's homes, and public health officials. Drawing on psychoanalytic vocabulary, Robertson claimed that film 'pierced the resistance' of adults who worked with children in clinical settings, forcing them to acknowledge a disavowed reality.[15] This turning point in the perception of infant suffering demonstrates that what can be 'seen' in psychiatric practice, and what others can be taught to see, is shaped by theoretical parameters, by what is being looked for. In other words, vision itself is historically constructed.

A final epistemological function of film that is specific to psychiatry is its therapeutic potential. Early psychiatric photographers, such as Hugh Diamond, used carefully curated images of their patients as mediating objects, allowing them to cast a moralising gaze upon their own behaviour (on photography, see Beatriz Pichel's chapter in this volume).[16] Hungarian psychiatrist Leopold Szondi created a pack of cards depicting deviant 'archetypes' to startle his patients into self-awareness.[17] Experimentation with film and video's formal possibilities during the post-war period led to more complex representations of patients' behaviour. Film historian Carmine Grimaldi has shown how, in 1960s San Francisco, radical psychiatrist Harry Wilmer encouraged his patients to create autobiographical videos to 'cultivate objective self-reflection', and to reimagine their relationship with the doctor as a dynamic feedback system.[18] Today, video-feedback continues to be used extensively in the field of infant psychiatry and psychotherapy. Mothers suffering from depression or trauma, for example, are encouraged to watch split-screen footage of their interactions with their babies so as to bring buried emotions to consciousness, and re-model their mothering style.[19]

Films made by psychiatrists capture, incidentally or implicitly, worlds we have lost. In this sense they are documents of social history, preserving physical environments, forms of social relationship and 'atmospherics' which are irretrievably past. Sometimes they provide new information about psychiatry's experimental tools, and patients' unpredictable reactions to them (usually providing a more ambiguous and nuanced account than written descriptions). In the 1952 TV film, *Autism's Lonely Children,* we see US psychiatrist Frank Hewett attempting to train a boy called Marty to speak by using negative and positive reinforcement within a 'teaching booth', a plywood box fitted with portcullis, sweet dispenser, and rotating chairs (Marty tries to bring the experiment to an end by showering Hewett with kisses). This little-known apparatus belongs to a family of 'cubicles of coercion' designed during this era, such as the Skinner Box, Harlow's wire rack, and the Milgram Obedience lab.[20]

The backdrop to a film's action also draws us in as viewers, whether it be furnishings, clothing, modes of expression, or framing devices which give us glimpses of the world beyond the therapy room. In *Camera Lucida*, Roland Barthes made a distinction between the *studium* – the intentional subject matter of a photograph – and the *punctum*, the poignant detail that escaped the photographer's notice but which gives the image its belated emotional power.[21] It is often the unintentional elements of a film – however tightly controlled its aims might be – which evoke tenderness in us towards the past, and a desire to translate these effects into historical research. These details may have less to do with psychiatric theory, and more to do with the social and material conditions in which it was practiced. Another TV film about autism, *This Year, Next Year, Sometime*, commissioned by British psychiatrist Joshua Bierer in 1953, shows a therapist communicating with a child by blowing long reels of cigarette smoke into the boy's mouth. He blows the smoke back to her, and in this way they have a 'conversation'. Uncontroversial at the time, it is now a moment of piercing historical counterpoint.[22]

Finally, psychiatry is always entangled with politics: through its policing of social and psychological norms, it defines the limits of community. Documentary film tells us a great deal about the utopian and dystopian visions that became bound up with psychiatric practice over the course of the twentieth century. The deadliest example of this was the profession's collusion with the Nazis' T4 extermination programme during the 1930s. Propaganda films such as *Das Erbe* (*The Inheritance*, 1935) and *Opfer der Vergangheit* (*Victims of the Past*, 1937, available intermittently online) played an important role in persuading the German public that the mentally ill were a threat to racial purity and social order.[23] The events of the Second World War and the Holocaust cast a long shadow on psychiatry's self-image during the post-war era. 'Anti-psychiatry' originated with visual exposés of the conditions inside mental hospitals, where patients – often so-called chronic schizophrenics – were herded naked around bare cells, or tied to posts.[24] As the cinematic evidence makes clear, the therapeutic communities and democratically-run asylums that emerged in the US and Europe in the following decades were not just humane alternatives to these warehouse-type asylums; they were experiments in new styles of observation. The objectifying gaze of the authoritarian expert was replaced by a fascination with intricate group dynamics and what R.D. Laing, borrowing from Gregory Bateson, termed 'the behavioural field'.[25] A 1969 film made by sociologists about Maxwell Jones's Dingleton Hospital in Edinburgh, pans back and forth between doctors, nurses, and patients set out in a circle in a series of lengthy meetings. Conflicts and alliances are brought to light and carefully disentangled, and the self-reflexive psychiatrist is shown to be in perpetual confrontation with his own prejudices and idiosyncrasies.[26] Democratic participation bleeds into managed anarchy in Peter Robinson's film, *Asylum* (1971, DVD), a study of Laing's 'psychotic community' in Archway, London. Director, cameraman, therapists, and patient-residents lived together as equals during the filming, in a celebration of both flattened social hierarchies and the collapse of 'critical distance'.[27]

These British experiments in turn inspired Italian radical psychiatrists Franco Basaglia and Giovanni Jervis to use photgraphy and film to press the anti-psychiatric case further, into the realm of political revolution. Their film colla-boration with Marco Bellocchio, *Matti da Slegare* (*Fit to Be Untied*, 1975), tells the story of various social misfits who escape oppressive institutions, but fail to find their place in capitalist society. The logic of psychiatric diagnostics and treatment are replaced here with a critique of the labour market and its measures of physical and psychological competence. Films from this particular era have explicit political and social agendas, but I suggest that every film source you will encounter on this subject is shaped by questions of power, progress and belonging.

Using sources: evidence, ethics, and empathy

We have discussed some of the explicit ways in which psychiatrists have used film to generate new knowledge; let us turn now to the practice of history, and some of the issues that face us when looking at a new film source. Our most basic task (and our first impulse, as readers and writers of texts) is to contextualise the film by looking for written accounts of it within the creator's publications and archival papers, where they exist. Can you find evidence for who made or commissioned the film, and why? Where was it screened? Private papers are more likely to contain information that relate to the messy and contingent process of directing and distributing films than polished, public-facing articles. Who reviewed the film, and in what disciplinary contexts? Did the film have an influence beyond psy-chiatry? What has been its afterlife (is this a 'canonical' film with a considerable historical literature, or is it obscure and uninterpreted?) Often you will discover the existence of a lost film, or evidence of film as clinical or documentary practice, solely through published descriptions and illustrations, from which it is possible to reconstruct a partial account of its significance. And it is of course important to think critically about words and texts within films, whether they are inter-titles, voiceovers, spoken dialogue, or background conversation. In what ways do they anchor the narrative? Do we see more or less when a film is silent? How do sound and images work together, or pull against one another?

Evidence

Films are amongst the most fragmentary and elusive type of evidence that his-torians of psychiatry can use. All types of film and video, not only early nitrate film stock, are subject to decay, destruction, and neglect in ways that textual material and still images are not. This is partly to do with film's bulkiness and material fragility, and partly to do with its dependence on a viewing apparatus. Although in principle you could visit an archive and hold a reel of 16mm film up to the light to look at its individual frames, you cannot experience it as a moving medium without a working projector, and the know-how to use it. Visual media were not highly prized as historical sources in past decades, and many films were thrown away by archives and libraries when the technology to watch them stopped working or became obsolete. Video, although an important experimental medium for the psychological sciences in the 1960s, 70s, and 80s, was designed to be a reusable technology, not a means of preservation. What has survived, and what you will be able to get your hands on, either physically or online, is mainly down to luck, confidentiality rules, and in some instances, the influence of particular archivists or estates with a moral or intellectual stake in their survival. Rare and undocumented mental health films appear on YouTube from time to time, only to disappear within a matter of weeks. The onus therefore lies with a new generation of critically-informed researchers to persuade institutions to repair and digitise those surviving reels and tapes which promise to broaden our understanding of psychiatric practice. Digitisation programmes are already taking place in well-endowed institutions such as the US National Library of Medicine, which acknowledges a huge public, as well as academic, interest in films about mental illness.[28] There is a clear need for a twenty-first-century version of the Psychological Cinema Register (the first catalogue of experimental psychology and psychiatric research films, created by Adelbert Ford in the 1930s), and I have made a first attempt at the end of this essay.[29] It is also worth noting that even once you have watched and analysed your film source, it is difficult to 'quote' film in a written text. In this essay, I rely on stills to illustrate my argument, and only where I have gained permission to reproduce them (this is much easier if the film is already in the public domain). Your powers of description, or what the Ancient Greeks called *exphrasis*, come into play here: you will need to explain not only how and why the film was constructed, but evoke something of its atmospherics and its play of forms. Examples of how to cite a film are also included below.[30]

Ethics

The making and viewing of historical films about mental illness inevitably present us with ethical problems regarding privacy and consent, particularly in the case of institutional exposés. I have attended several screenings, for example of Bill Morrison's historical montage *Re:Awakenings* (2013, now available online) and Raymond Depardon's asylum study *San Clemente* (1982, DVD), where members of the audience regretted their own complicity as witnesses, bystanders of an intrusion into the most private and defenceless realms of experience. It can often appear that the camera is being used as a 'prod', to use Scott Curtis's term, to extract a performance of irrationality or the uncanny.[31] In *Regarding the Pain of Others* (2003), cultural critic Susan Sontag outlined the ways in which such images might fulfil the audience's psychological needs: 'There is the satisfaction of being able to look at the image without flinching. There is the satisfaction of flinching... To steel oneself against weakness. To make oneself more numb. To acknowledge the existence of the incorrigible.'[32] We must acknowledge the vicarious pleasure, as well as discomfort, to be found in the camera's transgressive power.

To what extent have psychiatrists and filmmakers exploited the vulnerability of their subjects for documentary effect? As viewers, where do we draw the line between disinterested intellectual research and sheer voyeurism? Does it matter, from an ethical point of view, where and with whom, we watch such films (on a laptop at home, under controlled conditions in an archive, as part of a professional audience, or in a public cinema)? And is the question of participan's' consent the only ethical issue at stake here, or must we also weigh up filmmakers' wider moral claims about institutional power? We can assume that in many cases, permission to film was granted on behalf of patients by doctors or other officials, on the basis that those patients did not have the capacity to consent (though there is no correlation between schizophrenia and intellectual impairment, for example), or that participants only had the vaguest sense of how the footage might be used. The very notion of consent in the case of already powerless populations within institutions, is in any case a moot point. The film historian Brian Winston argues that Direct Cinema of the 1960s – which sought to portray American society's gritty underside – did nothing to improve the conditions of the marginalised, but merely exposed their degradation to public view. This he described as 'the tradition of the victim'.[33] Attempts to anonymise subjects often underscore their impotence: patients in *Symptoms in Schizophrenia*, for example, are clumsily disguised in bandit masks and bandages, preventing them from returning the camera's gaze.

The most prominent battle that has taken place over these issues was the 1967 *Wiseman vs Massachusetts* case, in which the state government sought an injunction over the release of Frederick Wiseman's documentary about Bridgewater State Mental Hospital, *Titicut Follies* (1967, DVD). Bridgewater governors claimed that Wiseman had not acquired the necessary release forms, and had shown patients, staff, and the fabric of the institution in the worst possible light. This included a scene in which a patient is force-fed (he later dies and is buried in the hospital grounds) and another where an elderly man, having been humiliated by staff, is hosed down naked in a decrepit cell. Wiseman countered that he had received oral permission from hospital officials and had always claimed full editorial rights over the final product, which he obliquely described as 'reality fictions'.[34] By 1991, when *Titicut Follies* was finally made available to the general public, the families of some patients claimed that the ban on screenings (and the reckoning that might have followed) led to their relatives' unlawful deaths at the hands of hospital personnel. The film's critique of power finally trumped any privacy concerns. In the words of film historians Carolyn Anderson and Thomas Benson: '*Titicut Follies* demonstrated the ethical paradox: good films are sometimes made for bad rules.'[35]

Today, it would be much harder, if not impossible, to make a film like Wiseman's. This is largely because of fear of litigation, declining trust in the accountability of institutions, and an increased awareness of the promiscuity of images. Film is no longer seen as a politically emancipatory technology, as it was in the 1960s and 70s, and laws on consent and mental capacity have been redrawn.[36] However, the question of who ultimately benefits from a greater anxiety about individuals' exposure to the public gaze remains open. A recent report about the global practice of shackling mental patients in hospitals and their own homes suggests that there is still a need for film exposés produced by journalists and psychiatrists working in unison, as occurred in the decades following the Second World War, as a first push towards legal reform.[37] 'Anti-psychiatric' documentaries of the post-war period, such as *Asylum* or Fernand Deligny's documentary about the wanderings of an autistic boy, *Le Moindre Geste* (1971, DVD) (or even *Trance and Dance in Bali*) can also educate us about the phenomenology of 'altered states' and what is now called neurological difference. Such films advance an ethics grounded in the idea that psychological experience is heterogenous and strange, and cannot always be neatly classified into 'illness' or 'health'.

Empathy

Are films 'indexical'; do they bear the stamp of reality? Documentaries do not of course provide a transparent window onto their subjects' feelings or mental states; like written texts, they are carefully edited constructions which seek to elicit particular reactions in the viewer. The images on the filmstrip may be formed by the indifferent play of light upon chemicals, but the positioning of the camera, and sculpting of the final product, is a highly subjective and prejudicial process. Even the barest forms of clinical footage are interpretive by virtue of what they include or exclude from the frame. An important part of your analysis will involve examining how aesthetic choices such as setting, lighting, camera position, close-ups, music, and depth of field make a film more emotionally effective and intellectually persuasive. Nevertheless, we should not let our critical awareness make us too cynical about film's testimonial power. Moving images do have a unique power to move and disturb us, to make us witness to the action in ways that other media cannot. Film theorists have recently drawn on mirror neuron theory (we experience emotions simply by observing them in others) and 'haptic visuality' (physical sensations can be evoked through watching close-ups of touch and movement) to describe a new empathic, rather than manipulated, film viewer.[38] Historians can use their emotions analytically when they watch films about psychological illness, as a response to the ethical quandaries outlined in the preceding section. This relates also to ideals of objectivity within psychiatric practice, to the status of both the psychiatrist and historian as feeling subjects.[39] We must reflect carefully on how emotions, and empathy, function as documentary content, as clinical strategy, and as viewer effects. Our own curiosity, fear, shame, and disgust can tell us, in refracted fashion, about the director's vision and the film's original reception, as well as something about the history of normal and pathological affect. I have discussed elsewhere how the camera became an arbiter of authenticity in mother-infant psychiatry, capturing at source the composite elements of emotional sincerity and artifice.[40] When I first watched Spitz's 1948 film *Grief*, a study of motherless babies, it was from behind my hands, and I felt physically shaken afterwards; from what we know of its history, many of its early audiences had similar reactions. Spitz claimed that he used the camera as a distancing device, to protect himself from the strength of his own feelings during observations, although he frequently enters the frame to comfort his subjects, and to look the audience in the eye. Emotions circulate here between patient, doctor and viewer, raw anguish transmuting into professional concern and moral outrage. Audience responses form an integral part of a film's history.[41]

Looking forward

Current psychiatric orthodoxy, with its emphasis on micro-cerebral structures, blood flow, and pharmacology, has banished many of these cinematic visions (and their fascination with tics, posture, relational selves, or political revolution) to obscurity. The discipline now stands on the firm foundation of evidence-based medicine, and in an echo of early twentieth-century psychiatric practice, is realigning itself with neurology.[42] But historical research involves not so much casting off from steady ground (into the murky waters of the past), as a shuttling back and forth between ever-shifting shorelines. The past enriches our under-standing of the present and reminds us of what we have jettisoned in the laudable, and often productive, pursuit of scientific truths. Within current psychiatric diagnostics, brain scanning – a combination of still and moving image technologies (fMRI, MEG, PET) – offers patients and their families a new form of 'mediating object' to which social and psychological sufferings can be at-tached.[43] Private narratives about living with mental illness, and the vicissitudes of psychiatric treatment, are available on online vlogs and mainstream TV.[44] This is an age of increasing loneliness – itself leading to an increase in psychiatric interventions – and psychological homogeneity, underpinned by the mediating presence of digital technology and the affective flattening that is a well-documented side effect of mood-stabilizing medications. The politics of the 'behavioural field' have largely retreated from view within psychiatric practice, with some notable exceptions.[45]

Although the stigma of (milder, if not severe) mental illness is fading, the ex-perience of depression, mania, psychosis, and autism, and most importantly, their social and political meanings, have become increasingly resistant to visualisation, and in effect, invisible to public scrutiny. Learning to watch historical documents like *Grief*, *Titicut Follies*, or *Asylum* carefully, critically, and with compassion, can therefore help us reflect on both the limits of interpretation, and the limits of intervention, in psychiatric practice, as well as the social contexts within which mental illness proliferates.

Funding

The author disclosed receipt of the following financial support for the research, authorship and/or publication of this article: This research was funded by the Wellcome Trust, grant 103344/Z/13/Z.

Notes

1 Alison Winter, 'Screening Selves: Sciences of Memory and Identity on Film 1930–1960', *History of Psychology*, 7, 4 (2004), pp. 367–401: p. 397.
2 Lorraine Daston and Peter Galison, *Objectivity* (New York: Zone Books, 2007), p. 187.
3 National Institute of Mental Health, 'Films on Schizophrenia: A Directory', *Schizophrenia Bulletin*, 1, 6 (1972), pp. 66–95; Adolf Nichtenhauser, *Films in Psychology, Psychiatry and Mental Health* (New York: New York Health Education Council, 1953); Adelbert Ford, *Psychological Cinema Register*, 1940–1944.
4 On war neuroses: Winter, 'Screening Selves'; Alison Winter, 'Film and the Construction of Memory in Psychoanalysis', *Science in Context*, 19, 1 (2003), pp. 111–36; Edgar Jones, 'War Neuroses and Arthur Hurst: A Pioneering Medical Film about the Treatment of Psychiatric Battle Casualties', *Journal of Medical and Allied Sciences*, 67, 3 (2012), pp. 345–73; Julie Powell, 'Shock Troupe: Medical Film and the Performance of "Shell Shock" for the British Nation at War', *Social History of Medicine*, 30, 2 (2016), pp. 323–45. On attachment theory and infant observation: R. Duschinsky, M. Greco, and J. Solomon, 'The Politics of Attachment: Lines of Flight with Bowlby, Deleuze and Guattari', *Theory, Culture & Society*, 32, 7–8 (2015), pp. 173–95; R. Duschinsky, and S. Reijman, 'Filming Disorganized Attachment', *Screen*, 57, 4 (2016), pp. 397–413; Katie Joice, 'Mothering in the Frame: Cinematic Microanalysis and the Pathogenic Mother 1945–67', *History of the Human Sciences*, (2020), https://doi.org/10.1177/0952695120924266, accessed 16 Mar. 2021. On cybernetics and family research: Seth Watter, 'Scrutinizing: Film and the Microanalysis of Behaviour', *Grey Room*, 66 (2017), pp. 32–69; Bernard Geoghegan, 'The Family as Machine: Film, Infrastructure and Cybernetic Kinship in Suburban America', *Grey Room*, 66 (2017), pp. 70–101; Deborah Weinstein, *The Pathological Family: Postwar America and the Rise of Family Therapy* (Ithaca, NY: Cornell University Press, 2013). On anti-psychiatry and film: Des O'Rawe, 'The Politics of Observation: Documentary Film and Radical Psychiatry', *Journal of Aesthetics and Culture*, 11, 1 (2019), https://doi.org/10.1080/20004214.2019.1568791, accessed 16 Mar. 2021; Katie Joice, 'Reviewing Laing's "Asylum" in the Age of Neuroscience', http://www.bbk.ac.uk/hiddenpersuaders/blog/reviewing-laings-asylum-in-the-age-of-neuroscience/ (2015), accessed 28 Mar. 2021; David Forgacs, *Italy's Margins: Social Exclusion and Nation Formation Since 1861* (Cambridge: Cambridge University Press, 2014), Ch. 4.
5 For academic analyses of mental health vlogs, see Irina Sangeorzan, Panoraia Andriopoulou, and Maria Livanou, 'Exploring the Experiences of People Vlogging about Severe Mental Illness on YouTube: An Interpretative Phenomenological Analysis', *Journal of Affective Disorders*, 246 (2018), pp. 422–8; Vera Woloshyn and Michael J. Savage, 'Features of YouTube Videos Produced by Individuals Who Self-Identify with Borderline Personality Disorder', *Digital Health*, 6 (2020), pp. 1–11.
6 Glen Gabbard and Kris Gabbard, *Psychiatry at the Cinema* (Chicago, IL: University of Chicago Press, 1995); Ron Roberts, *Real to Reel: Psychiatry at the Cinema* (Ross-on-Wye: PCCS Books, 2011); Martin Halliwell, *Therapeutic Revolutions: Medicine, Psychiatry and American Culture* (New Brunswick, NJ: Rutgers University Press, 2014); Homer B. Petty (ed.), *Mind Reeling: Psychopathology on Film* (Albany, NY: SUNY Press, 2020); Janet Bergstrom (ed.), *Endless Night: Cinema and Psychoanalysis, Parallel Histories* (Berkeley, CA: University of California Press, 1999); Marcia Holmes, 'Brainwashing the Cybernetic Spectator: The Ipcress File, 1960s Cinematic Spectacle and the Sciences of the Mind', *History of the Human Sciences*, 30, 3 (2017), pp. 3–24.
7 On the concept of 'the cognitive empire' see Boaventura de Sousa Santos, *The End of the Cognitive Empire: The Coming of Age of Epistemologies of the South* (Durham, NC: Duke University Press, 2018). On early Russian psychiatry see Ivan Pavlov, *Mechanics of the Brain* (1926), available on Vimeo, and Albert Maysles, *Psychiatry in Russia* (1955), excerpts on YouTube. The Czechoslovakian film *Children Without Love* (1963, Kratky films) is not currently available online, but has been discussed at length by Sarah Marks

in 'Bowlbyism Behind the Iron Curtain' (unpublished paper). Films about Japanese and African psychiatry in the 1960s, *Invisible Barrier: Japan and Psychiatric Patients* (1968) and *Tradition and Progress in African Psychiatry* (1960), are available on request from the US National Library of Medicine. Akira Kurosawa's *I Live in Fear* (1955), a drama about Japanese nuclear anxiety and mental illness, is on BFI DVD.

8 Sander Gilman, *Seeing the Insane* (New York: J. Wiley: Brunner/Mazel Publishers, 1982); Andreas Killen, 'Psychiatry and Its Visual Culture in the Modern Era', in Greg Eghigian (ed.), *The Routledge History of Madness and Mental Health* (London: Routledge, 2017), pp. 172–90.

9 Scott Curtis, 'Between Photography and Film: Early Uses of Medical Cinematography', *REMEDIA* (2016), https://remedianetwork.net/2016/01/19/medicine-in-transit-between-photography-and-film-early-uses-of-medical-cinematography/, accessed 16 Mar. 2021.

10 The term 'optical unconscious' was first used by cultural critic Walter Benjamin in his essay 'A Short History of Photography', in *One-Way Street and Other Writings* (Harmondsworth: Penguin Books, 2009). Hollis Frampton, *On the Camera Arts and Consecutive Matters: The Writings of Hollis Frampton* (Cambridge, MA: MIT Press, 2009), p. 47.

11 Available online at https://collections.nlm.nih.gov/catalog/nlm:nlmuid-9505462-vid, accessed 16 Mar. 2021.

12 Sylvia Brody, *Patterns of Mothering: Maternal Influence during Infancy* (New York: International Universities Press, 1956), p. 242.

13 Arnold Gesell, 'Cinematography and the Study of Child Development', *The American Naturalist*, 80, 793 (1946), pp. 470–5. See also Scott Curtis, '"Tangible as Tissue": Arnold Gesell, Infant Behavior, and Film Analysis', *Science in Context*, 24, 3 (2017), pp. 417–42.

14 See for example, René Spitz, *The First Year of Life* (New York: International Universities Press, 1965).

15 James and Joyce Robertson, *Separation and the Very Young* (London: Free Association Books, 1989), p. 4.

16 Sander Gilman (ed.), *The Face of Madness: Hugh W. Diamond and the Origins of Psychiatric Photography* (New York: Brunner/Mazel, 1976).

17 Lipot Szondi, Ulrich Moses, and Marvin Webb, *The Szondi Test in Diagnosis, Prognosis and Treatment* (Philadelphia, PA: Lippincott, 1959).

18 Carmine Grimaldi, 'Televising Psyche: Therapy, Play and the Seduction of Video', *Representations*, 139, 1 (2017), pp. 95–117: p. 105.

19 See for example Beatrice Beebe, 'Video Feedback with a Depressed Mother and her Infant: A Collaborative Individual and Psychoanalytic Mother-Infant Treatment', *Journal of Infant, Child and Adolescent Psychotherapy*, 2, 3 (2002), pp. 1–55.

20 Frank Hewett (with the National Educational Television and Radio Center), *Autism's Lonely Children* (1952), https://archive.org/details/autismslonelychildren, accessed 16 Mar. 2021. The teaching booth is described in Frank Hewett, 'Teaching Speech to an Autistic Child through Operant Conditioning', *American Journal of Orthopsychiatry*, 35, 5 (1965), pp. 927–36.

21 Roland Barthes, *Camera Lucida* (London: Vintage Books, 2000), pp. 27–59.

22 This film was briefly on YouTube but is no longer available at the time of writing.

23 *Opfer der Vergangheit* is available on YouTube, https://www.youtube.com/watch?v=J9Nwu1P8vGg (alternatively, search under 'Aktion T4'). A clip of *Das Erbe* can be found at https://www.youtube.com/watch?v=PMRc55nHuE4. Links last accessed 16 Mar. 2021. On this topic, see Ulf Schmidt, *Medical Films, Ethics and Euthanasia in Nazi Germany* (Husum: Matthiesen Verlag, 2002).

24 For example, Albert Deutsch, *The Shame of the States* (New York: Harcourt, Brace and Co., 1948) and Albert Q. Maisel's 'Bedlam 1946' in *Life* (6 May 1946).

25 R.D. Laing, *The Divided Self* (London: Penguin, 2010 [1960]).

26 John Mack (1969) [Video] Dingleton Hospital: A series of five films made by the University of Glasgow Television Service on behalf of and with the participation of the University's School of Social Studies.
27 For more on Robinson's *Asylum*, see Joice, 'Reviewing Laing's "Asylum"'; O'Rawe, 'Politics of Observation'.
28 Thanks to Carmine Grimaldi for sharing his experience of using video archives, and to Sarah Eilers from the National Library of Medicine for explaining its preservation policy.
29 For more information on the PCR, see Amanda Maple and Sarah Eilers, 'Psychological Cinema', *Circulating Now* (2019), https://circulatingnow.nlm.nih.gov/2019/08/22/psychological-cinema/, accessed 16 Mar. 2021.
30 This question is discussed in W.J.T. Mitchell, *Picture Theory: Essays on Verbal and Visual Representation* (Chicago, IL: University of Chicago Press, 1995).
31 Curtis uses this concept in the context of Charcot's work on hysteria.
32 Susan Sontag, *Regarding the Pain of Others* (London: Penguin, 2013), p. 34.
33 Brian Winston, 'The Tradition of the Victim in Griersonian Documentary', and Carolyn Anderson and Thomas W. Benson, 'Direct Cinema and the Myth of Informed Consent: The Case of *Titicut Follies*', in Larry Gross, John Stuart Katz, and Jay Ruby (eds), *Image Ethics: The Moral Rights of Subjects in Photographs, Film and Television* (Oxford: Oxford University Press, 1988), pp. 34–57, 58–90.
34 Barry Keith Grant, 'Ethnography in the First Person: Frederick Wiseman's *Titicut Follies*', in Barry Keith Grant and Jeannette Sloniowski (eds), *Documenting the Documentary: Close Readings of Documentary Film and Video* (Detroit, MI: Wayne State University Press, 1998), pp. 238–53: p. 240.
35 Anderson and Benson, 'Direct Cinema'.
36 See the 2005 Mental Capacity Act https://www.legislation.gov.uk/ukpga/2005/9/contents, accessed Feb. 2021; Joel M. Geiderman and Gregory L. Larkin, 'Commercial Filming of Patient Care Activities in Hospital', *Journal of the American Medical Association*, 288, 3 (2002), pp. 373–9.
37 Human Rights Watch, 'Living in Chains', available at https://www.hrw.org/report/2020/10/06/living-chains/shackling-people-psychosocial-disabilities-worldwide (2020), accessed 16 Mar. 2021.
38 Laura Marks, *The Skin of the Film: Intercultural Cinema, Embodiment and the Senses* (Durham, NC: Duke University Press, 2000); Vittorio Gallese and Michele Guerra, *The Empathic Screen: Cinema and Neuroscience*, trans. Frances Anderson (Oxford: Oxford University Press, 2019).
39 For a detailed discussion of these issues see Elizabeth Lunbeck, 'Empathy as a Psychoanalytic Mode of Observation: Between Sentiment and Science' in Lorraine Daston and Elizabeth Lunbeck (eds), *Histories of Scientific Observation* (Chicago, IL: Chicago University Press, 2011); Tyson Retz, *Empathy and History* (New York: Berghahn Books, 2018); Mark Salber Phillips, *On Historical Distance* (New Haven, CT: Yale University Press, 2013).
40 Joice, 'Mothering in the Frame'.
41 Spitz's colleague, Robert Emde, also remarked that reactions of physicians and psychiatrists to the film included 'teary agony', anxiety, laughter, and distraction. Robert N. Emde (ed.), *René A. Spitz: Dialogues from Infancy* (New York: International Universities Press, 1983), pp. 426–7. I have noticed a similar mixture of reactions when showing the footage to audiences today.
42 The first manifesto for this realignment was Bruce H. Price, Raymond D. Adams, and Joseph T. Coyle, 'Neurology and Psychiatry: Closing the Great Divide', *Neurology*, 54, 1 (2000), pp. 8–14.
43 For an anthropological analysis of these visual technologies, see Joseph Dumit, *Picturing Personhood: Brain Scans and Biomedical Identity* (Princeton, NJ: University of Princeton Press, 2004).

44 Recent documentaries about celebrities with mental illness include *What's Wrong with Tony Slattery?* (2019) and *Being Gail Porter* (2020), both BBC.
45 A less scientistic account of psychiatric practice can be found in Tom Burns, *Our Necessary Shadow: The Nature and Meaning of Psychiatry* (London: Penguin, 2013).

Further guidance

Citing a film

Director(s) last name, Initial (where known). (Year). *Title of film in italics*. [Film]. Production or Distribution company (where known). If there is no obvious director, use the name of the producer, writer, or institution where the film was made.
For example: Spitz, R. (1947). *Grief: A Peril in Infancy* [Film]. New York University Film Library.
If the format is a DVD: Wiseman, F. (1967). *Titicut Follies* [DVD]. Zipporah Films.
In-text citation (description or paraphrase of the film's contents): (Spitz, 1947)
In-text citation of image, dialogue, voiceover or inter-titles (direct quote with timestamp): (Spitz, 1947, 02:12 or 02.12:34)
If you wish to include a film still in a print or online publication, it is strongly recommended that you request permission from the copyright holder (in the case of many historical films, your first enquiry should be directed to the archive where the films are now held, such as the US National Library of Medicine).
The film resources which I have encountered during my research are listed below and organised by location. Online availability of some films will inevitably change over time.

Film Collections

National Library of Medicine (Bethesda, Maryland, US).
https://www.nlm.nih.gov/ and https://www.youtube.com/user/NLMNIH
Wholey, C.C. (1923). Case Study of Multiple Personality [Film].
Pierce Clark, L. (1930). *Child Analyses, Psychoanalytic Sanatorium* [Film].
Page, J.D. and Pennsylvania State College (1938). *Symptoms in Schizophrenia* [Film].
Gesell, A. (1939). *Life Begins* [Film].
Bishops Clarkson Memorial Hospital (1943). *Convulsive Shock Therapy in Affective Psychoses* [Film].
Bishops Clarkson Memorial Hospital (1944). *Prefrontal Lobotomy in Chronic Schizophrenia* [Film].
Bishops Clarkson Memorial Hospital (1944). *Narcosynthesis* [Film].
US Navy (1944). *Combat Fatigue* [Film].
Spitz, R. (1947). *Grief: A Peril in Infancy* [Film]. New York University Film Library.
Page, J.D. (1949). *Treatment in Mental Disorders* [Film]. The University of Rochester.
Aubry, J. and Appel, G. (1951). *Maternal Deprivation in Young Children* [Film].
US Navy (1954). *Combat Psychiatry: the Battalion Medical Officer* [Film].
Menninger, W. (1956). *Out of Darkness* [Film]. Columbia Broadcasting System. Documents the therapy of a young woman with schizophrenia.
The Maudsley Hospital (1957). *Approach to Objects by Psychotic Children* [Film]. New York University Film Library.
Brody, S. (1967). *Mother Infant Interaction* [Film]. New York University Film Library.
US Department of Health, Education and Welfare (1969). *Involuntary Hospitalization of the Psychiatric Patient* [Film].

Mental Health Film Board (1974). *Full Circle* [Film]. On group therapy in a psychiatric hospital.

Available on request:

Spitz, R. (1956). *Shaping the Personality* [Film]. New York University Film Library.

Director unknown (1960). *Tradition and Progress in African Psychiatry* [Film].

Director unknown (1968). *Invisible Barrier: Japan and Psychiatric Patients* [Film].

Library of Congress (Washington, US)

https://www.loc.gov/ and https://www.youtube.com/user/LibraryOfCongress

Mead, M. and Bateson, G. (1952). *Trance and Dance in Bali* [Film].

Wellcome Collection (London, UK)

https://wellcomecollection.org/

Spectator Films for the Central Office of Information (1943). *Neuro-Psychiatry* [Film]. Wartime documentary film showing the neuro-psychiatric treatment of neurotic civilians and soldiers.

Speed, F. and Prince, R. (1963). *Were ni! he is a madman: a study of the management of psychiatric disorders by the Yoruuba of Nigeria* [Film]. Royal Anthropological Institute.

Da Silveira, N. and Le Gallais, P. (undated, 1960s). *Painting in Psychiatry* [Film]. A study of painting therapy for schizophrenia in Brazil.

Prelinger Archives

https://archive.org/details/prelinger

Bateson, G. and Kees, W. (1951). *Communication in Three Families* [Film]. Kinesis Films.

Hewett, F., with the National Educational Television and Radio Center (1952). *Autism's Lonely Children* [Film].

Internet Archive

https://archive.org/

Spitz, R. (1952). *Psychogenic Disease in Infancy* [Film].

Confidential Telepictures, Central Intelligence Agency, and Bercel, N.A. (1955). *Schizophrenic Model Psychosis Induced by LSD 25* [Film].

Anthony, E.J. and the Maudsley Hospital (1960). *Natural History of Psychotic Illness in Childhood* [Film]. New York University Film Library.

Robert Anderson Associates (1961). *The Disordered Mind: Paranoid Schizophrenia* [Film].

Jensen, G.D. (1963). *Development of an Infant Psychosis* [Film]. University of Washington School of Medicine.

McGraw-Hill Films with Smith, H. (1977). *Madness and Medicine* [Film]. An ABC News Close-Up taking a critical look at mental institutions and their treatment programmes.

Eric Duvivier Films for Sandoz Pharmaceuticals

https://www.canal-u.tv/producteurs/cerimes/les_films_realises_par_eric_duvivier/psychologie_psychiatrie

Duvivier, E. (1961). *Images du Monde Schizophrenique* [Film]. ScienceFilm for Sandoz.

Duvivier, E. (1967). *La Femme 100 Tetes* [Film]. ScienceFilm for Sandoz.

Neurovision (a selection of short but historically important early twentieth-century neurological films, including those of Kurt Goldstein).
https://neurovision.org.uk/

Cummings Center for the History of Psychology, University of Akron (Ohio, US)
https://www.uakron.edu/chp/archives/
The Center preserves film footage from the most important psychological experiments of the twentieth century, as well as the original film reels of Arnold Gesell, René Spitz, Sylvia Brody, and Kurt Lewin. However, these are not available to view online.

Planned Environment Therapy Archives, Mulberry Bush Third Space (Gloucestershire, UK) https://mulberrybush.org.uk/the-mulberry-bush-third-space-mb3/archives/
(currently by appointment only)
Mack, J. (1969). *Dingleton Hospital: A series of five films made by the University of Glasgow Television Service on behalf of and with the participation of the University's School of Social Studies* [Video].

United States Holocaust Memorial Museum
https://collections.ushmm.org/search/catalog/irn1003150
Hartmann, C. (1935). *Das Erbe* [Film].

Commercial DVDs
Robertson, J. (1952). *A Two Year Old Goes to Hospital* [DVD]. Concord Media.
Robertson, J. (1967). *Young Children in Brief Separation* [DVD]. Concord Media.
Wiseman, F. (1967). *Titicut Follies* [DVD]. Zipporah Films.
Deligny, F. (1971). *Le Mondre Geste* [DVD]. Editions Montparnasse.
Robinson P. with R.D. Laing (1972). *Asylum* [DVD]. Kino Classics.
Depardon, R. (1982). *San Clemente* [DVD]. Double D Copyright Films.

YouTube (available at the time of writing in Feb. 2021).
Watson, J. (1920). *The Little Albert Experiment* [Film].
Bock-Stieber, G. (1935). *Opfer der Vergangheit.* [Film] Nazi propaganda film, search under 'Aktion T4'.
Maysles, A. (1955). *Psychiatry in Russia* [Film] (excerpts).
Harlow, H. (1959). *Mother Love* [Film].
King, A. (1967). *Warrendale* [Film]. CBC Films documentary about the Warrendale hospital for emotionally disturbed children.
Agosto, S. and Bellocchio, M. (1975). *Matti da Slegare* [Film]. An Italian documentary about the social and political problems surrounding the deinstitutionalisation of the mentally ill.
Deligny, F. and Victor, R. (1975). *Ce Gamin la* [Film]. A study of Deligny's 'anti-institution' for autistic boys in the Pyrenees.

Facebook (available at the time of writing in Feb. 2021).
Morrison, B. (2013). *Re:Awakenings* [Film]. https://www.facebook.com/OVIDtv/videos/re-awakenings-a-short-film-by-bill-morrison/216241493155825/

Vimeo (available at the time of writing in Feb. 2021).
Pavlov, I. (1926). *Mechanics of the Brain* [Film]. https://vimeo.com/20583313

Select bibliography

Cartwright, L., '"Emergencies of Survival": Moral Spectatorship and the New Vision of the Child in Post-War Child Psychoanalysis', *Journal of Visual Culture* 3, 2004, pp. 35–49.

Curtis, S., 'Between Photography and Film: Early Uses of Medical Cinematography', *REMEDIA: The History of Medicine in Dialogue with Its Present* (2016), https://remedianetwork.net/2016/01/19/medicine-in-transit-between-photography-and-film-early-uses-of-medical-cinematography/, accessed 28 Mar. 2021.

Duschinsky, R. and Reijman, S., 'Filming Disorganized Attachment', *Screen* 57, 2016, pp. 397–413.

Gallese, V. and Guerra, M., *The Empathic Screen: Cinema and Neuroscience*, trans. F. Anderson, Oxford: Oxford University Press, 2019.

Grimaldi, C., 'Televising Psyche: Therapy, Play and the Seduction of Video', *Representations* 139, 2017, pp. 95–117.

Joice, K., 'Mothering in the Frame: Cinematic Microanalysis and the Pathogenic Mother 1945–67', *History of the Human Sciences* (OnlineFirst, 2020), https://doi.org/10.1177/0952695120924266.

Jones, E., '"War Neuroses and Arthur Hurst": A Pioneering Medical Film about the Treatment of Psychiatric Battle Casualties', *Journal of Medical and Allied Sciences* 67, 2012, pp. 345–373.

Killen, A., 'Psychiatry and its Visual Cultures in the Modern Era', in G. Eghigian (ed.), *The Routledge History of Madness and Mental Health*, Milton Park, Abingdon, Oxon and New York: Routledge, 2017.

O'Rawe, D., 'The Politics of Observation: Documentary Film and Radical Psychiatry', *Journal of Aesthetics and Culture* 11, 2019.

Winter, A., 'Screening Selves: Sciences of Memory and Identity on Film 1930–1960', *History of Psychology* 7, 2004, pp. 367–401.

14

ORAL HISTORY IN THE HISTORY OF PSYCHIATRY

Victoria Hoyle

Oral history has been called 'the oldest and the newest form of the historical method'.[1] It has its roots in oral tradition, the word-of-mouth transmission of memory and story that humans have practised for millennia.[2] Stories have long been used in the production of history. Herodotus captured first-person testimony in his account of the Persian Wars in the fifth century BCE, and griot praise-singers have transmitted the histories of West African peoples across centuries.[3] However, it was not until the 1930s and 1940s that oral history practices were formally adopted by western historians, when oral history was defined as the deliberate collection of individual accounts of the past for the purpose of analysis and preservation. Such accounts call on a person's memory and interpretation of the past to explore histories that would be unavailable through the traditional archival methods that have been central to the discipline since the nineteenth century. One of the earliest oral history projects, for example, sought to capture the life stories of formerly enslaved people in the southern states of the USA.[4] Subsequently, oral history has been closely associated with 'history from below', and with local and community history, as a point of access to the voices of people who are less likely to be represented in archives, museums, and other repositories of historical knowledge. For example, women, LGBTQ+ communities, people of colour and Indigenous peoples, the working class, and those who have been marginalised and oppressed within dominant systems of power.

Psychiatry is one such system of power, which intersects closely with complex, overlapping indexes of oppression such as race, class, disability, gender, and sexuality. Oral history has become an established technique for exploring and making visible the experiences and perspectives of those who have been silenced or erased by this system. This includes patients, survivors, family members, activists, nurses, and non-medical workers. It has also been used to supplement, nuance, and critique histories generated from archival sources, through the collation of interviews with

DOI: 10.4324/9781003087694-15

psychiatrists, psychologists, and policy-makers. Recently the intersection of oral history with participatory action and co-productive research methodologies has broadened its scope and potential, contributing to reparative and social justice processes. But it is not just the preserve of academic or professional historians. Many oral history projects have been generated and led by lived experience communities, with the aim of empowering people who, through remembering and interpreting their own pasts, can work to address the impact of psychiatry on their lives and produce resources for individual and collective action. These can, as Steffan Blayney explores further in his chapter in this volume, offer valuable new perspectives on the history of psychiatry.

This chapter considers the value and potential benefits of using oral history for the history of psychiatry and mental health and discusses the challenges that this kind of research presents. Engaging directly with personal experiences, memories, and stories provides unique opportunities, but questions of subjectivity, power, and trauma must be acknowledged. Although oral history is a well-established technique, best practice continues to develop as notions of trust, sensitivity, and the position of the researcher are foregrounded. As oral historian Michael Frisch has said, 'the central issues in oral history are confronted first and most deeply in practical application', which is why this chapter discusses practical and technical as well as ethical challenges, such as interviewee recruitment, transcription, and analysis.[5] It concludes by reflecting on the therapeutic significance of oral history for people who have been marginalised within medical and psychiatric systems and by society. Its aim is to provide a theoretical, technical, and ethical framework, as an entry point to a broad and diverse field.

Defining oral history

The term 'oral history' can be used to describe both a methodological process (oral history) and the records that the process creates (oral histories). The process is a type of qualitative interviewing, which involves speaking and listening to people who were involved in (or have direct knowledge of) a subject of study or interest. It has been pithily described as 'the interviewing of eye-witness participants in the events of the past for the purposes of historical reconstruction'.[6] It draws on a hybrid of archival and social science methodologies, including traditions of source analysis (history), ethnographic observation (anthropology), and semi-structured interviewing (sociology). Interviews can take a variety of forms, being more or less structured, short or long, specific or broad. However, the defining feature of an oral history interview is that interviewees are invited to remember and discuss some aspect of the past, in conversation with the interviewer. This format provides opportunities to explore a period in a person's life, an event, or a theme over time, with a focus on living memory and personal experience. For example, in the context of psychiatric history, interviews might focus on a particular type of treatment (such as electroconvulsive therapy), an institution (such as a hospital), or a life experience (such as being an LGBTQ+ young person in psychiatric care).[7]

Interviews not only describe places and events from particular points of view, but also encourage reflection on how and why things happened, what a person thought and felt, and the impact on their present and future. As a result, every oral history interview produces a unique narrative, because individuals decide how to share their stories, the language they use, and the elements that are emphasised.

Oral histories are the records that are created during and after the interview, generally in the form of audio-visual recordings and transcriptions for future use. In this way the oral history process converts what would otherwise be ephemeral and transient – spoken words, memories, opinions, thoughts – into something that can be interpreted and referenced as a historical source. They are distinct from other genres of first-person account, such as autobiography or letters, because they are produced through the interaction between the person being interviewed and the researcher. This interaction fundamentally alters the relationship between the historian and their source, as both parties are intellectually and emotionally implicated in its production.[8] Issues of power, voice, and politics are centralised. Who has authority over what is said? How does the perspective of the interviewer shape the interviewee's narrative? How should stories be interpreted and presented? Who is the oral history for? How will it be used, not only in the first instance but thereafter? What is the relationship between the past as it was and as it is being remembered? Critical reflection on these questions is fundamental to the enterprise of oral history.

Memory and the past

Memory is the central theoretical component of oral history practice. Historians have traditionally been wary of memory as a historical source in comparison to archives, material culture, and the built environment.[9] Unlike a textual document, memory is unfixed, selective, personal, sociable, and in a constant state of change, defying empiricist notions of the relationship between the past 'as it happened' and the present. Interviews take place in the present, and reflect on events or experiences retrospectively, generating reconstructions of the past overlaid by interpretations and feelings. An interview is a unique and dialogic encounter, as interviewees speak and elaborate on their stories in the moment, often contradicting their own earlier accounts and the accounts of others. The past changes as it is shared. If you asked the same person the same questions in a week or a year's time, their contribution would be subtly different. It would also be changed by speaking with a different interviewer. This is because we remember in relation to others and to context. Thereafter the historian exercises their own subjectivity, implicating their own perspectives, interests, and political positions in how they choose to interpret the recording and transcription of the encounter. If oral histories are archived they become available for new uses, purposes, and interpretations that may not have been imagined by the original creators. As Geoffrey Cubitt explains:

The circumstances of oral historians' research are … ones which repeatedly prompt them to think about memory less as a process accomplished in the past that has bequeathed products, in the form of documentary evidence, that are there to be critically scrutinized *than as a process whose outcomes are always fluid, mutable, provisional, responsive to changing conditions and to human interventions, and therefore open not just to textual scrutiny but to probing and interrogation…*[10]

In other words, oral history cannot supply a linear, chronological, and externally verifiable account of the past. While people often reference names, dates, and places in interviews, they are not the primary characteristics of an oral history account. Indeed, leading oral historian Luisa Passerini suggests that oral history's 'faithfulness to reality' is the least interesting thing about it: 'Memory narrates with the vivid tones of actual experience. […] what attracts me is memory's insistence on creating a history of itself…'[11] The value of oral history, then, is its emphasis on the subjective, intimate experiences of the individual, and how they have interpreted those experiences in broader social and cultural terms. What was life like for people of colour living in mental health institutions in the 1980s and 1990s?[12] How did nurses and other carers feel about adults with learning disabilities before and after the emergence of community care?[13] What was the impact of psychiatric practices on LGBTQ+ communities in the 1960s and 1970s?[14] Questions like these, which ask people to remember with reference to their shifting perceptions and emotions, lend themselves to oral history inquiry.

Subjectivity, experience, and storytelling

The postmodern turn of the late twentieth century underpins the value of oral history within histories of psychiatry. In his influential book *The Wounded Storyteller* (1995), sociologist Arthur W. Frank suggests that 'The postmodern divide is crossed when people's own stories are no longer told as secondary but have their own primary importance'.[15] He is speaking here about the acknowledgement of personal experience, narrated by individuals about themselves, as an authentic and valid source for understanding physical and mental illness, its treatment and aftermath. His study of this 'embodied knowledge' challenged interpretations based on the scientific paradigm of publications, medical records, and expert opinions. Frank highlighted the epistemic inequality in the way illness had been historically constructed, arguing that technical stories about what it means, for example, to have a mental health diagnosis, discount the social, cultural, personal, and emotional experience of being a 'patient'. *The Wounded Storyteller* is representative of a shift of attention from the 1980s onwards, away from the study of the structures and systems of healthcare towards the subjective, multiple, and personal experiences of individuals.

The same shift was evident amongst historians, who acknowledged that histories of health and medicine had obscured the varied experiences of patients and their families in deference to the 'physician-centred account'.[16] This gave rise to histories that refocused on the perspective of the 'mad', including Roy Porter's *A Social History of Madness: Stories of the Insane* (1989) and Dale Peterson's *A Mad People's History of Madness* (1987).[17] Much of this research sought out and un-covered patient experience and testimony using archival methods, but oral history was also employed. Work by Diana Gittins, Jocelyn Goddard, and Caroline Knowles pioneered the capture of voices of lived experience, providing both micro and macro histories of psychiatry, institutions, and systems of 'care'.[18] These oral histories provided insights that reframed the experience of 'madness' and 'treatment', not as accumulations of historical facts but as relational concepts that could be understood and situated in new ways. Gittins, for example, described how the twentieth-century landscape and space of Severalls lunatic asylum in Essex – its wards, padded rooms, and gardens – were transformed by her inter-views with former patients. The 'material space', which she could see in extant photographs, maps, and archives held by the North East Essex Mental Health NHS Trust, was overlaid with 'another space: the space of imagination, vision, madness...' She explained: 'Patients I interviewed often described their experi-ences of visions/delusions/epileptic fits as if they were quite distinct landscapes they inhabited...'.[19] The centring of subjective experience enabled the emergence of this alternative asylum landscape, in which the patient rather than the doctor was the expert navigator. Archives did not (and perhaps could not) contain or delineate knowledge of this landscape – it was only available through the words of individuals who had been there. The authenticity and value of Gittins' interviews arose not from the authorised context of production, as it would in the archive, but from an epistemological claim that what a person thinks, feels, and remembers is a valid form of historical knowledge. Radical historian Raphael Samuel de-scribed this kind of knowledge as 'history's netherworld – where memory and myth intermingle, and the imaginary rubs shoulders with the real'.[20]

As well as memory and lived experience, concepts of storytelling are central to the practice of oral history. Interviews provide rich, descriptive, and exploratory narratives, constructed not only from recollections but from a range of social norms and established stories that help a person to understand how they fit into a bigger picture. Caroline Knowles suggests that the ways in which different nar-ratives diverge from and converge with one another in oral history is particularly revealing in the context of psychiatry. In her work with people diagnosed with schizophrenia she describes how stories about episodic and traumatic events in the past reveal not only an individual's personal reality but how their understanding of the world and themselves has been constructed in relation to narrative conven-tions, cultural stereotypes, collective expectations, and the cultural and social systems of mental health.[21] Alistair Thomson suggests:

> In our storytelling we identify what we think we have been, who we think we are now and what we want to become. The stories that we remember will not be exact representations of our past, but will draw upon aspects of

that past and mould them to fit current identities and aspirations... Memories are 'significant pasts' that we compose to make a comfortable sense of our life over time, and in which past and current identities are brought more into line.[22]

The identification of 'significant pasts' through the analysis of themes and ways of thinking in interviews can help in understanding the relationship between past experiences or actions and present circumstances.

In order to navigate the challenges of memory and story, oral historians deploy analytic strategies to contextualise, historicise, and interpret the interviews they collect. In her work on the psychology of working-class people in Fascist Italy Luisa Passerini explored how interviewees used pre-existing cultural forms and notions to translate their personal experiences into historical narratives. Thematic analysis of interviews revealed how people connected their own beliefs and feelings to broader events and socio-cultural expectations.[23] Tommy Dickinson found in his work *Curing Queers* (2015), that the recollections of former mental health nurses and survivors of gay conversion therapies were in a constant process of reconfiguration as they constructed their past, present, and imagined selves with reference to what they understood about the wider world. For example, nurses used stories about the absolute authority of doctors in the 1960s and 1970s, and emphasised a culture of obedience to hierarchy, in order to explain and justify how things were. Some mitigated their individual roles in administering treatments for 'sexual deviance' by describing moments of subversion, which they framed as stories of underground resistance. This enabled them to understand what had happened in the past in ways that aligned with the recognition of LGBTQ+ rights in the present.[24] Kerry Davies applied similar analysis to interviews with psychiatric patients from late twentieth-century Oxfordshire. She identified three key narrative frames: stories of loss, stories of survival and self-discovery, and stories of 'the self as patient'.[25] The interaction of individual experience with these established story-forms brought together inner worlds with 'the outer world of the changing experience of being ill'.[26] As Gittins had also found, the complexity of these inner worlds was not evident in the archive of the same hospital.

Archival deficits

Oral history is often conceived as filling an archival deficit. There are numerous instances where no archival traces survive, because they have been lost or destroyed, or because archives cannot be accessed. The absence of records is particularly acute for historians of the later twentieth century, where many archives (especially patient and case records) are not widely available. They may remain in the closed custody of current medical services and administrative centres, or have been destroyed in line with records management and patient confidentiality policies.[27] In many countries around the world data protection legislation now strictly limits access to medical and other highly sensitive information during the lifetime of the subjects.[28] This complicates access not only to case records but to any archives which may contain references to patients or staff. In such cases lived experience can fill the gap, with oral history providing a means of documenting and studying periods and places that would otherwise be closed to scrutiny. In time oral histories may come to form part of an archive themselves, establishing a long-term resource for future researchers.

However, even in cases where an archive survives and is available for use, it is still unlikely to provide direct access to the experiences, feelings, and perceptions of patients. The development of psychiatric medicine, institutionalism, and societal prejudice has persistently marginalised and silenced psychiatric service users and survivors. Those in positions of influence, with societal claims to expertise, have controlled recordkeeping. The creation, form, and preservation of documents, and access to them, has been shaped by medical practitioners and policy-makers. This includes the use of genres such as asylum casebooks or case notes (explored further in Sarg et al.'s chapter in this volume). Within such documents, patient experiences may be described using technical language or terminology that does not represent their own perspective or experiences.[29] Similarly, the accounts of nurses and non-medical staff are often omitted. When records are transferred to archives and become available to historians, the point of view of the psychiatrist and the institution is the view that is projected into the future.[30]

Leavy argues that oral history is particularly valuable in these contexts where key historical actors are obscured or paradigmatically voiceless.[31] Oral histories can provide insights that are otherwise unavailable, which can either be used on their own terms or in order to critique, contrast, and supplement documentary sources. For example, they can offer creative entry points to a particular research question or problem as, for example, in Fiona Byrne's exploration of cultures of mental health hospitals in mid twentieth-century Ireland through the eyes of the children of staff members.[32] It can also give access to intersecting issues of gender and sexuality, which may only emerge through the lens of contemporary values and understandings: Sheena Rolph, Jan Walmsley, and Dorothy Atkinson's work with Mental Welfare Officers explores the gendered landscape of disability and mental health community care in the 1950s and 1960s.[33]

However, oral histories need not reject the archive or other sources of historical knowledge. They are generally predicated on some other form of research, either secondary or primary, which contextualises interviews as part of a mixed methods approach. Interviewees sometimes encourage this themselves, by using their own case notes, photographs, or material cultures as reference points or scaffolding for their narrative. The Memory-Identity-Rights in Records-Access (MIRRA) project (2017–2019), which examined the lifelong memory and identity needs of care-experienced adults in England, found that this relationship between lived experience and archives was critical.[34] While a person's recollection of their past often conflicted with what social workers, psychiatrists, and foster parents had written about them, social care and mental health records nevertheless played an important role in structuring and justifying their personal narratives.

Indeed, friction with absent or inhospitable records can be productive and empowering, providing a perspective to defy or argue against. The Mental Health Recovery Archive (2012–2013) was co-created by academic Anna Sexton and a team of contributors with lived experience of mental health recovery, in response to the deficit of patient perspectives in the Wellcome Library collection in London. The archive, available online, is compiled of oral histories, images, art, videos, poems, and other creative responses to past experiences, constructed around narratives of each person's recovery journey.[35] This includes Sexton's own experience of researching mental health recovery, as a person without lived experience, but with a commitment to deeply reflective and auto-ethnographic historical practice.[36]

Practices, technologies, and practicalities

The first step in planning an oral history project is to reflect on whether it is an appropriate method. Taking into account the potential benefits and challenges, is it the best way to explore your research interest? Questions to be asked include: What other source materials exist? Do you have a personal, political, or social agenda in pursuing oral history? How difficult will it be to interview people? What questions will you ask them? How will the interviews be collected, managed, and used, in the immediate and long term? The answers to these questions, and many others, will inform ethics applications to universities, and other institutions such as hospitals or the NHS, from whom you will need to gain permission before you begin.

Although oral history may appear expansive and intuitive, given the wide-ranging content it produces, the method requires close planning as part of time-limited projects. A clear research focus will enable the identification of potential interviewees, as well as routes for making contact with them. Some research lends itself to interviewing specific individuals (such as Gittins' research on Severalls) while other projects require a cohort that is representative of a particular experience (such as Dickinson's oral history of LGBTQ+ experience in the 1960s and 1970s). Studies can have a significant number of interviewees, like Knowles' work with schizophrenia survivors, while others have as few as one. An example of this is Patricia Leavy and Lauren Sardi Ross's examination of anorexia nervosa through a single life story.[37] In either case, recruitment may be targeted, with interview requests sent directly to identified people; or self-selecting, by advertising the opportunity to participate through newsletters, social media, or word of mouth. Making initial contact with potential interviewees can be difficult, depending on pre-existing relationships and the number of people you would like to speak to. If the topic is a sensitive or highly personal one, as is often the case in mental health research, there are challenges relating to trust, privacy, and the use of language. Few people will volunteer to speak to a stranger without some prior contact. It may be helpful to begin by building rapport with advocacy or support organisations, or with public activists, who are able to verify your credentials and recommend individuals to approach. For example, in the case of the MIRRA project a partnership with The

Care Leavers' Association, a care leaver-led charity, helped researchers to make contact with people with relevant experience.[38] Organisational partners or colla-borators can also provide additional support, both to interviewees and to researchers, as they will have expertise of working with clients' issues and may be able to signpost to specialist services, such as counselling if it is required.

Communication before, during, and after an interview is vital. Informed consent is a pillar of oral history practice, and almost universally required by local ethics processes for research involving people. This means that all interviewees should be fully informed about the subject of the research and what will happen to their contribution, including whether it will be preserved in the long term. They should know they are being recorded, and how you will transcribe that recording. It is good practice to give interviewees the opportunity to check and amend their contribution before you use it. They should also know that they have the right to withdraw from the research at any time, at which point records of their interview would be destroyed. Data protection legislation (e.g. the General Data Protection Regulation, or GDPR, within the EU) requires that researchers clearly state how any personal information collected will be used, handled, and managed, as well as how long it will be kept.[39] If you are affiliated with a higher education institution they will act as the 'data controller' for the interviews that you collect and use as the 'data processor', and will have guidance about how the law applies to your specific project. Finally, the language and format of the information provided should be accessible and inclusive, accounting for differences in literacy and comprehension. Sensitivity about the use of labels and medicalised terms show contributors that you understand their perspective and will be respectful of their needs and feelings.[40]

Oral history also requires equipment, and the technical expertise to use it. Increasingly interviews can be recorded using commonly owned devices, such as mobile phones or computers. However, issues such as sound quality, output format, reliability, and privacy are still important. Needs will differ depending on a number of factors. Will you use audio or video, and why? Who will listen to the recordings? Will they be published online, or archived? Who else has access to the equipment you are using? Whatever equipment is used it is important to know how it works and to test it beforehand, so as not to cause delays or problems during or after an interview. A failed or partial recording does not only impact the research, but is also upsetting or hurtful to the interviewee who has given their time and made an emotional investment in order to contribute.

The venue in which interviews take place is also a consideration. As with many aspects of the interview process, it has a relation to power. Interviewees may be uncomfortable speaking in institutional settings, such as hospitals, universities, and office buildings, particularly if they have negative associations with such spaces. In these cases, it may be most convenient to meet in a neutral public space like a library or coffee shop. A partner organisation may also be able to provide a venue. However, there are practical implications to external locations, such as background noise, and the difficulty in maintaining privacy and confidentiality. Some inter-viewees may feel most comfortable speaking in familiar surroundings that are local to where they live. Tommy Dickinson described his decision to interview retired nurses and former patients in their own homes, to maintain 'informality' and encourage easy conversation.[41] Yet others may prefer to speak on the phone, where they feel less observed, or to meet in an open public place like a park, which they can readily leave. Consequently, it may be necessary to be flexible and responsive to the needs and preferences of individuals. However, the safety of both interviewee and interviewer is always paramount and risk has to be carefully assessed if travelling alone to unfamiliar or isolated locations.

Interviews are different to other types of conversation, in that two strangers talk about experiences and perspectives which may be deeply personal and specific. Individuals respond to this scenario differently, depending on their personalities and circumstances. If interviewees have rehearsed their memories and opinions frequently in analogous circumstances, such as to the media or as part of advocacy work, then they may speak with confidence. Similarly, if they feel they are in a position of authority or expertise, i.e. as a medical professional speaking to a non-professional, they may share more freely. Others may not have spoken to anyone about a topic before and therefore be reticent. These circumstances shape not only what a person says, but how they say it. In both cases, the approach and attitude of the interviewer helps in establishing a rapport through eye contact, and visual or audible feedback, such as nodding, smiling, and making affirmative noises. Using a pre-interview checklist and prompt phrases can be helpful in ensuring the interviewee knows what to expect. The role of the interviewer is to listen and to participate only insofar as it is necessary to elicit information and guide the interviewee to explore relevant aspects of their story in greater depth. Nevertheless, during the course of an interview the interviewer may be called upon to respond. This could be in the course of regular conversation, such as being asked an opinion, or it might be to support a person who has become distressed or upset. Revisiting the past can be traumatic and difficult, evoking unexpected memories and emotions.[42] It is not unusual for interviewees to become angry, to cry, or to struggle to articulate themselves. Ethics procedures will require you to consider these possibilities and to prepare strategies to cope with situations in advance. This includes knowing where to refer people who need additional help, for example to counselling or support organisations, and what to do if an interviewee appears to be at risk of harming themselves or others.

Interviews vary in length, by design, and by interviewee preference. However, for practical reasons it may be helpful to agree a time limit on an encounter, keeping in mind that transcribing, analysing, and interpreting oral histories is time intensive. As a rule, depending on the speed at which a person speaks, an hour's recording produces 10,000–15,000 words of written content. This takes between four and six hours to transcribe, again depending on factors such as the experience of the transcriber, talking speed, use of specialist language (i.e. technical medical and pharmaceutical words), accent, and the coherence of the interviewee's sentences. Transcription can be outsourced to a third party, but this may not be feasible for cost reasons or because of the sensitive content of the material.

Transcription is another specialist practice and skill implicated in oral history. Interpretive decisions (what is transcribed?) and representational decisions (how is it transcribed?) have wide-ranging implications for the interpretation and analysis of an interview's content. As Willow Robert Powers explains, 'Transcribing any recorded speech is a form of translation', in which the oral is fixed as text.[43] Whereas written language is an idealised system of grammar, word choice, and order, spoken language is messy, broken, and syntactically confused. Interviewees will abandon and restart sentences, rephrase themselves, lose their train of thought, contradict themselves, repeat words, misuse words, and communicate using gestures and non-verbal sounds such as laughs, sighs, and groans. Translating this onto the page or screen is necessarily interpretative. It may be considered a subjective act that 'reflects transcribers' analytic or political bias and shapes interpretation of the relationships and contexts depicted in the transcript'.[44] For example, the extent to which the transcriber decides to retain errors, repetitions, dialect words, contractions, linguistic tics, and confused expressions changes perceptions of the narrative.

Mary Bucholtz defined two principal approaches to transcription, with different potentials and capacities.[45] 'Denaturalised' transcription gives oral discourse primacy over written language, and attempts a verbatim depiction of speech. This may include, for example, the inclusion of stutters, pauses, word repetitions, features of oral expression such as 'erm' and 'ah', and non-verbal signals such as laughter. Features of written language, such as punctuation or paragraphing, are omitted. 'Naturalised' transcription, in contrast, applies the conventions of written language to spoken talk, inserting full stops, commas, and paragraphs, and may also standardise sentence structures to prioritise sense-making over what was literally said. Naturalised transcription focuses on the substance and content of *what* is said, while denaturalised transcription focuses on *how* it is said. These modes of transcription reflect different ways of locating importance in an interview. Whereas the latter is suited to approaches like critical discourse analysis, which seek to reveal an interviewee's subjectivity by analysing features of their speech (such as word choice and features like hesitations), the former serves approaches such as thematic content analysis or narrative analysis, which focus on meanings and broader context.[46]

Transcription highlights the paradox of oral histories, which is that they are not purely oral. Both recordings and transcript continue to exist beyond the moment and outside of the context of the interview itself. The future preservation and accessibility of an oral history project in an archive is often seen as a benefit of the method, in supplementing and enhancing the documentary record – filling the archival deficit. Specialist sound and oral history archives actively collect content from local and national projects. For example, the Mental Health Testimony Archive at the British Library is the largest collection of its kind in the UK.[47] The Essex Sound and Video Archive holds a number of oral histories relating to Severalls and other local institutions.[48] University archives and data repositories also store and provide access to oral histories generated by research projects, like the Scottish Oral History Centre at the University of Strathclyde.[49] If your oral histories are intended for long-term preservation this should be decided at the outset, as it may shape some of the decisions that are made during recruitment and transcription.

Ethics, empowerment, and co-production

All research has ethical implications, but research involving people who may have experienced trauma or systemic oppression, and who may have mental health challenges, brings these implications into sharp focus. Before the oral history interview occurs memories, narratives, and stories may not have consciously existed or been articulated. Even where an individual is relatively practised at telling their story, a new configuration of their history is brought into being during the encounter between interviewee and interviewer. Thoughts and meanings that were previously dynamic and unfixed are turned into something which can be repeated and revisited, so that memory and story become available for analysis. In oral history the researcher and the interviewee collaborate on this production of knowledge, which emerges out of the specific circumstances of their encounter. That encounter is structured by the practical arrangements discussed – the venue, the recording equipment, the questions asked – and by the power dynamics that impact on what is said and shared. No oral history takes place in a vacuum. Frisch used the term 'shared authority' to describe this relationship, in which the interplay between the interviewer and the interviewee produces the final recording, transcript, and interpretation of the past.[50] However, the extent to which authority is truly shared varies and is debatable, depending on the design and implementation of the oral history project. Navigating shared authority presents a particular challenge where there is a significant differential of power between the parties, as may exist between an academic researcher and someone who identifies as a mental health survivor. Indeed, the very concept of the interview may recall the doctor/patient relationship, in which a person is observed and has their testimony recorded, written up, and analysed by someone in a position of power. Negative associations with these types of encounters may have emotional implications for some interviewees, impacting on their willingness to take part and what they feel able to share.

The structures and systems of research itself can maintain and exacerbate these existing power imbalances, for example in projects where all decisions about a project are made by an academic researcher and the contribution of interviewees is limited to the interview itself. Historians operating in analogous areas of marginalised, community, and identity history have advocated models of co-production that reduce distance between the researcher and the researched. They seek to address inequalities of power by collaborating with lived experience co-researchers throughout the research process.[51] For example, Elizabeth Pente and Paul Ward have argued that notions of 'shared authority' be expanded beyond the creation of the primary source (the interview) to include a 'sustained contribution' to the creation of new knowledge about the past (the oral history process).[52] In oral history this might involve working together with those with lived experience to co-produce a project, from the design of the questions to the interviewing, interpretation, and analysis. This is a model that has already been widely adopted in local and community history projects that take place outside universities. However, this work requires significant personal and emotional investment over time from all members of the co-production team. Researchers have discussed how these approaches generate new challenges, in relation to the maintenance of boundaries; the development of friendships with lived-experience co-researchers; and the emergence of conflicts within the team.[53]

Some, though by no means all, oral history work is oriented towards justice and aligns to the broader context of critical mental health scholarship and activism. The emergence of Mad Studies as a field of enquiry over the last decade has contested dominant forms of research and knowledge production, particularly those that have traditionally been the focus of psychiatric histories, such as treatments, illnesses, and institutions.[54] Oral history methodologies intersect with Mad Studies when they contribute towards 'survivor research', through the centralisation of experiential knowledge. Where projects focus on the testimonies of patients and those who have been subject to the mental health care system, they may be seen to contribute towards the ongoing work of redistributing power. The interactional and demo-cratising nature of oral history works against the objectivist distance between re-searcher and researched that Mad Studies considers actively harmful.[55]

Nevertheless, the potential to do harm is ever-present. By their nature, oral histories of psychiatry are highly likely to engage with subjects that are important to a person's sense of self and wellbeing. This is not only the case with former patients and survivors, but can also be true of medical and mental health practitioners whose reputations, legacies, and emotions are implicated in remembering their past work. The potential impact on an interviewee of taking part in research, in the immediate and long term, is considerable. On the one hand, being asked to tell their own stories, in their own words, may be validating. Having previously dismissed or ig-nored experiences and feelings acknowledged as part of a piece of research can be empowering – the act of sharing may also be therapeutic. However, it may also be distressing, especially if it takes place in the context of ongoing mental health challenges. Being asked to recall painful memories can lead interviewees to revisit trauma, generating difficult and negative emotions in the present. As Glenn Smith, Annie Bartlett, and Michael King found in their interviews with LGBTQ+ survi-vors, the past is not over but continues to impact on mental health in the present.[56] Retraumatisation is a risk and it is important to provide support for participants that can be accessed afterwards.[57] This may be in the form of access to specialist mental health and counselling services. However, the provision of support should account for concerns and issues of trust which some survivors and former patients may have with traditional mental health care services. Instead it may be appropriate to refer interviewees to peer support networks and community organisations, outside of formal healthcare structures. At the same time researchers must be mindful of caring for their own physical and mental wellbeing, given the emotional labour of researching difficult subjects and the possibility of vicarious trauma.[58]

Conclusion

Oral history has the capacity to transform perspectives on psychiatric and mental health histories, by acknowledging the multiplicity and inconsistency of experiences and understandings of the past. Interviews produce unique sources that can help to fill gaps because archives do not exist or are inaccessible. They can provide access to points of view that have been erased, marginalised, or silenced. Where oral history practices seek to redistribute the power in psychiatric systems by centralising the voices of former patients, survivors, and 'mad people', they can also play a role in empowerment and validation. The intersection of oral history with 'survivor research' and Mad Studies, through participation and co-production, can contribute towards socially just approaches to history. These potential benefits arise from the collaborative production of knowledge, which is generated from the 'shared authority' between the researcher and those who take part in the research.

However, theoretical and ethical challenges are particularly acute. In her work on community care, *Bedlam on the Streets* (2000), Caroline Knowles writes: 'In involving ourselves in the lives of others in the course of research, we change them and we change ourselves: we help them write *their* story in specific terms and we rewrite our own in the process.'[59] Political and cultural subjectivities frame every oral history – from the selection of interviewees to the questions we ask, the way we transcribe and analyse, and how we interpret and present the past to external audiences. A grounding in oral history theory, an attentiveness to practical and technical questions, and ethical self-reflection are important tools to avoid harm and produce histories that serve and tend to the needs of all involved.

Notes

1 Richard Cándida Smith, 'Analytic Strategies for Oral History Interviews', in Jaber F. Gubrium and James A. Holstein (eds), *Handbook of Interview Research* (London: Sage, 2001), pp. 711–32: p. 712.
2 For the disputed and changing status of oral tradition in history as a discipline, see Jan Varsina, *Oral Tradition as History* (Madison, WI: Wisconsin University Press, 1985); Julie Cruikshank, 'Oral Tradition and Oral History: Reviewing Some Issues', *The Canadian Historical Review*, 75, 3 (1994), pp. 403–18; Alistair Thomson, 'Four Paradigm Transformations in Oral History', *The Oral History Review*, 34, 1 (2007), pp. 49–70.
3 Rebecca Sharpless, 'The History of Oral History', in Thomas L. Charlton, Lois Myers, and Rebecca Sharpless (eds), *Thinking About Oral History: Theories and Applications* (Lanham, MD: Altamira Press, 2008), pp. 7–32: p. 7.
4 Benjamin A. Botkin (ed.), *Lay Down My Burden: A Folk History of Slavery* (Chicago, IL: University of Chicago Press, 1945).
5 Michael Frisch, *A Shared Authority: Essays on the Craft and Meaning of Oral and Public History* (Albany, NY: State University of New York Press, 1990), pp. xv–xvi.
6 Ronald J. Grele, 'Directions in Oral History in the United States', in D.K. Dunaway and W.K. Baum (eds), *Oral History: An Interdisciplinary Anthology*, 2nd edn (Walnut Creek, CA: Altamira, 1996), pp. 62–84: p. 63.
7 See for example John Adams, 'British Nurses' Attitudes to Electroconvulsive Therapy, 1945–2000', *Journal of Advanced Nursing*, 71, 10 (2015), pp. 2393–401; Verusca Calabria,

---

'Insider Stories from the Asylum: Peer and Staff-Patient Relationships', in Joanna Davidson and Yomna Saber (eds), *Narrating Illness: Prospects and Constraints* (Oxford: Inter-Disciplinary Press, 2016), pp. 1–12; Tracy N. Hipp, Kayla R. Gore, Amanda C. Toumayan, Mollie B. Anderson, and Idia B. Thurston, 'From Conversion toward Affirmation: Psychology, Civil Rights, and Experiences of Gender-Diverse Communities in Memphis', *American Psychologist*, 74, 8 (2019), pp. 882–97.

8 Robert Perks and Alistair Thomson, *The Oral History Reader*, 3rd edn (Oxford: Routledge, 2016), pp. xii–xiv.

9 Geoffrey Cubitt, *History and Memory* (Manchester: Manchester University Press, 2007), p. 33.

10 Italics mine. Cubitt, *History and Memory*, p. 71.

11 Luisa Passerini, *Fascism in Popular Memory: The Culture of the Turin Working Class* (Cambridge: Cambridge University Press, 1987), p. 23.

12 For example, John Wainwright, Mick McKeown, and Malcolm Kinney, '"In These Streets": The Saliency of Place in an Alternative Black Mental Health Resource Centre', *International Journal of Human Rights in Healthcare*, 13, 1 (2019), pp. 31–44.

13 Bob Gates and Debra Moore, 'Annie's Story: The Use of Oral History to Explore the Lived Experience of a Learning Disability Nurse in the Twentieth Century', *International Journal of Nursing History*, 7, 3 (2002), pp. 50–9; Gail Thomas and Elizabeth Rosser, 'Research Findings from the Memories of Nursing Oral History Project', *British Journal of Nursing*, 26, 4 (2017), pp. 210–5.

14 Tommy Dickinson, *'Curing Queers': Mental Nurses and Their Patients, 1935–1974* (Manchester: Manchester University Press, 2015).

15 Arthur W. Frank, *The Wounded Storyteller: Body, Illness and Ethics*, 2nd edn (Chicago, IL: University of Chicago Press, 2013), p. 7.

16 Roy Porter, 'The Patient's View: Doing Medical History from Below', *Theory and Society*, 14, 2 (1985), pp. 175–98: p. 175.

17 Dale A. Peterson (ed.), *A Mad People's History of Madness* (Pittsburgh: University of Pittsburgh Press, 1987); Roy Porter, *A Social History of Madness: Stories of the Insane* (London: Weidenfeld and Nicholson, 1989).

18 Diana Gittins, *Madness in Its Place: Narratives of Severalls Hospital, 1913–1997* (London: Routledge, 1998); Jocelyn Goddard, *Mixed Feelings: Littlemore Hospital – An Oral History Project* (Oxford: Oxfordshire Department of Leisure and Arts, 1996); Caroline Knowles, *Bedlam on the Streets* (London: Routledge, 2000).

19 Gittins, *Madness in Its Place*, p. 5.

20 Raphael Samuel, *Theatres of Memory: Past and Present in Contemporary Culture* (London: Verso, 1994), p. 8.

21 Knowles, *Bedlam on the Streets*, p. 100–33.

22 Alistair Thomson, *Anzac Memories: Living with the Legend* (Melbourne: Oxford University Press, 1994), p. 10

23 Passerini, *Fascism in Popular Memory*.

24 Dickinson, *'Curing Queers'*, p. 12.

25 Kerry Davies, '"Silent and Censured Travellers"? Patients' Narratives and Patients' Voices: Perspectives on the History of Mental Illness since 1948', *Social History of Medicine*, 14, 2 (2001), pp. 267–92.

26 Ibid, p. 268.

27 Records of this period may also be less likely to survive in the future, due to the increased formalisation of records management practices, including disposal policies. See for example the current policy and model retention schedules, NHS Digital, *Records Management Code of Practice for Health and Social Care 2016*, https://digital.nhs.uk/data-and-information/looking-after-information/data-security-and-information-govern-ance/codes-of-practice-for-handling-information-in-health-and-care/records-manage-ment-code-of-practice-for-health-and-social-care-2016, accessed 15 Mar. 2021.

28 In the EU and UK data protection legislation is permissive, and there are access exemptions for statistical and historical purposes which may be relevant to some researchers. See The National Archives website for the latest advice: https://www.nationalarchives.gov.uk/archives-sector/legislation/archives-data-protection-law-uk/gdpr-faqs/, accessed 15 Mar. 2021.

29 Sally Swartz, 'Asylum Case Records: Fact and Fiction', *Rethinking History*, 22, 3 (2018), pp. 289–301.

30 Anna Sexton and Dolly Sen, 'More Voice, Less Ventriloquism – Exploring the Relational Dynamics in a Participatory Archive of Mental Health Recovery', *International Journal of Heritage Studies*, 24, 8 (2008), pp. 874–88: p. 874.

31 Patricia Leavy, *Oral History* (Oxford: Oxford University Press, 2011), p. 24.

32 Fiona Byrne, 'Growing up in "The Mental": Childhood Experiences at Cavan and Monaghan Mental Hospital on the Irish Border, 1930–1950', *Oral History*, 46, 2 (2018), pp. 87–96.

33 Sheena Rolph, Jan Walmsley, and Dorothy Atkinson, '"A Man's Job"? Gender Issues and the Role of Mental Welfare Officers, 1948–1970', *Oral History*, 30, 1 (2002), pp. 28–41.

34 Victoria Hoyle, Elizabeth Shepherd, Elizabeth Lomas, and Andrew Flinn, 'Recordkeeping and the Lifelong Memory and Identity Needs of Care-Experienced Children and Young People', *Child and Family Social Work*, 25, 4 (2020), pp. 935–45.

35 Anna Sexton, Andrew Voyce, Dolly Sen, Stuart Baker Brown, and Peter Bullimore, *Archive of Mental Health Recovery Stories* (2013), https://mentalhealthrecovery.omeka.net/, accessed 15 Mar. 2021.

36 Anna Sexton and Dolly Sen, 'More Voice, Less Ventriloquism – Exploring the Relational Dynamics in a Participatory Archive of Mental Health Recovery', *International Journal of Heritage Studies*, 24, 8 (2018): 874–88.

37 Patricia Leavy and Lauren Sardi Ross, 'The Matrix of Eating Disorder Vulnerability: Oral History and the Link between Personal and Social Problems', *The Oral History Review*, 33, 1 (2006), pp. 65–81.

38 Hoyle et al., 'Recordkeeping'.

39 The Oral History Society provides extensive guidance on how GDPR applies to oral history research: https://www.ohs.org.uk/advice/data-protection/, accessed 15 Mar. 2021.

40 The Oral History Society provides information on pre-interview preparation: https://www.ohs.org.uk/advice/ethical-and-legal/2/. This includes a sample of a recent easy-to-read information sheet for the NHS at 70 project: https://www.ohs.org.uk/wordpress/wp-content/uploads/NHS-at-70-Participant-Information-Sheet-Revised-April-2019-BL.pdf. The Health Research Authority also has an interactive guide, with examples, which relates more generally to research with patients and medical practitioners: http://www.hra-decisiontools.org.uk/consent/. All links last accessed 15 Mar. 2021.

41 Dickinson, '*Curing* Queers', p. 12.

42 There is an extensive literature on managing trauma in oral history. As a starting point, see Emma L. Vickers, 'Unexpected Trauma in Oral History Interviewing', *The Oral History Review*, 46, 1 (2019), pp. 134–41.

43 Willow Roberts Powers, *Transcription Techniques for the Spoken Word* (Oxford: Altamira Press, 2005), p. 9.

44 Alexandra Jaffe, 'Introduction: Non-Standard Orthography and Non-Standard Speech', *Journal of Sociolinguistics*, 4, 4 (2000), pp. 497–513: p. 500.

45 Mary Bucholtz, 'The Politics of Transcription', *Journal of Pragmatics*, 32, 10 (2000), pp. 1439–65.

46 Daniel G. Oliver, Julianne M. Serovich, and Tina L. Mason, 'Constraints and Opportunities with Interview Transcription: Towards Reflection in Qualitative Research', *Social Forces*, 82, 2 (2005), pp. 1273–89.

47 For more information see the British Library Collections Guide for Disability and Personal and Mental Health: https://www.bl.uk/collection-guides/oral-histories-of-personal-and-mental-health-and-disability#. Transcripts of the interviews can be found on the original project website, *Testimony: Inside Stories of Mental Health*, available via the Web Archive: https://www.webarchive.org.uk/wayback/archive/20121113104457/http://www.insidestories.org/. Links last accessed 15 Mar. 2021.

48 Information on these collections can be found on the Essex Record Office website: https://www.essexrecordoffice.co.uk/research/sound-video-archive, accessed 15 Mar. 2021.

49 See https://www.strath.ac.uk/humanities/schoolofhumanities/history/scottishoral historycentre/, accessed 15 Mar. 2021.

50 Michael Frisch, *A Shared Authority: Essays on the Craft and Meaning of Oral and Public History* (Albany, NY: State University of New York Press, 1990).

51 See Sarah Lloyd and Julie Moore, 'Sedimented Histories: Connections, Collaborations and Co-Production in Regional History', *History Workshop Journal*, 80, 1 (2015), pp. 234–48; Paul Ward, *Britishness since 1970* (London: Routledge, 2004); Elizabeth Pente, Paul Ward, Milton Brown, and Hardeep Sahota, 'The Co-Production of Historical Knowledge: Implications for the History of Identities', *Identity Papers: A Journal of British and Irish Studies*, 1, 1 (2015). Available at https://doi.org/10.5920/idp.2015.1132.

52 Elizabeth Pente and Paul Ward, 'Let's Change History! Community Histories and the Co-Production of Historical Knowledge', in Lyndon Fraser, Marguerite Hill, Sarah Murray, and Greg Ryan (eds), *History Making a Difference: New Approaches from Aotearoa* (Cambridge: Cambridge Scholarly Publishing, 2017), pp. 94–112: p. 94.

53 Sexton and Sen, 'More Voice'; Hoyle et al., 'Recordkeeping'.

54 Helen Spandler and Dina Poursanidou, 'Who Is Included in the Mad Studies Project?', *The Journal of Ethics in Mental Health*, 10 (2019). Available at http://clok.uclan.ac.uk/23384/8/23384%20JEMH%20Inclusion%20iii.pdf, accessed 15 Mar. 2021.

55 Alison Faulkner, 'Survivor Research and Mad Studies: The Role and Value of Experiential Knowledge in Mental Health Research', *Disability and Society*, 32, 4 (2017), pp. 500–20: p. 505.

56 Glenn Smith, Annie Bartlett, and Michael King, 'Treatments of Homosexuality in Britain since the 1950s – An Oral History: The Experience of Patients', *British Medical Journal*, 328, 7434 (2004), pp. 427–9.

57 For an example of managing retraumatization in the oral history process, see David Palmer, '"Every Morning before You Open the Door You Have to Watch for that Brown Envelope": Complexities and Challenges of Undertaking Oral History with Ethiopian Forced Migrants in London, U.K.', *The Oral History Review*, 37, 1 (2010), pp. 35–53. For more information on the dynamics of retraumatization, see Robert Reynolds, 'Trauma and the Relational Dynamics of Life-History Interviewing', *Australian Historical Studies*, 43, 1 (2012), pp. 78–88.

58 There is a small but growing literature on the emotional labour of oral history work, and the risk of vicarious trauma. A good starting point is Virginia Dickson-Swift, Erica L. James, Sandra Kippen, and Pranee Liamputtong, 'Researching Sensitive Topics: Qualitative Research as Emotion Work', *Qualitative Research*, 9, 1 (2009), pp. 61–79.

59 Knowles, *Bedlam on the Streets*, p. 9.

Select bibliography

Adams, J., 'British Nurses' Attitudes to Electroconvulsive Therapy, 1945–2000', *Journal of Advanced Nursing* 71, 2015, pp. 2393–2401.

Byrne, F., 'Growing up in 'The Mental': Childhood Experiences at Cavan and Monaghan Mental Hospital on the Irish Border, 1930–1950', *Oral History* 46, 2018, pp. 87–96.

Calabria, V., 'Insider Stories from the Asylum: Peer and Staff-Patient Relationships', in J. Davidson and Y. Saber (eds), *Narrating Illness: Prospects and Constraints*, Oxford: Inter-Disciplinary Press, 2016, pp. 1–12.

Davies, K., "Silent and Censured Travellers'? Patients' Narratives and Patients' Voices: Perspectives on the History of Mental Illness since 1948', *Social History of Medicine* 14, 2001, pp. 267–292.

Dickinson, T., *'Curing Queers': Mental Nurses and their Patients, 1935–1974*, Manchester: Manchester University Press, 2015.

Hipp, T.N., Gore, K.R., Toumayan, A.C., Anderson, M.B., and Thurston, I.B., 'From Conversion toward Affirmation: Psychology, Civil Rights, and Experiences of Gender-Diverse Communities in Memphis', *American Psychologist* 74, 2019, pp. 882–897.

Leavy, P. and Ross, L.S., 'The Matrix of Eating Disorder Vulnerability: Oral History and the Link between Personal and Social Problems', *The Oral History Review* 33, 2006, pp. 65–81

Pente, E., Ward, P., Brown, M., and Sahota, H., 'The Co-Production of Historical Knowledge: Implications for the History of Identities', *Identity Papers: A Journal of British and Irish Studies* 1, 2015.

Sexton, A. and Sen, D., 'More Voice, Less Ventriloquism – Exploring the Relational Dynamics in a Participatory Archive of Mental Health Recovery', *International Journal of Heritage Studies* 24, 2018, pp. 874–888.

Sharpless, R., 'The History of Oral History', in Thomas L. Charlton, Lois Myers, and Rebecca Sharpless (eds), *Thinking About Oral History: Theories and Applications*, Lanham, MD: Altamira Press, 2008, pp. 7–32.

INDEX